Pediatric Consultation-Liaison Psychiatry

Anthony P. S. Guerrero • Paul C. Lee
Norbert Skokauskas
Editors

Pediatric Consultation-Liaison Psychiatry

A Global, Healthcare Systems-Focused, and Problem-Based Approach

Springer

Editors
Anthony P. S. Guerrero
Department of Psychiatry
University of Hawai'i John A. Burns
School of Medicine
Honolulu, HI, USA

Paul C. Lee
Department of Psychiatry
University of Hawai'i John A. Burns
School of Medicine
Honolulu, HI, USA

Norbert Skokauskas
Faculty of Medicine and Health Sciences,
NTNU
Department of Centre for Child and Youth
Mental Health, Institute of Mental Health
Trondheim, Norway

ISBN 978-3-030-07784-6 ISBN 978-3-319-89488-1 (eBook)
https://doi.org/10.1007/978-3-319-89488-1

Printed on acid-free paper

This Springer imprint is published by the registered company Springer International Publishing AG part of Springer Nature.
The registered company address is: Gewerbestrasse 11, 6330 Cham, Switzerland

Foreword by Aimee M. Grace

"No man is an island, entire of itself;
Every man is a piece of the continent, a part of the main..." (John Donne, as read to me by my grandfather, Robert A. Nordyke, MD)

The increasing interconnectedness of the world and its profound implications on health and human well-being is increasingly evident, from Ebola to public shootings to the Syrian refugee crisis. *"Any man's death diminishes me, because I am involved in mankind..."* continues the Donne poem. The ability of each person, family, community, state, and nation to thrive depends on our mutual commitment to investing in the comprehensive well-being of others. Perhaps, the experience of childhood bullying led a future mass shooter to harbor bitterness toward the world. Perhaps, the understanding smile of a pediatric health provider turned one adolescent with an aim of suicide to reconsider, avoiding a family and community's lifetime of devastation. Perhaps, one state's laws allowed children with developmental disabilities to access critical services, thus eventually allowing them to work and thereby save costs for the public. Perhaps, one nation's lack of public health infrastructure resulted in the spread of disease around the world. We as a global society are interconnected in boundless and powerful ways, and our youth are not only the future of this society, but they are also continually impacted by it directly and indirectly. Ensuring a strong foundation of mental health in our children is essential for ensuring a stable, positive, and economically productive future for the world.

The phrase "children are not just little adults" is common in pediatrics, and particularly so regarding pediatric mental health. The complex developmental and socio-emotional processes that children and adolescents undergo are a wonder to behold. When development proceeds at an appropriate pace, with strong supports throughout the ups and downs of daily life, children can become young adults and then older adults that are well-grounded emotionally; that thrive in home, at school, and at work; and that contribute positively to society.

Yet far too often stressors strike our youth, which — without adequate buffering and support — can negatively alter their trajectories over a lifetime. The burgeoning field of understanding Adverse Childhood Experiences, or ACEs, has yielded profound insights into the complex interaction of physiology and adversity that lead to poor outcomes over the life course, with profound implications on society. With increasing numbers of ACEs — such as the death of a parent, abuse or drug use in the home, parental divorce, and incarceration of a family member — growing youths too often experience dose-proportional long-term poor health outcomes. Without adequate buffering and support from a health systems approach involving parents and families, health professionals, schools, communities, government, and more, these adverse outcomes can result in a nation and world whose members are thwarted from becoming thriving, contributing members of society. These impacts are profound: a stifled next generation of Albert Einsteins or Steve Jobses; decreased economic productivity; increased costs in the justice or welfare systems; decreased military readiness; and damaged lives.

Pediatric consultation-liaison psychiatry is a critical field that recognizes the inherent stressors associated with childhood illnesses and that seeks to engage and support the health system to bring understanding and healing to medically ill individuals and their families in ways that maximize their human potential. From addressing constipation in a scared youngster to facilitating family therapy for an adolescent with suicidal thoughts to collaborating with other pediatric health professionals on overall plans of care, the field of pediatric consultation-liaison psychiatry is rich with high-touch, high-impact processes and results. It plays an important role in the context of pediatric primary and specialty healthcare as a liaison between patients' mental health and overall health; between hospitals and outpatient health systems; and between the patient in the "patient" role versus in the family member, student, friend, and citizen roles. Pediatric consultation-liaison psychiatry also reminds policymakers that robust communities and nations result from healthy children that have the comprehensively strong support and care they need to grow into their full potential as adults.

Drs. Anthony Guerrero, Norbert Skokauskas, and Paul Lee here set out critical principles in the practice of pediatric consultation-liaison psychiatry as well as lessons that transcend the field. Beyond its clinical excellence, the text beckons the child and adolescent psychiatrist toward an approach to individuals and families affected by psychosomatic conditions that is holistic, grounded in evidence, thoughtful, engaging, and thorough. Their work offers a global lens through which to approach human well-being: holding others' medical illness and its socio-emotional impacts in skilled hands that are gentle and clinically excellent.

I can hardly imagine a better leader in this effort than Dr. Guerrero, whom I have admired since he taught psychiatry and pediatrics at our University of Hawai'i John A. Burns School of Medicine, where I graduated in 2009. His sharp intellect and leadership in these fields combined with his warmth, holistic approach to medicine, and the aloha spirit make him a leader of the best sort.

Perhaps most importantly, this work reminds us of the profound interconnectedness of us all. We are all only one step away from illness, from disaster, or from tragedy. Channeling our systems approaches to invest in the psychosocial foundations of our youth will require all hands on deck, but the prospects are great. The future is now.

Director of Health Science Policy
University of Hawaiʻi System,
Honolulu, HI, USA

Aimee M. Grace

Foreword by Bennett L. Leventhal

The task of writing the foreword to a text is a complex matter. There are any number of approaches and many possibilities for its content and function. One might assume that the principal function of the foreword is to be in the "fore" and come before the body of work that follows. But, it could serve other functions, such as "leading the charge forward" into an interesting scholarly work that will energize the field. In the present instance, it is my privilege to serve both functions simultaneously. Even more importantly, this volume is leading the charge forward in a contemporary approach to what were, traditionally, "psychosomatic medicine" and "consultation-liaison psychiatry" for children and adolescents.

Pediatric Consultation Liaison Psychiatry: A Global, Healthcare Systems-Focused, and Problem-Based Approach offers a novel approach to an old topic. It is rich with evidence that the field of psychosomatic medicine has evolved greatly from the times of Weiner, Minuchin, and others, when psychosomatic illness was limited to asthma, diabetes, hypertension, and others with underlying etiological models embedded in defective psychological structures, psychic distress, and family dysfunction. Rather, Guerrero, Skokauskas, and Lee, along with their multinational team of authors, offer a model that focuses on the interactions between cognitive, emotional, and behavioral function in health and disease. This approach is a revolution in that it provides directions for integrating psychiatric care in the general healthcare setting, where it properly belongs, and for optimizing global access to a specialty universally in short supply.

Why is this such a revolution? Well, perhaps, it is not. Rather, it is recognition that there are fundamental principles of child and adolescent psychiatry that are intrinsic to healthcare:

The first of these principles is that all human function and illness must be placed in a developmental context. Even before conception, developmental factors are playing a role in the creation and function of the gametes that lead to the zygote and then to the complex human fetus. The genetic activity, epigenetic effects, and gene–environment interactions that take place at each stage along the entirety of the human lifespan shape who we are and how we function. Without sensitivity to these ongoing processes and their impacts on development in health and disease, there is no compass to direct our work.

The second principle at work is that most disruptions in health are syndromes – a cluster of symptoms that tend to cluster together and share a common natural history. As a result, not all illnesses look precisely the same, their impacts may be very different on any given individual, and they often represent a spectrum of health and dysfunction across the population.

The third principle is that the brain is the epicenter of health and disease. The principal functions of the brain are to maintain homeostasis and foster adaptation: when there is time and energy left over, other unique functions, like creativity, come to the fore. Subcortical areas focus primarily on basic self-preservation and physiologic homeostasis, while cortical areas manage behavior, cognition, and emotion.

The fourth principle is that humans live and function in complex systems (biological, psychological, social, cultural, political, etc.) Therefore, for any intervention (prevention, early intervention, or treatment) to be effective, it must be intrinsically connected or exquisitely sensitive to the relevant systems. In the case of healthcare, these systems include all the above plus the practitioners and contexts in which they provide care.

Are any of these principles novel? No. But, integrating them into a care model is the way forward in children's healthcare. Going beyond a more limited consultation and liaison model, this model embraces the integration of psychiatric medicine in general healthcare for youth. It also responds flexibly to specific disease states as well as to the needs of children, family, and practitioners. Further, it is sensitive to cultural diversity in the experience of illness and its treatment for each of the individuals involved.

Modern child and adolescent psychiatry is well-suited to meet the challenges requiring its full participation in the care of children, adolescents, and their families. It is inherently developmental, and it is the home of a systems-driven model of care that appreciates the incredible capacity of brain function.

So, I am pleased to come before the body of *Pediatric Consultation Liaison Psychiatry: A Global, Healthcare Systems-Focused, and Problem-Based Approach*. It provides a fresh view of children's healthcare by offering general principles, exposure to common scenarios, examination of values, and exploration of healthcare systems as well as global perspectives. And, this textbook is capped off with practical and useful teaching and screening tools. This information is all helpful but will mean nothing if it is not put into practice as a part of modern child and adolescent psychiatry.

The eminent physician, Sir William Osler, had book plates that read:

"He who studies medicine without books sails an uncharted sea,
but he who studies medicine without patients does not to go to sea at all."

Read this book, absorb its wisdom, and then go see the patients who need our care.

Division of Child & Adolescent Psychiatry,
Department of Psychiatry,
Langley Porter Psychiatric Institute
University of California San Francisco,
San Francisco, CA, USA

Bennett L. Leventhal

Foreword by Calvin C. J. Sia

It is my privilege to provide a Foreword for this textbook, which is very timely, given the urgent importance of psychosocial well-being in children's health. I have the humble distinction of being recognized as the "grandfather" of the medical home concept system of care, which strives for comprehensive primary care through partnerships between patients, clinicians of all specialties, medical staff, families, and their communities.

It is an essential component of healthcare's present and future and I fully applaud the authors' efforts to describe how knowledge of the psychiatric aspects of pediatric conditions and enhanced pediatric/psychiatric collaboration in all healthcare settings can ensure that children's care is truly accessible, family centered, coordinated, comprehensive, continuous, compassionate, and culturally effective.

In the last half-century, we have made significant strides in improving children's health through home visiting programs, early intervention programs, and other multidisciplinary training and workforce-focused programs for at-risk children and youth. Currently, with growing recognition of the social environment's impact upon health and healthcare costs, the lifelong and trans-generational effects of adverse childhood experiences and toxic stress, and the continued significant morbidity and mortality associated with environmental and psychosocial issues, we need to further strengthen a healthcare system that is integrated, comprehensive, coordinated, and collaborative in support of good health, strong families, positive learning experiences, and early childhood systems. Toward this goal, we as primary care physicians value a strong relationship with child psychiatrists and all developmental, mental, behavioral, and social health providers serving children and youth for the twenty-first century.

"Every child and youth deserves a medical home." I sincerely hope that readers of this book will provide well-informed and comprehensive care for children and — in partnership with other colleagues — embrace their role in helping to make this mandate a reality.

Department of Pediatrics
University of Hawai'i
John A. Burns School of Medicine,
Honolulu, HI, USA

Calvin C. J. Sia

Contents

Part I
Basic Principles

Chapter 1
General Principles of Pediatric Consultation-Liaison Psychiatry

Anthony P. S. Guerrero, Norbert Skokauskas, Paul C. Lee, H. Charles Fishman, Cathy K. Bell, and Jason R. Keifer

Introduction

Orientation to This Textbook

Welcome to "Pediatric Consultation-Liaison Psychiatry: A Global, Healthcare Systems-Focused, and Problem-Based Approach!"

This textbook brings together practitioners from around the world to explore essential concepts in pediatric consultation-liaison psychiatry (also known as pediatric psychosomatic medicine) utilizing a problem-based approach. Shaw et al. (2010) define pediatric psychosomatic medicine as the "subspecialty of child and adolescent psychiatry that is dedicated to providing mental health services to

A. P. S. Guerrero (✉) · P. C. Lee
Department of Psychiatry, University of Hawai'i John A. Burns School of Medicine, Honolulu, HI, USA
e-mail: GuerreroA@dop.hawaii.edu; paul.c.lee23.civ@mail.mil

N. Skokauskas
Department of Centre for Child and Youth Mental Health, Institute of Mental Health, Medicine and Health Sciences, NTNU, Trondheim, Norway
e-mail: norbert.skokauskas@ntnu.no

H. C. Fishman
Department of Psychiatry, University of Hawai'i, John A. Burns School of Medicine, Honolulu, HI, USA

Reconnect Family Services, Auckland, New Zealand
e-mail: charles@fishman.co.nz

C. K. Bell · J. R. Keifer
Kahala Clinic for Children & Family, Honolulu, HI, USA

A. P. S. Guerrero et al. (eds.), *Pediatric Consultation-Liaison Psychiatry*
https://doi.org/10.1007/978-3-319-89488-1_1

youngsters with physical illness." The United States' Accreditation Council for Graduate Medical Education (ACGME) describes psychosomatic medicine as "the discipline encompassing the study and practice of psychiatric disorders in patients with medical, surgical, obstetrical, and neurological conditions, particularly for patients with complex and/or chronic conditions" (ACGME 2016). Likewise, a consensus paper from the European Association of Consultation-Liaison Psychiatry and Psychosomatic Medicine (EACLPP) and the Academy of Psychosomatic Medicine (APM) considered "psychosomatic medicine" and "consultation-liaison psychiatry" to be interchangeable and described the specialty's scope as inclusive of consultative, collaborative, or integrated care participation for patients being treated in the nonmental health setting. It specifically outlines that "The scope necessarily includes psychiatric collaboration or integration in support of mental healthcare services provided in primary care and specialty care settings" (Leentjens et al. 2011). While much of the content of this textbook focuses on traditional inpatient consultation-liaison psychiatry, it includes chapters and case vignettes (even in this chapter) that take place in outpatient and community settings.

The editors enthusiastically believe that pediatric psychosomatic medicine, or pediatric consultation-liaison psychiatry, is the single most important specialty in the future of healthcare, nationally and globally for two reasons. First, it plays a major role in preventively addressing the psychiatric and psychosocial comorbidities affecting a vulnerable population that adversely impact healthcare outcomes throughout the lifespan and that lead to potentially avoidable healthcare spending. Second, it has a potential role in optimizing access to child and adolescent mental healthcare through its collaboration with other healthcare specialties.

Targeting a broad audience, the editors have chosen to include illustrative vignettes throughout the textbook. These cases were developed based on scenarios commonly encountered by both psychiatrists and referring professionals from other disciplines working in a variety of settings, ranging from the traditional inpatient and tertiary care settings to the community. The editors are especially delighted that this book is a global collaboration, involving authors from various parts of the world, including North and South America, Europe, Asia, Africa, and New Zealand.

The chapters are structured around the study of case vignettes that demonstrate the value of psychiatry in various contexts and settings. In the spirit of problem-based learning, or PBL, and with the hopes of simulating real-life clinical problem-solving, cases are structured, where appropriate, around a progressive disclosure model, to allow for further reflection and reading in between the parts of the vignette. The reader is encouraged to learn more about applications of PBL in teaching and learning psychiatry (see Alicata et al. 2016). We strongly believe that pediatric consultation-liaison psychiatry is particularly well suited to PBL, which promotes multidimensional thinking, collaboration, and lifelong learning: all essential aspects of the specialty.

Terminology

Across countries, different terminologies may be used to describe common elements within pediatric consultation-liaison psychiatry. For the sake of clarity, the term "fellow" or "resident" or "junior doctor" describes a physician who is completing specialty training in psychiatry or child and adolescent psychiatry or other subspecialty. The term "attending psychiatrist," "psychiatrist consultant," or "senior doctor" describes the senior, supervising psychiatrist who specializes in pediatric consultation-liaison psychiatry. The term "referring physician/provider" or "attending physician/provider" describes the nonpsychiatrist physician/provider who is referring the patient for psychiatric consultation. Finally, where applicable, the term "parent or guardian" includes the child's caregiver or anyone else with legal responsibility for the child.

Without further delay, let us begin studying a fictitious case, to illustrate general principles of pediatric consultation-liaison psychiatry.

General Principles Relevant to Children and Adolescents on a Consultation-Liaison Service

Preparing for the Pediatric Consultation-Liaison Encounter

Case Vignette 1.1

You are a relatively new fellow/junior doctor on the pediatric psychiatry consultation-liaison service. You receive the following new consult request from the newborn nursery: "please evaluate and provide support for the 17-year-old mother of a new baby with congenital clubfoot." You wonder how to approach this somewhat unfamiliar situation.

This case illustrates the importance, in pediatric consultation-liaison psychiatry, of maintaining an open mind and embracing inquisitiveness and lifelong learning. In the above scenario, many questions arise: Who is really the patient, the newborn or the mother? Is it the consultant's role to be seeing the parents of pediatric patients, even though the mother is also in the pediatric age group? Do we need the mother's parent or guardian to agree to the consult, or is the mother able to consent for herself? Is "providing support" a typical role for a consulting psychiatrist?

While the actual answers to these questions may differ, based on country or local statute or practice, they are nonetheless important to think through. Many other questions often arise. One key practice to address some initial questions is to discuss the case with the referring provider before seeing the pediatric patient. This discussion will allow one the opportunity to ask the referring provider their understanding of some of the initial questions and aid in developing a clear idea of the issues to address in the consultation. Where applicable, one should get an idea of the prognosis of the patient's medical condition. More fundamentally, it is important to ascertain who is the most appropriate "identified patient" to facilitate appropriate registration and documentation. In the vignette, it is not immediately obvious who is the "patient."

If the identified patient is a child or adolescent or other person without legal autonomy, it is advisable (except in unusual circumstances) to ensure that the parent(s) and/or guardian(s) have been informed about, and have agreed to, the consultation. Indeed, the effectiveness of the consultation-liaison psychiatrist is limited if the initial encounter with the patient and family is awkward or confrontational merely because they had not been informed that a psychiatric consultation was requested. Along these lines, and for the purposes of documenting medical necessity, the consultant should ensure that the referring medical team has either written an order for the consultation or documented that a consultation is necessary and therefore being requested.

Case Vignette 1.2

Following a discussion with your attending psychiatrist/senior doctor, you call the referring physician to discuss the team's specific concerns and to learn more about the baby's prognosis. You learn that the neonate's prognosis beyond the clubfoot is otherwise very positive. You ensure that a consult has been formally requested for the mother as the identified patient. You also confirm that her own legal guardian (the baby's maternal grandmother) will be agreeably involved in the initial interview. You then ponder what your approach should be to the initial meeting with the patient.

In the interests of maintaining optimal relationships with the system of care surrounding a pediatric patient, the consultant should always remember this advice: all consultation requests should be regarded with respect and full consideration. Even if the identified patient were to seem "fine," or if the referral question were "vague," every consultation request suggests that someone in the system – whether a family member, healthcare professional, or other stakeholder – is concerned and therefore potentially able to benefit from a timely, systems-sensitive intervention. In one of the author's institution's consultation-liaison service, residents and fellows are encouraged to take the perspective of bright and eager new physicians who are grateful for the privilege to work in the medical center and who are always pleased to find work that can support their practice. Adopting such an attitude improves the overall quality of the consultation-liaison service and, ultimately, the care the patients and families receive.

Case Vignette 1.3

You meet with the patient, the nursing baby, and the patient's mother at bedside. Before beginning the formal assessment, you politely introduce yourself, discuss your understanding of the reason why you are meeting, and share what you know about her history thus far. You congratulate her on the birth of her new baby. Sensitive to the realities of what it must be like to be in the hospital and to just have given birth, you ask general questions about how she is doing now and whether it is a good time to do an interview. Although not denying that she is quite exhausted and sleep-deprived, she confirms that the time is convenient and that she wants her own mother to be present, to help her with the baby.

You identify some symptoms of anxiety related to family tensions involving concerns over having to care for a child at too young an age, the responsibilities involved with parenthood, and the unexpected outcome of the congenital clubfoot. You consider a possible adjustment disorder and take the opportunity to provide education about the signs and symptoms of depressive and anxiety disorders, for which you feel she has some risk factors. In working with the staff, you strengthen your collaborative relationship. Finally, you insure that your documentation is concise and reflective of the impressions and recommendations that you conveyed, using understandable language, to the patient and staff.

The Developmental Perspective: Understanding and Empathizing with Children

Case Vignette 1.4

You consult on a five-year-old male who has been admitted for constipation, encopresis, and fecal impaction. Outpatient interventions, including behavioral interventions and medications for constipation, have been unsuccessful. You think about your initial differential considerations for why outpatient interventions have been unsuccessful up to this point and the additional information that you would seek.

Children and adolescents are continually developing, so it is very important to consider the developmental level of the patient. A comprehensive review of child and adolescent development is beyond the scope of this chapter. However, this chapter will review key aspects of development and particularly how development affects the impact of, understanding of, and adaptation to general medical illnesses. Development will also be recurring theme in future chapters.

Case Vignette 1.5

In speaking to the child, you discover that he is fearful of sitting on the toilet and has been holding in his stool because he was afraid that "if my poop fell into the hole of the toilet, I could fall in there too." Together with the rest of the healthcare team, you help him overcome his fear of getting flushed down the toilet, and prior to discharge, he successfully defecates into the toilet. The parents, who are committed to helping him sustain this progress, are very appreciative of your help.

One key principle is that development is a continuous process that builds on success in earlier stages. The consultation-liaison psychiatrist working in pediatric settings should therefore recognize the potential disruption that medical illnesses may have on normal child development.

Table 1.1 summarizes key developmental stages. Emphasis has been placed on social and cognitive domains that may be of clinical importance in the context of medical illnesses. Children's developmental levels are important to consider in

Table 1.1 A summary of the key stages of development

Age	Social development	Cognitive development	Clinical implications
4–6 months	Increasing awareness and recognition of people, development of attachment		Potential reactive attachment disorders, failure to thrive if inadequate attention to these issues in the context of general medical illness and separation from family
12–15 months		Object permanence	Stranger anxiety; important to consider impact of hospitalization and separation from caregivers
3–6 years	Improved separation (the age when children usually start school)	Preoperational thinking; possible "magical" or otherwise erroneous beliefs	If there is ongoing severe separation anxiety, need to consider differential possibilities, for this child's reactions and emotions are still very much connected to the family's
7–11 years	Generally good coping with separation	Concrete thinking	Relatively favorable age for elective surgery; increasing ability to be involved in explanations of illness and treatment, though need to adjust to concrete thinking
11–20 years	Challenging authority	Formal operations: morals, ethics, self-control, humanitarian/global concerns	Need to anticipate/address potential impacts on compliance; may be able to give more detailed explanations of illness and implications

understanding their illness, in discussing coping with their illness and the associated treatments, and in addressing issues related to death and dying. For example, 6-year-olds may have erroneous (though developmentally age-appropriate) beliefs about human physiology and may believe that they can lose all their blood from a blood draw or injection, despite well-meaning reassurances that the pain will not be severe. As another example, unknown to a parent or caregiver, a 6-year-old might believe that justice can emanate from inanimate objects and might blame him or herself for a personal illness or otherwise be afraid of reporting symptoms. Older children, despite more accurate perceptions about the causation of illness, may still not be able to appreciate all the mechanisms that lead to illness. Hence, relatively straightforward explanations about the need for certain treatments may be most appropriate.

Beyond the cognitive understanding of illness, the emotional adjustment to illness is heavily influenced by developmental level. For example, it is likely that a preadolescent who must cope with a physical deformity may be more vulnerable to emotional difficulties compared to a younger child, who may have a less developed body image, or an older adolescent, who may be more cognitively mature.

For children to optimally adjust to issues related to death and dying, they need to understand that death is irreversible, final, inevitable, and causally explained. When children who have not yet reached the developmental stage to understand these principles must face death, whether it is their own death, or the death of a loved one, they are vulnerable to experiencing adjustment difficulties. For example, a child who does not realize that death is inevitable or causally explained may consider death to be a punishment for wrongdoing. Parents or guardians are often able to gauge their child's cognitive development. However, they frequently benefit from briefings about how to discuss challenging topics, such as death and illness, in a manner that best matches that cognitive development.

The Systems Perspective: Collaborating and Appreciating Role in a Larger Context

Case Vignette 1.6

Right after returning home from work, you are called back to the hospital to assess a 16-year-old female who has been referred by the school counselor to the emergency department for expressing suicidal thoughts while at school. The parents/legal guardians are not currently at bedside. The charge nurse reports that the parents left just a few moments ago, "probably to take a break." You think about what your next step should be. Should you begin interviewing the patient?

Children, both legally and developmentally, are not autonomous beings. They are part of a complex system that includes their family and other professionals involved in a child's care. While local laws may differ somewhat on the degree to which adolescents can consent to certain aspects of medical care (e.g., often related to family planning, sexually transmitted diseases treatment, and substance abuse treatment), most locales require parental consent for most types of behavioral healthcare, except in emergency situations. Additionally, conscientious, system-sensitive involvement of the family in the care of a child or adolescent, whether legally mandated or not, usually constitutes the most optimal clinical care.

Consultants often ask what the best way is to approach child or adolescent patients and their family for the initial consultation. Should the patient or caregivers be interviewed separately first, or should the patient and caregivers be initially interviewed together? The editors believe that there is no one correct answer to this question and recommend that ideally (1) the patient and available family at bedside be introduced to the context of the consultation and then asked about how they would like to proceed (in part, to assess how they view – accurately or otherwise – the relative contributions of the people and the interactions between the people); (2) time be set aside to interview the patient and parents separately, particularly if there are concerns about abuse or other sensitive issues; and (3) a comprehensive biopsychosocial formulation with attention to the child's age and development and the family and systems perspectives guide the titration of the amount of time spent with the patient or parents alone and with the patient and parents together (for instance, if improving communication between the patient and parents is an important focus of the intervention).

Case Vignette 1.7

You call the parents on their cellular phone, and they report that they had gone to the cafeteria to eat dinner. "We were sitting in the emergency department for the last couple of hours. We both had just gotten off from work and had not eaten the whole day. They gave a meal tray to our daughter, but we were not so lucky, so we went to the cafeteria before it closed."

You empathize with how the parents must be feeling, and you encourage them to finish their meal. Knowing that you need to be alert, focused, and calm to do a competent job with the consultation (not to mention drive back home later in the night), you are glad that you made sure to eat a nutritious meal and to reasonably take care of your own well-being before seeing the family.

The parents soon return to the emergency department. You gather basic information from the youth and the parents. In the individual portion of the history-gathering, she denies that there is any problem. You discuss your understanding of why she is in the emergency department and empathize with what appears to be the reality: that she was not the one who asked to be brought to the emergency department.

She subsequently becomes more open to discussion. She states, "when I told my teacher that all my classmates' drama was making me think of suicide, I wasn't really serious, but then the teacher made the school counselor and my parents all scared, so now I'm here." She had never attempted suicide. While she has some symptoms of depression, she does not meet full criteria for a major depressive episode. There is no history of substance use, and the remainder of the psychiatric history and mental status examination were unremarkable. Based upon your findings, you are inclined to discharge her, but you realize that there are other steps you must take before doing so.

Children and adolescents rarely request psychiatric consultations on their own. The requests for psychiatric assistance and the reporting of psychiatric symptoms are therefore often seen through the lens of the family, healthcare providers, or other concerned individuals. It is also essential to determine why the consultation is being requested. The consultation reason facilitates deciding which aspects of the system warrant attention and intervention. For example, if someone other than the child or family requested the consultation, an effective approach must include directly addressing that person's concerns. Consultation-liaison psychiatry is the perfect venue to practice the biopsychosocial formulation (discussed in more detail in Chap. 10), which can guide interventions and healing on multiple levels beyond just the psychiatric "diagnosis," which has the risk of overemphasizing individual illness and undervaluing strengths and resources within the family and larger system.

Many requests for consultation arise from concerns about emotional or behavioral symptoms in a parent or other family member involved in the child's care. These are entirely appropriate reasons to consult psychiatry, since the family is part of the whole system affecting the child's health. Therefore, while it is certainly appropriate to clarify the intent of the consultation with the referring provider, we recommend against becoming resistant to a medical team's request for help. In such situations, it is important to document consultations from the perspective that the child is the identified patient, even though observations about the parent or other caregiver may also be included. If a parent or other family member needs their own follow-up as a separately identified patient, then this can be part of the recommendation.

Case Vignette 1.8

You meet with the parents, who describe their daughter's many strengths, including her overall good achievement in school and extracurricular activities, but who are concerned with some of her "moodiness" and "irregular sleep habits." The father is especially concerned, because he recalls experiencing some of these symptoms as a teenager. He was later diagnosed with major depression as a young adult, and although, at one point in his life, he was hospitalized for a suicide attempt, he is currently doing well on antidepressant medications. "I feel bad that, of all of the things that our daughter could have inherited, she might have inherited my depression." You provide appropriate education to the parents, who are grateful for the follow-up resources that you have offered.

In addition, because it was the school counselor who recommended the referral (the "why now?" that led to the emergency room visit), you then involve the parents and patient in a phone call to the school counselor, who left her cellular phone number with the parents. She explains that the school is taking any statements of suicide very seriously, particularly because of a recent serious suicide attempt among one of the high school seniors. The school counselor is grateful for your prompt assessment, your involvement of the family, and your phone call, and she requests a doctor's note providing clearance to go back to school. You recognize that calling the school counselor was an important step in completing the consultation; if the school did not have the reassurance that a proper evaluation had been done, then the patient might be referred again for an emergency assessment.

This vignette describes a consultation with a reasonably positive outcome and a reasonably satisfied group of interested adults. Other situations may have additional complexities that can be effectively approached by paying attention to one's role and relationship with the family and system surrounding the patient. Common family and systems-related situations and the potential role for the consultation-liaison psychiatrist are summarized in Table 1.2.

In the next sections, we discuss how optimally caring for patients in pediatric consultation-liaison psychiatry means challenging ourselves to broaden the ways in which we think.

The Psychosomatic Family Model, Insuring the Right Approach, and Empowering the Primary Care Team

Case Vignette 1.9

The patient is a 10-year-old female who is hospitalized for migraine headaches with significant pain and nausea requiring intravenous medications and fluid. Laboratory tests did not indicate any other medical problems. It was felt that her degree of pain was significantly more than what would be expected for this condition. Nursing staff reported that the patient seemed to most be in pain when her mother and stepfather were in the room together. She otherwise would seem "fine."

It had been noted that there were recent family stressors, including marital conflict between the mother and stepfather and the birth of a new sibling, who is now 3 months old. The mother had reported that, particularly in the last few months, the patient had been crying more, arguing more, and complaining more of headaches. A psychiatric consultation was suggested to evaluate for "adjustment difficulties," to rule out a psychological component to the headaches, and to provide "therapy" if indicated.

The identified patient and her family were interviewed. The mother and stepfather report that they are somewhat concerned that patient's symptoms might indicate the presence of an "aneurysm," which the maternal great grandmother, who was close to the patient, died from 5 months ago. Patient was not worried that the headaches represent anything other than her migraines.

The family noted that, in the past few months, there have been multiple stressors, including the birth of the patient's half sister (who is the only other child in the family); loss of the stepfather's job; increased marital conflict, probably related to the financial pressures of the stepfather's job loss; and the beginning of a new academic year in a new school. Per the family's report, there are no previous behavioral concerns. She has had a history of migraines from an early age that was usually well controlled with prophylactic medication. There are also no other medical problems, and there was no pattern of recurring somatic complaints other than the migraines. There is a strong family history of migraines, and mother notes that her own migraines began during childhood.

The patient admitted that she has been feeling sad, "bummed out," and "a little worried" over all the "money problems" their family had been having. She believed that her migraines may be worse whenever she feels stress. While she says that she likes the new baby, she "never really liked the idea of mom getting re-married." She recalled that in the previous marriage, "my real dad was always drunk, and he used to hit her, so that's why they got a divorce." While she reports being afraid whenever she witnessed violence, she denies any nightmares, flashbacks, or significant distress upon re-exposure to reminders of previous trauma. She denied any past or present history of physical or sexual abuse. She denied excessive worry about her mother's safety or anxiety upon separating from her family to attend school and other activities. While she has had poor appetite and sleep for the past 2 days since the migraine difficulties began, she denied any previous sleep, appetite, or energy level changes and denied any definite anhedonia or suicidal or homicidal ideations. While cooperative on interview, she did appear uncomfortable, and she preferred the lights off. Vital signs were significant for mild tachycardia.

While a complete discussion of family-based treatments (on which we highly recommend further reading) is beyond the scope of this textbook, it is important to recognize the importance of applying the appropriate model for treatment. Otherwise, instinctively selected interventions or intervention combinations (e.g.,

Table 1.2 Common family-related situations and the potential role for the consultation-liaison psychiatrist

Consultation-liaison scenario	Potential tasks for the consultation-liaison psychiatrist	Possible pitfalls
Family adjustment (e.g., depression, anxiety, "denial") to a child or adolescent's illness	Provide family-oriented support and psychoeducation	Providing long-term or in-depth care for a specific family member, without making it explicit to the family or in the medical record, that you have assumed this role, separate from your consultation/liaison role to the identified patient
	Evaluate for the need for further mental health services for family members and provide referrals as appropriate	Not adequately recognizing that initial adaptive "denial" may interfere with optimal medical care and possibly constitute medical neglect
	Educate the medical team on possible emotional reactions to a child's illness, including what may be initial "denial"	
History or possibility of mental illness (including substance abuse) in the parent and/or other caregiver adult	Evaluate for any acute dangerousness in the parent, or possible abuse/neglect of the child	Providing long-term or in-depth care for a specific family member, without making it explicit to the family or in the medical record that you have assumed this role, separate from your consultation/liaison role to the identified patient
	Evaluate for the need for further mental health services for family members and provide referrals as appropriate	Giving the appearance of having performed a forensic assessment of the adult's parenting capacity, whereas such a function might better be performed by another mental health provider using standardized assessment tools and usually affiliated with child protective services
Possible parental abuse/neglect, including Munchausen-by-proxy	Evaluate for the need for further mental health services for family members and provide referrals as appropriate	Providing long-term or in-depth care for the parent (see above). Giving the appearance of having performed a forensic assessment of the adult's parenting capacity whereas such a function might better be performed by another mental health provider using standardized assessment tools and usually affiliated with child protective services
	Assist the team in making referrals to child protective and hospital risk management services, where indicated	
	Assist the team in formulating a crisis plan (e.g., with hospital security) where indicated	

(continued)

Table 1.2 (continued)

Consultation-liaison scenario	Potential tasks for the consultation-liaison psychiatrist	Possible pitfalls
Angry, abusive, potentially litigious family	Listen closely to parents' concerns, including what they are most concerned about with their child's condition	Not adequately helping the medical team to avoid unnecessary medicolegal risk via:
	Consider all possible reasons for the family's anger, including factors that may be within the medical team's control	"Splitting"
	Evaluate the need for further mental health services for family members and provide referrals as appropriate	Inappropriate documentation Indiscreet conversations
	Evaluate the need for other referrals (e.g., domestic violence help)	
	Assist the team in making referrals to child protective and hospital risk management services, where indicated	
	Assist the team in formulating a crisis plan (e.g., with hospital security) where indicated	
Failure to thrive	Provide a thorough assessment that considers child variables (e.g., temperamental and other behavioral conditions), caregiver variables, and interactional variables; encourage multidisciplinary approaches	Failing to recognize the multifactorial nature of failure to thrive or inadequately managing general medical conditions coexisting with psychosocial conditions
	Evaluate the need for further mental health services for the child or family members and provide referrals as appropriate	

vague or haphazardly planned "individual plus family" approaches) that are not grounded in a coherent, evidence-based model may be counterproductive.

From the family system's perspective, the dynamics seem obvious from the nursing staff report that the patient seemed to be most in pain when her mother and stepfather were in the room together. Given the history, it would be important to treat this youngster and her family using the *psychosomatic family model*.

In 1962, Princeton professor T. S. Kuhn published the landmark book: *The Structure of Scientific Revolutions*. The book documented the discontinuity between paradigms. For example, Einsteinian theory could not be reduced into Newtonian mechanics. Similarly, $E = mc^2$ was not reducible into Quantum Mechanics (Kuhn and Hawkins 1963).

Edgar Levenson (Levenson 1972) described the progression of models in psychiatry and psychology. In the late-nineteenth century, a problem such as this patient's would be seen as being within her mind, and she would be referred for individual counseling. The metaphors with this first model, the individual approach, were based on the technology of the time: the steam engine. Terms like "displacement" and "repression" described a patient's psychological manifestations. The second model was the communication model. The symptoms developed because this patient was not communicating her feelings. This model came into vogue during World War II. The technological metaphor was a guided missile system: if the missile gets the appropriate feedback, it hits its target. The third model, and the model on which this work is based, is the organismic model. The locus of the patient's problems is in social ecology. The metaphor is biological. The problem is in her social ecology, its structure.

The Psychosomatic Family Model

The term "psychosomatic family" first entered the literature in the early 1970s, when child psychiatrist Salvador Minuchin, psychologist Bernice Rossman, and pediatrician Lester Baker published their book: *Psychosomatic Families: Anorexia in Context* (Minuchin et al. 1978). The model is based on their work at the Children's Hospital of Philadelphia in the early 1970s. Minuchin and colleagues treated three school-aged girls, all with labile diabetes, whose ketoacidosis was exacerbated in one context: while at home with their families. They posited the psychosomatic family model based on their family interactional patterns. The model consisted of four interactional patterns: triangulation, involving the symptomatic child caught between the parental split (such that the resulting diffusion of parental conflict becomes associated with symptom exacerbation), rigidity, conflict avoidance, and perfectionism.

The patient in the vignette is a 10-year-old with a history of migraines accompanied by significant pain and nausea. Her symptomatology manifested most severely when she was with her parents during the evening. Her family system is complex, with father's job loss, economic difficulties, and birth of a new child. These are important factors, adding stress. From the psychosomatic family perspective, however, the pivotal issue to be addressed is an interactional pattern: the split between the parents. To the extent that mother and stepfather cease triangulating their 10-year-old daughter, the symptoms should ameliorate. Note that the tenets of the psychosomatic family model are recursively connected: with a change in one tenet, the others also change.

In the psychosomatic family model, once tests determine that there is no other medical etiology, the clinicians assess the patient's social context, especially interactional patterns within the family. In this case, the crucial step is dealing with the parental unit. In this model, there is a distinction between etiology and maintenance. In the systems model, focus is on the contemporary interactional patterns that are maintaining the symptomatology. The etiology is lost in history and irretrievable;

what *is* retrievable and imminently visible is a conflict between the parents and a temporal connection to the exacerbation of her symptoms.

In the case above, the psychosomatic family model should guide the overall approach. Clearly, working collaboratively is crucial. With this approach, however, individual or supportive counseling would not be a priority and would be counter-productive. Families could get confused when different mental health paradigms are introduced: "is the problem in their daughter's mind or is the problem in her context." "Do we have to change," families ask, or "will you professionals change her?" Instead, the focus should be on dealing with the split in the system, normalizing this girl's behavior, and enriching her life with her peers such that she would be less adversely influenced by the family dynamics.

In terms of the primary care provider's (PCP's) role, rather than immediately involving other consultants for direct care, the PCP might meet with the family and address the triangulation. The provider would discuss the essentiality that they agree on whatever steps are necessary in parenting their child. Disagreements must be resolved away from their daughter. They need to realize that the crucial step is de-triangulating their child.

In the authors' experience in working with PCP's, such interventions can powerfully illustrate family transformation and mitigation of presenting symptomatology and can be especially effective in the context of PCP's often long-term relationships with families.

Case Vignette 1.10
You work collaboratively with the pediatric team to optimize medical management of acute pain. A family-based treatment model is applied, and several months later, her headaches are under stable control, and there are no further hospitalizations.

Interventions based on the psychosomatic model are widely supported in the literature and applied worldwide. In one of the authors' clinical audit of patients with eating disorders, followed for up to 20 years, self-starving behavior ceased within weeks, and the anorexia nervosa had not recurred after the initial treatment (Fishman 2005).

The Family Development Perspective: Appreciating Adaptiveness, Equilibrium, and Potential Resistance to Change

Case Vignette 1.11
During team rounds, a family physician in an integrated primary care/behavioral health setting asks for your help on a complex patient, an almost 18-year-old female "with what I think is bulimia nervosa... I started her on fluoxetine two months ago, but she still isn't getting better."

The patient recently entered a prestigious university and had always been a perfectionistic high achiever. Toward the end of her senior year, she and her friends made a pact to lose weight before a class field trip that involved a visit to the beach.

She lost 5–8 pounds through food restriction and purging. Even after the event was finished, she continued to binge and purge, to the point where she is at risk of not being able to continue in college because of health reasons.

You recognize the potential complexities and seriousness of the case, and you agree to see the patient, together with the primary care team.

Essential pediatric consultation-liaison skills include maintaining an attentive, nonjudgmental, and clinically discerning ear when listening to referring providers; thinking comprehensively and according to biopsychosocial formulation principles (to be further discussed in Chap. 10); and triaging according to levels of risk and severity (in this case, appreciating the potential morbidity and mortality associated with eating disorders, which are also discussed in more detail in Chap. 6).

Case Vignette 1.12

The patient, who is an only child, currently lives with relatives who live closer to the university that she is attending. Through interviewing the patient and the family, you learn that just recently, she began questioning her competence and career choice, worrying significantly about disappointing her parents, and recognizing how much her parents had sacrificed. As she was growing up, the parents, who were busy business owners, tended to not ask much of her since she did well in school and had many extracurricular activities. She tended to be an "intense" child, and when she would get emotionally overwhelmed, upset, or angry, the parents tended to decrease expectations and step in and help her. Mindful of how busy her parents were, however, she tried as much as possible to not to "bother them" with her "issues."

However, she currently does not perceive that her parents validate her feelings. She is currently quite upset (1) that her parents are in the process of semi-retiring and moving to be closer to her university, (2) that they did not ask permission from her to do so, and (3) that her parents have recently told her that she is "spoiled" and "disrespectful." She notes that her symptoms tend to worsen when she feels upset or stressed, especially when she feels "judged and unsupported" and as she hears her parents giving "mixed messages," such as "you're such a smart girl and you're essentially an adult now, but we don't want you to be a college dropout."

You complete your initial evaluation and communicate, to the primary care team, your recommendations that (1) in addition to medical monitoring and treatment, family-based treatment and intensive structural psychotherapy should also be provided and (2) there are practical interventions that are informed by knowledge of family development and structure that the primary care team can implement and that are likely to be beneficial.

Again, it is important to highlight certain family principles that are particularly relevant to pediatric consultation-liaison psychiatry, which involves working with children and adolescents and their families, usually around an acute or chronic medical problem of some variety.

The first principle is that behavioral or other health-related challenges need to be understood in terms of social context, beyond just a diagnosis with an associated treatment (such as fluoxetine for binging and purging in Bulimia Nervosa). The context, behaviors, and patterns of interaction have evolved over time and generally have a basis in what was once adaptive. Failing to appreciate the system's adaptiveness and consequent potential resistance to change often leads to unsuccessful treatment, even with what is supposed to be effective and evidence-based. The second principle is that, just as individuals (as discussed in the previous section) undergo development, families also undergo development, and transitions between developmental stages (such as the launch from adolescence to adulthood, as described in the vignette) can often disrupt the equilibrium achieved in previous stages and lead to stress and associated symptoms. The third principle is that effecting meaningful change often requires addressing issues with the family structure, as evident from the conclusion of this case.

Case Vignette 1.13

Successful family-based treatment for this patient included regular, developmentally appropriate communication between the parents and the patient, where feelings that otherwise could fester could be openly and non-judgmentally discussed; appropriate empathy and understanding for the parents, without previous experience in launching an adolescent toward adulthood and relying on nurturing instincts that previously were adaptive; and encouragement for the parents, in their semi-retirement, to pursue their interests and hobbies that they otherwise were planning to put on hold "so that we could be busy again, not with the business this time, but with taking care of our daughter in college."

After a few weeks, the patient felt more confident in communicating her self-doubts to her parents, who in turn, provided developmentally appropriate reassurance, support, and mentorship for their daughter to take on more adult roles. Correspondingly, her binging and purging improved significantly.

The primary care physician was grateful for your intervention and for your teaching about family principles, especially as relevant to supporting the patient's recovery and preventing relapse in a primary care setting.

Relationships: The Foundation of Effective Pediatric Consultation-Liaison

In closing this chapter, we emphasize that relationships – with patients, families, and healthcare team members – are the foundation upon which effective consultation-liaison work must be built.

Case Vignette 1.14

You are a senior doctor in pediatric consultation-liaison psychiatry, about to do weekly rounds with a child and adolescent psychiatry fellow (junior doctor). Your fellow reports that it is an unusually quiet time of the year and that there are no known new active cases to round on. You therefore have a free hour in the morning, and you wonder how your time should best be spent.

For pediatric consultation-liaison work to be effective, it is of utmost importance to build and maintain solid working relationships with the healthcare team. This goal can be accomplished through collaborations during rounds and other interprofessional meetings with involved providers.

Case Vignette 1.15

You remind your fellow that, even without specific patients to see, doing "walk rounds" in the hospital can be helpful in emphasizing availability of the consultation-liaison service to all units, in learning about new cases who may benefit from consultation, in providing educational debriefings about past consultations, and in strengthening relationships with healthcare team members who will inevitably be important partners for future consultations and even the viability of the consultation-liaison service.

You and your fellow visit several units in the hospital and in doing so encounter:

- *A general pediatrician, who is glad that you stopped by to allow for a face-to-face discussion of a new patient who is being referred for a consultation.*
- *Another general pediatrician, who confirms with you that a mutual patient is currently in reasonably good spirits, even though his bupropion dose has been held, while his renal function tests remain elevated following a significant ibuprofen overdose.*
- *A pediatric hematologist-oncologist, who provides follow-up on several patients who are mostly being seen in the outpatient chemotherapy service and who confirms that a new chemotherapy regimen does not include medications that may interact with one patient's antidepressant.*
- *A pediatric intensive care nurse manager, who provides positive feedback about a delirium screening protocol that your team has recently implemented.*
- *The neonatal intensive care unit multidisciplinary rounding team: they are pleased to tell you that the new building to where the unit is moving will have more space for your family meetings, but they are all a bit anxious about having to adapt to a larger unit.*
- *The hospital chief executive officer, who is grateful for your team's services and who asks whether it may be possible to work with the outpatient team on an integrated behavioral health grant proposal.*
- *And finally, something that is new to you notwithstanding your years of experience in the specialty: a 16-year-old patient on the obstetrical service, who is readmitted to the hospital with preeclampsia, signs of organ failure, and symptoms of delirium; in addition, the referring team is interested to hear your advice on how the hospital should handle calls from advocates who believe that the patient is a victim of sex trafficking.*

You realize that the "downtime" earlier in the morning has now ended, and you encourage your fellow to embrace the day's challenges and all the associated learning.

Thinking of how exciting our work can be (even with just 1 h of fictitious rounding), we welcome you to the rest of this textbook.

Overview of Chapters and Sections

The editors are pleased to include three forewords from eminent leaders in pediatrics, global child and adolescent psychiatry, and healthcare systems. The first four chapters discuss basic principles, provide somewhat ambitious overviews of the specialties of pediatrics and psychiatry, and introduce an approach to psychopharmacology (often complex) in pediatric consultation-liaison psychiatry. The subsequent five chapters discuss common scenarios – not necessarily associated with a single diagnosis or diagnostic category – traditionally encountered in inpatient pediatric consultation-liaison psychiatry. The subsequent six chapters build on the foundation of the previous chapters and illustrate the value that pediatric consultation-liaison approaches – including biopsychosocial formulation, psychological testing and preprocedure evaluation, promotion of adherence and behavioral change, and thoughtful management of complex situations – can bring to multiple specialties and healthcare settings. These chapters also include specific discussion of neurological conditions (which, in some settings, may be initially managed by a psychiatrist as the available physician with specialized knowledge about the brain) and psychiatric genetics. The final seven chapters extend the discussion of pediatric consultation-liaison psychiatry to include global and healthcare systems perspectives. Through the chapter vignettes, we have attempted to cover all major organ systems and all settings where consultation-liaison psychiatrists may practice. At the end of the textbook, quick-reference appendices are provided on the topics of screening tools, teaching tools, and talking points for making the case for pediatric consultation-liaison psychiatry.

Through the chapter vignettes, the editors hope to illustrate the richness of pediatric consultation-liaison psychiatry and stimulate learning around fictitious but realistic scenarios. We sincerely hope that you will enjoy this textbook and gain knowledge and practical wisdom from the authors, to whom we are deeply indebted for their generous contributions of time and talent.

Further Reading

Accreditation Council for Graduate Medical Education (ACGME). (2016). https://www.acgme.org/Portals/0/PFAssets/ProgramRequirements/409_psychosomatic_med_2016_1-YR.pdf. Accessed 26 Jan 2017.

Alicata, D., Jacobs, N., Guerrero, A., & Piasecki, M. (2016). *Problem-based behavioral science and psychiatry* (2nd ed.). Cham: Springer.

Fishman, H. C. (2005). *Enduring change in eating disorders: Interventions with long-term results*. New York: Routledge.

Koli, R. L., & Guerrero, A. P. (2015). Chapter 32: Consultation-liaison with children and adolescents. In *Handbook of consultation-liaison psychiatry* (pp. 497–519). New York: Springer.

Kuhn, T. S., & Hawkins, D. (1963). The structure of scientific revolutions. *American Journal of Physics, 31*(7), 554–555.

Leentjens, A. F., Rundell, J. R., Wolcott, D. L., Diefenbacher, A., Kathol, E., & Guthrie, E. (2011). Psychosomatic medicine and consultation-liaison psychiatry: Scope of practice, processes, and competencies for psychiatrists or psychosomatic medicine specialists A consensus statement of the European association of consultation-liaison psychiatry and the academy of psychosomatic medicine (vol 52, pg 19, 2011). *Psychosomatics, 52*(3), 301–30 .

Levenson, E. A. (1972). *The fallacy of understanding*. Hillsdale: Analytic Press.

Minuchin, S., Rosman, B. L., & Baker, L. (1978). Psychosomatic families: Anorexia nervosa in context. Cambridge, MA: Harvard University Press.

Shaw, R. J., Bassols, A. M. S., Berelowitz, M., Bowden, M., Eapen, V., Frank, R., Gao, H., Kamaraju, Y., Mardini, V., Omigbodun, O. O., Schieveld, J. N. M., & The Dutch Study Group on Pediatric Consultation/Liaison Psychiatry. (2010). Chapter 1. Pediatric psychosomatic medicine. In R. J. Shaw & D. R. DeMaso (Eds.), *Textbook of pediatric psychosomatic medicine* (p. 3). Washington, DC: American Psychiatric Publishing.

Chapter 2
Pediatric Medicine for the Child Psychiatrist

Amanda Schroepfer O'Kelly

Introduction

A functional knowledge of general pediatric principles is essential for pediatric consultation-liaison (C-L) providers. While a review of the full breadth of pediatrics is beyond the scope of this textbook, this chapter endeavors to cull relevant issues often encountered in a pediatric C-L service and to examine them through a general pediatrics lens. Familiarity with the pediatrician's rationale and approach adds depth to the pediatric C-L providers' care and provides insight and allows for more collaboration with pediatric colleagues. Links and references to convenient charts, tables, and patient handouts are provided throughout the chapter. Current treatment guidelines (e.g., for obesity and diabetes), with acknowledgement that they can and will change over time, are referenced with links to principal regulating agencies for the most up-to-date information available to the reader.

Growth

Case Vignette 2.1 As part of your work with a primary care integration team, you collaborate with and provide psychiatric consultation for a local pediatric group practice. One of your pediatric colleagues calls regarding her new patient, Sam, a 10-year-old male who was previously diagnosed with severe oppositional defiant disorder (ODD) and other specified attention-deficit/hyperactivity disorder (ADHD) and who has been taking risperidone 1 mg twice daily for the past year. The pediatrician is concerned that Sam is being treated with an atypical antipsychotic despite having no psychotic disorder and is eager to have you provide a second

A. S. O'Kelly (✉)
Departments of Psychiatry & Pediatrics, UH-JABSOM, Honolulu, HI, USA
e-mail: okellya@dop.hawaii.edu

A. P. S. Guerrero et al. (eds.), *Pediatric Consultation-Liaison Psychiatry*,
https://doi.org/10.1007/978-3-319-89488-1_2

opinion on his diagnoses and management before she prescribes the medication. She forwards the collateral information she has received from the previous treating psychiatrist, and you schedule an appointment to assess the child.

You meet with Sam and his stepmother Susan via a video teleconference (VTC) connection to the pediatric clinic. They both report that the patient's symptoms have improved dramatically on risperidone. This history is corroborated by the previous psychiatrist's notes. Susan enthuses, "We tried everything with him, and nothing worked, but now he's like a different kid!" She goes on to describe the high levels of aggressive and disrespectful behavior across all settings that led to constant conflict with his parents and school personnel, a series of school suspensions and failing grades prior to beginning the medication. A review of the past medical records reveals two failed trials of stimulants as well as an α-agonist to treat the patient's diagnosis of other specified ADHD, with rating scales documenting several persistent symptoms of distractibility, interrupting others, and difficulty sitting still without meeting full criteria for a more specific ADHD presentation. His aggressive and disruptive behaviors were rated as very impairing, and rating scales from both parents and teachers reveal high levels of disruptive behavior symptoms. "He got in too much trouble and he was going to be expelled; that's when his old doctor suggested we try this medication." The patient and stepmother deny trials of family or individual therapy, aside from meeting with a school counselor through his individualized education program (IEP). Susan states unequivocally that she desires continuing the risperidone given the positive changes she has observed in her son's behavior. On individual interview, Sam is ambivalent about his medication, but willing to continue taking it as it has been "helpful for keeping calm." They both note that Sam's appetite has been "very large" since beginning the medicine, but otherwise deny side effects. Susan has no concern about the increased appetite and notes that "growing boys eat a lot." They recall bloodwork being done at the initiation of the risperidone roughly 1 year ago, but report that no labs have been done since. You obtain vital signs today. Sam's vital signs appear unremarkable at first glance. His height is 57 inches and his weight is 100 pounds. His past medical history is unremarkable, without developmental delays or medical problems. His family history is positive for maternal postpartum depression and a cousin with ADHD.

With evidence-based child psychiatry practice guidelines in mind, you conduct a thorough assessment and conclude that ODD is indeed the most appropriate diagnosis for the patient, confirm that he does not currently meet full criteria for ADHD, conduct disorder, or a mood disorder. There is no history of exposure to trauma; however, the patient's biological parents divorced when he was in kindergarten. He has little contact with his biological mother and appears to have a conflicted relationship with both his father and stepmother. In school, he has a history of oppositionality with authority figures and poor relationships with peers. These problems have detracted from his performance and enjoyment of school. However, he was able to pass all his classes and was promoted to the sixth grade. Everyone, including Sam, is hoping for a fresh start at his new middle school.

As you discuss your assessment and treatment options, Susan interrupts nervously to ask, “You're going to refill his risperidone, aren't you? I am going to have to find another doctor if you won't. It is the only thing that has helped, and we just can't go back to how it was before.” While you recognize the risks of atypical antipsychotic treatment and are knowledgeable of the evidence-based, non-pharmacologic interventions for disruptive behavior disorders (in particular, multi-systemic therapy, parent management training, and functional family therapy), you also recognize the need to establish rapport with the patient and family and to gather important information such as laboratory studies, to best care for the patient. You agree to refill the patient's risperidone prescription once with a follow-up appointment scheduled for next month. Sam and his stepmother are willing to get the fasting bloodwork that you order, and are amenable to your recommendation to return with Sam's father for the follow-up, to review the lab results and discuss additional treatment options.

While entering your note in the electronic health record (EHR), you are somewhat surprised to see that Sam's body mass index (BMI) is in the 95th percentile for his age and diagnostic of obesity. On presentation, he seemed slightly older than his age, but he did not strike you as obese at the time of the visit. You are somewhat embarrassed that you did not recognize his obesity at the initial encounter and you wonder how best to address it with the family. You plan to collaborate with the pediatrician, as you are unaware of the current assessment and treatment recommendations for overweight and obese children.

What are the recommendations for monitoring growth parameters in children, both in general and when using medications that may impact growth? What is the child psychiatrist or primary care provider's responsibility in tracking growth?

In pediatrics, growth parameters (height, weight, and BMI) for healthy toddlers, school-aged children, and adolescents are generally tracked annually and are best assessed using comparative age and gender norms. They are frequently plotted on a growth curve, comparing the values with those of other children of the same age and gender, yielding a percentile for age (% for age). The most commonly utilized growth charts are produced by the Centers for Disease Control and Prevention (CDC) and the World Health Organization (WHO): https://www.cdc.gov/growthcharts/cdc_charts.htm. Since the growth of children with certain conditions, such as prematurity, Down syndrome, and achondroplasia, is known to deviate substantially from the general population, several specialized growth curves are available for these subpopulations.

As children's fat and muscle mass ratios vary considerably at different ages and stages of development, simple measurements of weight, height or even BMI do not tell the full story. Preschoolers, for example, are not only shorter, but generally thinner and leaner than babies or school-aged children, and the average BMI for a 4-year-old female is just 16 kg/m^2. In fact, a BMI of 25 kg/m^2, the upper range for “normal” body mass index in adults, would be considered obese for any female <12 years of age. With the increasing obesity epidemic, there are now charts denoting how many standard deviations above normal range a child's BMI has become. Prior to this epidemic, percentile for age was the only clear reference point, which becomes less meaningful in parsing out risk level in a population with high rates of obesity. Height or weight parameters above the 95 percentile or below the 5 percentile for age are considered abnormal, and providers may wish to begin an investigation or treatment. In addition to monitoring for growth parameters outside of the normal range, providers also track changes in the percentiles for age over time. Changing from 90 percentile to 40 percentile for age in height over the course of 2 years would be concerning, as the child is not growing as his or her previous measurements would predict. Pediatricians often refer to "crossing growth curves" or failing to track along the growth curve as expected, when discussing a child's growth. An example of this would be moving from the 90 percentile to the 50 percentile for age curves for weight from one well-child visit to the next. For psychiatrists monitoring children on medications that may affect growth parameters, such as stimulants or atypical antipsychotics, current guidelines recommend monitoring height, weight, and BMI at least quarterly and more often upon initiation of the medication or if the provider detects changes in growth. Risks and benefits, including those related to growth, should be discussed with patients and families prior to initiating medications.

How is obesity diagnosed in children and adolescents? Are there evidence-based weight-management interventions for children and teens?

In children, obesity is measured using the BMI (weight in kg/height in meters squared), which varies markedly by age and gender. The BMI is then plotted on a growth curve and evaluated according to % for age.

Underweight: BMI <5 percentile for age
Normal weight: BMI 5 percentile to <85 percentile for age
Overweight: BMI 85 percentile to <95 percentile for age
Obese: BMI ≥95 percentile for age

The American Academy of Pediatrics (AAP) recommends that the evaluation for obesity includes laboratory testing for comorbidities such as diabetes mellitus and dyslipidemia for children ages 10 and older and those with clinical indicators of impaired glucose tolerance or other risk factors for morbidities related to obesity. These recommendations are in flux, as the current obesity epidemic worsens, and more children are diagnosed with type 2 diabetes. *Current guidelines for evaluation and treatment of obesity from the AAP Institute for Healthy Childhood Weight can be found at https://ihcw.aap.org.* As might be expected, those patients who develop young onset diabetes suffer higher rates of medical complications and poorer outcomes over the course of their lifetime (Wilmot and Idris 2014). Data support the commonly held belief that overweight children grow up to be overweight adults and that pediatricians must take a proactive approach to overweight children. It is generally believed that lifelong eating patterns and behavioral habits are established in childhood, and accordingly, diet and activity patterns are standard subjects evaluated at every well-child visit starting from birth.

Effective, evidence-based weight-management programs exist for children and teens, and the interventions with the highest level of evidence support for improving BMI involve the whole family. These programs are typically intensive, and they address multiple aspects contributing to obesity in a comprehensive fashion. They often include sessions focused on nutrition, cooking, exercise, activity, and psychological factors and may involve the use of motivational interviewing, mindfulness, and cognitive and behavioral techniques to promote and facilitate change.

Lower-intensity interventions, often employed in the pediatric setting as first-line strategies for overweight children without obesity or weight-related comorbidities, include referral to a dietician/nutritionist; regular follow-up with the primary care provider (PCP) to provide support, to set goals, and to monitor progress; and recommendations for diet and exercise changes. As mentioned, interventions that involve the entire family are generally most effective, and pediatricians will often recommend that extended family members become involved for success. For example, a PCP may recommend that parents hold a meeting with the extended family to discuss their concerns regarding their child's health and request that all family members support a "no soda or candy" rule with the preschooler. Motivational interviewing techniques are often employed, with a brief, primary care focused approach. One example of a broad-based recommendation for lifestyle modification is the 5-2-1-0 strategy (http://www.live5210.ca/about-live-5-2-1-0/the-live-5-2-1-0-message/Accessed 1/1/2018). This guideline lists four goals for a healthy lifestyle: consume five servings of fruits and vegetables daily, spend less than 2 h in front of a screen per day (including television and Internet-connected devices such as computers, smartphones, and tablets), be active for 1 h daily, and have 0 sugary drinks per day.

Over time, there have been some positive developments in public health efforts. As the childhood obesity epidemic continues to grow, public knowledge regarding obesity is also increasing, motivating some families to make changes. In many locations, schools now send parents information regarding a student's BMI and make efforts to remove "junk food" and increase access to healthy options on campus. Public health campaigns aimed at encouraging exercise and healthy diets are becoming commonplace in many areas.

Case 2.1 (continued) On review of your pediatric colleague's initial assessment of Sam, you learn that he has a family history of diabetes on both sides of the family, including his father. According to your colleague's assessment, laboratory tests are indicated based on the patient's BMI. The pediatrician has reviewed the patient's prior records and plotted his weight gain on a growth chart. You are dismayed to discover that Sam has gained 25lbs over the past year. While he also underwent a 3-inch growth spurt during that time, his BMI increased from 18 (84% for a 9-year-old boy) to 22 (95% for a 10-year-old boy). While his BMI is considered normal for adults, you can clearly see that he has become obese since initiating risperidone 1 year ago. Additionally, you note the greater than 10% increase in Sam's weight early during treatment and recall that this increase is a predictor of poor metabolic outcomes with atypical antipsychotics.

On further review of the initial pediatric evaluation, you note a pattern of delayed immunizations, well-child visits, and dental care. He has severe dental caries. It appears that the patient has not seen a pediatrician or dentist over the past 2 years. Because of multiple cancelations, he was only seen every few months by his previous psychiatrist. With this additional history, you wonder about Sam's future treatment adherence and overall health.

What is the recommended schedule for well-child checks in the pediatric setting? How are growth abnormalities assessed and treated in the pediatric setting?

Most children in the US are cared for in a pediatric setting (with a portion managed by family or internal medicine providers). The AAP recommends well-child checks every year from the ages of 2 to 10 years and every 2 years thereafter. These visits include a comprehensive assessment of physical, emotional, and social health and development. Most pediatricians (and insurance providers) recommend yearly well care visits even during the preteen and teen years to monitor growth, physical and mental health, school achievement, social concerns, and safety issues. Frequency of visits to a medical provider vary widely both individually and regionally, but 2012 data from the United States reveals only 1/3 of children ages 6–17 years old are seen for an annual well-child assessment (Uddin et al. 2016).

Depending on whether growth abnormalities are identified during well-child care or acute visits, the differential diagnosis can be wide, encompassing genetic, endocrine, central nervous system, gastrointestinal (GI), infectious, or psychosocial problems. Common screening done in primary care can include assays of thyroid-stimulant hormone/free thyroxine (T4) to screen for thyroid dysfunction or electrolyte or inflammatory markers. Assessments may include other hormone levels, such as sex hormone levels in suspected pituitary dysfunction, or insulin-like growth factor/fasting growth hormone in gigantism. Imaging studies can be considered, such as a bone scan to determine bone age, or a brain magnetic resonance imaging (MRI) to rule out a tumor if pituitary dysfunction is suspected, as in the case of pediatric growth hormone deficiency. Specific screening for infectious processes (e.g., purified protein derivative (PPD) skin test for suspected tuberculosis, stool ova/parasite examination for parasitic disease) or GI dysfunction (e.g., celiac panel, complete blood count (CBC), erythrocyte sedimentation rate) can help rule out additional causes. Turner syndrome (45, XO) is associated with short stature and delayed puberty in females and can be determined by karyotype analysis. After narrowing the differential via history and initial investigation, the provider can refer to specialists to help determine or confirm a suspected diagnosis and guide treatment options.

What are the implications of treatment nonadherence for a patient's overall health and prognosis?

Delaying or not following the recommended schedule for general pediatric care is a form of treatment nonadherence that may be associated with delayed dental and specialty care as well as financial and social stressors and that may lead to poorer outcomes, especially in children (Strickland et al. 2004). Thus, in the above case, the family's nonadherence with recommended medical care and screenings could be considered a negative prognostic indicator for Sam's overall health. However, it should be noted that this conclusion is rooted in the context of Western medicine's biomedical culture. Indeed, one of the tenets of providing culturally competent care is to create a treatment plan in conjunction with the patient and family. The phrases "compliance with medication" and "adherence to the schedule" underscore Western medicine's emphasis on following a medical professional's prescribed plan, oftentimes without input from the patient and family. Additionally, with less than half of school-aged children in the United States completing the recommended well-child visits every year, while Sam's medical care may not be ideal, it is, unfortunately, typical.

Case 2.1 (continued) Following up on Sam's labs, you are relieved to note his fasting glucose is within normal limits, but disappointed to learn he has developed hypercholesterolemia and his hemoglobin A1c (HbA1c or A1c) places him at increased risk for diabetes. The stakes are high, as you recognize the patient's current medication has likely caused this increase in weight, dyslipidemia, and impaired glucose tolerance, but you are also cognizant of the dysfunction and impairment in all areas of his life associated with his untreated psychiatric symptoms. Both the metabolic and the psychiatric concerns have huge implications for your patient's future, so you resolve to learn what you can to address the issue at the follow-up visit.

What are the criteria for diagnosing diabetes or pre-diabetes in young people? Is type 2 diabetes mellitus considered a disease of adults, or can it develop in children?

Once considered a disease of adults, type 2 diabetes is becoming more prevalent in children and adolescents as the obesity epidemic worsens. Diagnostic criteria for diabetes and pre-diabetes apply to people across all ages, including children. In fasting (defined as 8 h without calorie consumption), a blood glucose of ≥126 mg/dL is consistent with diabetes. A fasting glucose <100 mg/dL is considered normal, and results between 100 and 125 mg/dL are consistent with "pre-diabetes," also known as impaired glucose tolerance or IGT. HbA1c, which estimates the average blood glucose level over the 3-month lifespan of hemoglobin molecules, may also be used for diagnosis. A HbA1c of 6.5% or greater (normal <5.7%) is consistent with diabetes, and values between 5.7 and 6.4% reflect "pre-diabetes," with higher values representing a higher risk for the development of diabetes. The 2016 American Diabetes Association guidelines list an oral glucose tolerance testing (OGTT, where the patient ingests a 75-gram glucose load after fasting) value of ≥200 mg/dL measured 2 h after the glucose load or any non-fasting blood glucose of ≥200 mg/dL with symptoms of hyperglycemia as alternate diagnostic criteria. The guidelines recommend repeating the testing to confirm diabetes when hyperglycemia is equivocal. Testing in special populations can vary somewhat, such as the modified two-step OGTT often given to pregnant women who fail a one-step

OGTT. *Updated guidelines are available through the American Diabetes Association: www.diabetes.org/diabetescare.*

Are young people more at risk for growth-related side effects? Which psychiatric medications are most frequently associated with abnormal growth and weight-related laboratory test abnormalities in children and adolescents? What is the recommended frequency of laboratory testing for youth taking these medications?

Unfortunately, it has been demonstrated that children are at increased risk for growth-related side effects (Overbeek et al. 2010) and metabolic changes (Dori N and Green T 2011). Among prescription psychotropic medications, the atypical antipsychotics are most frequently associated with increased weight gain and metabolic abnormalities in youth. Meta-analyses of studies conducted with youth taking atypical antipsychotics report metabolic risks that vary with the medication used and that are similar to findings reported in adults (Almandil et al. 2013). Clozapine and olanzapine are consistently associated with significant weight gain, and multiple studies have noted statistically significant increases in triglycerides (TG), cholesterol, and prolactin (Correll et al. 2009). Risperidone has been associated with statistically significant weight gain (Loy et al. 2017) and increased prolactin. Although aripiprazole often causes less weight gain compared to the previously named antipsychotic medications, in meta-analysis it has still been consistently associated with statistically significant weight gain in children and adolescents. Although it is clear that children and adolescents on atypical antipsychotics are at risk for weight gain, determining their level of risk for developing weight-related laboratory abnormalities is more challenging. Many of the studies conducted with young people on antipsychotics do not have statistically significant data to report on changes in metabolic parameters. This absence is to be expected, as many of these studies were of short duration (e.g., 12 weeks). Longer-term studies examining the metabolic effects of atypical antipsychotics in youth are rarer and often limited by small sample size (Goeb et al. 2010). However, they have consistently demonstrated an increased risk for substantial weight gain, which is linked to many metabolic abnormalities including insulin resistance, diabetes, and dyslipidemia (Correll and Carlson 2006). Further research is clearly needed in this area.

Considering the substantial evidence regarding the risk for weight gain and metabolic changes, current guidelines recommend obtaining baseline weight, height, BMI, and fasting glucose and lipid panel for all youth prior to starting an atypical antipsychotic and repeating these laboratory studies at 3 months and every 6 months thereafter. Weight, height, and BMI measurements are recommended at every visit. Youth whose BMI becomes ≥95% for age, or who are at elevated risk for metabolic complications, should be monitored closely, including youth who experience an increase of >5% in weight during the first 3 months of treatment.

Additional medications associated with weight gain and metabolic abnormalities in youth include mood stabilizers such as lithium and divalproex sodium, and antidepressants such as mirtazapine. One meta-analysis of mirtazapine found a 15% rate of significant weight gain and an equal potential for liver enzymes or lipid level increases, which rarely but importantly can be rapid and substantial.

Vital Signs Are…Vital!

Case Vignette 2.2 Brittany is a bright 8-year-old girl whose medical home is a pediatrics practice that you collaborate with to provide integrated behavioral health (BH) services. Brittany's PCP diagnosed her with ADHD, combined presentation, helped the family to request an evaluation for school accommodations, and continued to provide medication management services. There is a family history of ADHD in Brittany's father and brother, but no history of learning disorders or other psychiatric comorbidities. The patient is overall healthy, without mental health or other comorbidities. Brittany has done very well with the combination of behavioral interventions at home, educational accommodations in school through *a 504 plan*, and the long-acting stimulant methylphenidate ER.

Near the end of the school year, it was noted that the patient's response to the medication was less robust than in the past, despite all interventions remaining unchanged and no additional stressors being identified. Thinking that the medication's decreased effectiveness was likely due to Brittany's growth, the PCP increased the long-acting stimulant's dose to the next available strength. Now, however, the patient complains of a significantly decreased appetite and two-pound weight loss over the past 2 months, so the PCP has consulted you for medication recommendations. Upon review of the case with the PCP, you note the patient's stimulant is currently dosed above the U.S. Food and Drug Administration's recommended maximum limit for her age. Given the patient's suboptimal response and adverse effect with the maximum recommended dosage of methylphenidate you recommend discontinuing it and starting a trial of mixed amphetamine salts (MAS). As the PCP has never prescribed other stimulants and expresses significant discomfort, you agree to temporarily manage the medication titration.

What is failure to thrive? When does a child or teen's weight loss or failure to gain weight become a concern?

Failure to thrive is the medical term for decelerated or arrested physical growth, often defined as height and weight below the 3 percentile or 5 percentile for age or a decline across two major growth percentiles. However, data points alone do not diagnose a growth problem. For example, 5% of all children would be expected to have heights in the 5% or less range, and only a fraction of them would have a pathological cause. Constitutional short stature is a common etiology for decreased height, so pediatricians will routinely ask for parental heights and monitor a patient's growth across time to determine if they are growing in an "expected" pattern (i.e., consistently tracking along the same growth curve and maintaining the increased height velocity normally seen during growth spurts). True failure to thrive is important to differentiate from nonpathologic causes of decreased growth, as it implies significant medical, psychological, social, or economic concerns that can impact a child's development, and it is sometimes associated with neglect or abuse. It is worth noting that in pediatric patients, acquired growth difficulties are often noted first in the weight (as opposed to height or head circumference) parameter.

The point at which weight loss in a child or teen becomes a concern depends on the specific circumstances. Acute weight loss (e.g., within days, as commonly seen with acute gastroenteritis) is most concerning for dehydration and should be evaluated by a medical provider if significant clinical findings are present, especially in young children. More commonly seen in psychiatric settings is subacute or chronic weight loss that develops over weeks to months, often after interventions such as the stimulant prescription described in this case. It is important to remember that it is not absolute weight that providers must monitor for decline, but weight and BMI percentiles, as all children would be expected to increase in weight as their height increases, until cessation of linear growth in late adolescence or, for some boys, early adulthood. Always consider prescription misuse or presence of an eating disorder as a potential cause of excessive weight loss in a patient being treated with stimulants. Failure to maintain at least 85% of expected/ideal weight for age and height is a concerning finding, which may be consistent with an eating disorder or other medical comorbidity and which indicates need for medical evaluation.

Patients who experience decreased appetite with weight loss or relative weight loss for age, but who are not underweight, are frequently encountered in the psychiatric setting. Unfortunately, clear guidelines for intervention in these situations are lacking. If no medication or intentional lifestyle changes are responsible for the weight loss, review of diet, inquiry into food security (defined as access to adequate, healthy food), and referral to the pediatrician should be considered. Interestingly, food insecurity has been frequently associated with being overweight, which is thought to relate to the availability of inexpensive and unhealthy foods in many industrialized countries. When medication is the likely cause of inadequate weight gain, a discussion of the weight changes and an updated discussion with the patient and family about the benefits, risks, and alternatives to the current treatment is indicated. In such cases, possible interventions include a trial of medication schedule adjustments (e.g., take after breakfast), formulation changes (e.g., multiple doses of short-acting medication to be taken after mealtimes), decrease in dosage, augmentation with (or switch to) a non-stimulant, medication holidays, or dietary changes (e.g., incorporation of healthy, high-calorie snack foods) to offset the side effect of decreased appetite in an otherwise effective treatment regimen. Consultation and collaboration with the patient's pediatrician or a nutritionist can be helpful in managing inadequate weight gain. Increasingly, children in all practice settings may commonly be overweight at baseline, and assessing weight loss in these cases is more nuanced. Most providers agree that weight loss in a significantly overweight child is not in and of itself a problem (indeed, it can be a positive finding in terms of overall health), unless the weight loss is significant or precipitous. Screening for eating disorders should not be overlooked, if indicated, at any weight, and weight loss should be evaluated to ensure that appropriate nutrition is provided to support continued growth and development and optimal functioning.

How is weight loss addressed in the pediatric setting? What are the basic nutritional guidelines for children, and how do they differ from adults?

When weight loss is evaluated in pediatric settings, the initial investigation involves determining the significance, etiology, and need for intervention. To ascertain significance, weight loss is quantified relative to previous measurements, age, height percentile for age, BMI percentile for age, and risk category. Pediatricians will inquire how much weight was lost, and over what timeframe? What is the change in BMI % for age? Is the problem restricted to weight, or has the height been affected? In infants and toddlers, is the head circumference also affected? Has the patient moved from obese to overweight? Normal weight to underweight?

To investigate etiology, medical providers will typically inquire about intentional versus unintentional weight loss, lifestyle changes, medication use, and food security, among other factors. Additionally, they will conduct a focused history and physical examination and potentially order laboratory studies, especially if a pathological cause is suspected (e.g., inflammatory bowel disease, malnutrition, eating disorder, thyroid dysfunction, depression, cancer, substance use).

Nutritional needs of children vary with age. Relative caloric intake requirements to maintain growth and proper nutrition are estimated at 1000 kcal/day from age 2–3 years and then in girls 1200 kcal/day from ages 4–8, 1600 kcal/day from 9–13, 1800 kcal/day from 14–18, and 2000 kcal/day for young adults. In boys, estimates of caloric needs are slightly higher: 1400 kcal/day from ages 4–8, 1600 kcal/day from 9–13, 1800 kcal/day from 14–18, and 2400 kcal/day for young adults. The above figures represent averages for sedentary children and adults and will increase by 200–600 kcal/day for highly active individuals (Dietary Guidelines for Americans 2005). Caloric intake requirements also vary by individuals' overall size and metabolism. Pregnancy, lactation, and chronic or acute illness also change an individual's nutritional needs, sometimes dramatically. Serving sizes for young children are smaller, for example, one fruit or vegetable serving is a quarter to a third cup for a toddler and half a cup for a preschooler. A broadly applicable guideline is that one serving size is roughly equal to the area of the palm of an individual's hand.

Regarding micronutrients, the recommended daily allowance (RDA) for most vitamins and minerals grows closer to adult requirements by age 14 years but is not fully equivalent until the age of 19 years. It is important to note that the RDA for various vitamins and minerals does not necessarily increase in linear fashion with age. For example, humans' requisite calcium intake increases in children with age, peaks in preadolescence/adolescence, declines during adulthood, and rises again after the age of 50 years to near peak levels.

Which psychiatric medications are most frequently associated with decreased weight velocity or weight loss?

Stimulants are the psychiatric medications most often associated with weight loss and, to a lesser extent, other medications that act on dopamine or norepinephrine, such as bupropion, atomoxetine, and venlafaxine. Similarly, medications that affect the gut, cause GI side effects or affect satiety signals can also cause weight loss.

Case 2.2 (continued) You titrate the dose of the MAS to the optimal dose, maximizing its positive impact while minimizing side effects. At her next follow-up appointment, Brittany and her parents report that they are very pleased with the effects on this dose of the medication. She can focus appropriately in class, and homework completion is very manageable after school. They have not noted any side effects. You note that her height and weight are appropriate. When you log in to your EHR to document the visit, you notice that the patient's blood pressure (BP) of120/78 mm/Hg is highlighted in a red font. Wondering why this seemingly normal BP has been flagged, you review her past vital signs, and you notice that her previous readings tended to be around 100/60 mm/Hg. Her pulse, while still within normal limits, is also higher today at 98 beats/minute (bpm) compared to previous pulse readings ranging 60–80 bpm. As a busy provider, you have time for only a quick internet search, and discover blood pressure charts for children developed by the National Institutes of Health. For your patient, an 8-year-old female of average height, a BP of 102/61 mm/Hg represents the 95% for age, and her current reading of 120/78 would be considered abnormal. Concerned, you decide that the best course of action is to contact the patient's pediatrician to ask a few questions.

Do normal vital signs (VS) vary by age?

Normal VS certainly vary by age, especially for young children (https://www.pedscases.com/pediatric-vital-signs-reference-chart). As a general guideline, adolescents typically have BP, pulse, and respiratory rates similar to adults. BP ranges consistent with hypertension in children are defined by age, gender, and height percentile for age (Falkner 2010). Hypotension for school-aged children is roughly defined as systolic BP <70 + (age ×2) and <90 for children aged 10 and older. For young people, BP is interpreted normed by age, sex, and height % for age. BP charts for boys and girls are freely available (http://pediatrics.aappublications.org/content/early/2017/08/21/peds.2017-1904), and some EHRs now include automatic interpretation of a child's BP with % for age/gender/height. For school-aged children, and even more so for preschool children, pulses of greater than 100 bpm may be normal. Bradycardia varies by age as well, and although athletic, older teens may have pulses as low as 50 bpm at baseline, school-aged children's usual pulse ranges from 70 to 115 bpm while awake. As with adults, VS ranges are presented merely as guidelines, and individual variation is important to acknowledge. Clinical response and patient presentation directs treatment. Symptoms of orthostasis that develop in a patient after initiating clonidine, for example, are more clinically significant than the isolated systolic BP value in an asymptomatic patient.

How is BP interpreted for children and adolescents?

In children, as in adults, BP is most accurately measured using a properly sized BP cuff, whose bladder length is ideally 80%, and width ≥ 40%, of the patient's arm circumference, with the patient seated and resting quietly. For overweight and obese children and teens, the most appropriate cuff may be the large child, small adult, adult or even large adult BP cuff. Use of an undersized BP cuff can result in a falsely high BP, while use of an oversized cuff results in the opposite. Young, uncooperative, or hyperactive patients that move or flex their arm muscles during assessment can also have inaccurate BP readings (frequently higher than actual). Anxiety and white coat hypertension (elevated BP values noted in doctor's office, but not outside of it) are additional causes of increased BP readings in patients without true hypertension.

What are the causes of elevated BP in youth? What are the criteria for diagnosis of hypertension (HTN) in a child? How is it evaluated, and how prevalent is it?

In addition to measurement errors, there are several medical causes for increased BP and HTN in youth. In preadolescent children, secondary HTN (HTN caused by a specific pathologic process) is most common and is usually related to renal disease. In addition, secondary HTN can be seen with cardiovascular abnormalities, adrenal and thyroid disease, sleep apnea, hyperaldosteronism, mineralocorticoid excess, and tumors. Like adults, adolescents more often have primary HTN, with obesity and family history of HTN among the main risk factors. As with adults, a single elevated BP does not constitute a diagnosis of HTN. HTN is diagnosed after a patient is found to have three separate, properly measured BPs for age/gender/height > 95 percentile. An assessment for pediatric HTN may include urinalysis (UA), CBC, blood chemistries, and/or blood hormones (e.g., plasma renin) to evaluate for renal disease and, if indicated, drug testing for substances that increase BP. Additional evaluation for less common but clinically important etiologies of hypertension may include laboratory screens for pheochromocytoma or neuroblastoma. Blood tests for lipids and glucose tolerance are recommended for all overweight children with HTN, as is polysomnography for overweight children with HTN and symptoms suggestive of sleep pathology. For youth in the United States, the prevalence of prehypertension (i.e., BP ≥ 90 percentile for age/gender/height, but <95 percentile) has been estimated to be 14% in boys and 6% in girls, while the prevalence of HTN (BP ≥95 percentile for age/gender/height) is estimated to be 3–4% (George et al. 2014).

Which psychiatric medications are most frequently associated with changes in blood pressure and pulse? What is the recommended frequency of monitoring VS of patients taking psychotropic medications?

Tachycardia and elevated BP are most commonly associated with medications that affect norepinephrine, such as stimulants, atomoxetine, and serotonin-norepinephrine reuptake inhibitors (SNRIs). Small increases in heart rate and BP of 3–6 bpm and 2–4 mmHg, respectively, are common side effects of stimulants. Uncommonly, patients taking stimulants, atomoxetine, or SNRIs may have clinically significant increases in pulse and BP and may require a reconsideration of the risks and benefits of the agent and potential discontinuation of the medication. The α-agonists clonidine and guanfacine increase α-2 activity, thereby reducing peripheral muscle tone and causing the associated side effects of decreased pulse and BP. These medications can be dangerous if used in patients with very low pulse rates (<50 bpm) or BP. Discontinuing α-agonists can be associated with significantly elevated pulse and BP, especially with the abrupt discontinuation of a long-standing, high-dose regimen. If a patient's BP and pulse are noted to become elevated as the α-agonist is discontinued, the previous dose should be resumed then tapered more slowly. In patients taking both a stimulant and α-agonist, while it is theoretically possible that the side effects of each will "cancel each other out," the potential combinations for medication dosages and time of action are innumerable, and careful monitoring of vital signs is still warranted.

Orthostatic hypotension is a potential side effect of atypical and conventional (especially low potency) antipsychotics and is thought to be due to α-1 antagonist activity. This side effect has been reported with increased frequency with clozapine and quetiapine, and it is one of the primary reasons cited for recommending slow titration of iloperidone, which has a relatively high affinity for α-1 receptors. In patients who have been stable on clozapine but experience a lapse in treatment of three or more days, slow re-titration is also recommended, in part due to the risk of orthostasis with rapid return to high dosages. Prazosin, an α-1 antagonist, also carries a risk of orthostatic hypotension, and it is prudent to monitor BP and query patients regarding symptoms of orthostatic hypotension upon medication initiation and with each subsequent visit.

Children taking psychotropic medications should have pulse and BP checked at least quarterly and more often if doses are changed, if high-risk medications are used, or if the patient experiences symptoms or has any other risks for side effects.

Development

Case Vignette 2.3 You serve as a BH consultant working closely with local pediatricians. Dr. Young, one of the PCPs, asks you about a 12-year-old patient whom she recently evaluated. This patient's father complained about his son's immature and clingy behavior and frequent avoidance of socializing with other kids. The PCP used the GAD7 (Generalized Anxiety Disorder 7-item scale) and PHQ9A (Patient Health Questionnaire-9 modified for Adolescents) to screen for anxiety and depression. Both were negative, and the boy denied having any difficulties with anxiety or socialization. He did acknowledge his preference to stay at home but denied any problem with school attendance, bullying, or peer interactions. His mother and maternal aunt have anxiety disorders, but there are no other mental health problems in the family. The patient is introverted, quiet, and high-achieving academically, but does not participate in organized sports, which is something that his parents value. He reports having a couple friends, and he spends a fair amount of time playing video games. The PCP stated, "I feel he is immature; after all, he is still Tanner stage one and short for his age, but I wanted to get your advice on any further questions or screenings to help rule out anxiety. Should I refer him to a therapist? He seems to be doing alright, but I don't feel entirely confident that I could assess him fully on my own without backup. His parents are concerned that there's something wrong with him, but he denies any problems." You note that anxiety is under-recognized in children and can be quite impairing. You inform her of more detailed anxiety screen-ers, including the open access Screen for Child Anxiety Related Emotional Disorders (SCARED). Additionally, you discuss some helpful questions to investigate the possibility of separation, social, generalized anxiety, and panic disorders, as well as community resources that are available. With the mismatch between the parent and patient concerns regarding socialization, you mention the possibility of an autism spectrum disorder (ASD) and encourage Dr. Young to review the patient's history and assess for signs of this diagnosis as well.

You ponder what the implications of physical development are for this young patient and mentally compare him to several similar aged boys in your own practice. You realize that you are not entirely confident in assessing pubertal development (psychiatry's lack of physical exam aside). You wonder if knowledge regarding puberty has changed since you were in medical school, and you recall hearing that puberty has been beginning earlier and that some articles have discussed the potential negative consequences for delayed puberty in boys. You ask the PCP about any updates on pubertal development in boys and girls.

What are the stages and timing of typical pubertal development for boys and girls? Have they changed over time, and do they vary across cultures? What are the ramifications for early or delayed pubertal development for children of both genders?

Over time, and despite longer lifespans, pubertal development in boys and girls has begun earlier across all cultures. Currently, girls in the United States enter puberty on average at 10.5 years old, compared to the average ages of 12 in 1980 and 13 in 1950. In the United States, the average age of menarche is 12.5 years old. There continues to be substantial individual variation in timing of pubertal onset and progression, as well as variation across cultures. For example, on average, African-American girls enter puberty earlier than Caucasian girls. Currently in the United States, boys typically begin puberty around 12 years old, an age which has also declined gradually over time. Early pubertal development compared to peers has been correlated with negative psychosocial effects on girls.

What about physical development in transgender, transsexual, and gender non-conforming children? What interventions are accepted as medical treatment for these individuals? What role do pediatricians and child psychiatrists play in advocating for lesbian, gay, bisexual, and transgender (LGBT) youth?

Current pediatric models of care for transgender youth emphasize the importance of supporting the child or teen's wishes regarding self-identification and transition to another gender and providing appropriate medical care and support for the patients and their families. Following standards in behavioral health, pediatricians use the patient's preferred name and gender pronouns in communication and use currently accepted terms (e.g., F2M or "female to male") in documentation. Due to the highly stigmatized and complicated nature of the issues that gender non-conforming youth face, referral to a physician who has experience working with transgender youth is ideal, and involvement of a BH specialist is also recommended. The process of gender affirming treatment or gender transition is not delayed until a patient reaches adulthood or late adolescence, as the physical changes associated with puberty can be very distressing for the individual, and delays make the transition process more complicated. For prepubertal children, gender transition is social, with the child adopting a preferred name and style. Clinicians can assist schools and families in affirming and supporting the child during this process. Medical stages of gender transitioning can be broadly broken down into three stages, the first of which is fully reversible, consisting of puberty-suppressing hormones (i.e., gonadotropin-releasing hormone analogs) also used in the treatment of precocious puberty (Hembree et al. 2017). The second stage consists of cross-gender hormone administration and is considered partially reversible. The last, "irreversible" stage, consists of transition surgery (Human Rights Campaign 2017). Desire of a youth to transition genders is respected and medical supervision strongly recommended. Youth without access to appropriate medical care may turn to hormones obtained illegally, which is a dangerous alternative.

As behavioral health providers trained in LGBT issues are aware, these youths are at higher risk of several psychiatric comorbidities, including suicidality, bullying, abuse, exploitation, and homelessness. An LGBT youth with psychiatric comorbidities faces the double stigma of mental illness and their sexuality and may face barriers accessing quality care. From a pediatric perspective, they are at risk for suboptimal medical care, with provider assumptions and implicit biases potentially contributing to gaps in care. Striking examples of this public health problem exist. For example, the clinician needs to ensure that adolescent women who identify as lesbian (and patients transitioning from female to male gender) who present with gynecologic symptoms are appropriately screened for pregnancy and sexually transmitted infections (Care for transgender adolescents 2017).

What are the general stages of cognitive, social, emotional, and motor development recognized in pediatrics (https://www.cdc.gov/ncbddd/actearly/pdf/checklists/all_checklists.pdf)?

From the pediatric perspective, what is the workup for delayed development?

In pediatrics, development is reviewed at every well-child check. Developmental screening, commonly done via parent-completed reports such as the Ages and Stages Questionnaire (ASQ) or the Parents' Evaluation of Developmental Status (PEDS), is conducted regularly throughout the child's life. Specific ASD screening is also recommended for all toddlers. Communication delay always warrants a formal audiological evaluation, which is available in various forms for all ages of children. Failed development screens should lead to further inquiry; continued monitoring; referral for early intervention services providing speech, occupational, and/or physical therapy; school referral; or referral to a developmental-behavioral pediatrician, pediatric neurologist, child psychiatrist, child psychologist, or other specialist for further assessment. Delayed pubertal development is a trigger to search for medical etiologies including hormonal or genetic causes. Consideration and/or assessment for Turner syndrome should occur in females without menarche by 16 years of age.

Case 2.3 (continued) In follow-up, Dr. Young has discovered that the patient prefers to be alone and has a very limited range of interests. He is obsessed with Pokémon, a multiplayer card game that is popular with much younger children but he rarely plays with anyone else. Overall, he has difficulty with transitions, for which reason he often stays home and frequently gets upset when his parents insist that they dine as a family at a restaurant. His speech, while appropriate and without history of delay, is somewhat monotonous, and his father endorses a history of the patient speaking in a didactic tone even as a young child. Some family members nicknamed him "the little professor," and he does not seem to grasp his cousins' jokes. The additional screenings for anxiety and depression were negative, and considering these new findings, Dr. Young is now mainly concerned about the possible diagnosis of ASD. You agree that this possibility needs to be evaluated further, and you inquire about the PCP's plans.

What are currently recommended diagnostic tests for autism spectrum disorder (ASD) and intellectual disability (ID)?

Current guidelines recommend incorporating laboratory studies including chromosomal microarray and Fragile X testing for all individuals diagnosed with autism or intellectual disability. If the patient appears to have syndromic features, has additional comorbidities suspicious for a specific syndrome, or a history consistent with known etiologies of developmental impairment (e.g., fetal alcohol syndrome), additional referrals or studies may be warranted. Additional investigations such as MRI or electroencephalogram (EEG) are indicated only if there are additional neurological concerns such as seizures or tuberus sclerosis. In some cases, the specific etiology is linked to comorbidities that warrant additional testing for common comorbidities (e.g., annual screening for hypothyroidism in Down syndrome). *Current Centers for Disease Control and Prevention (CDC) and American College of Medical Genetics (ACMG) Guidelines can be found at https://www.cdc.gov/ncbddd/autism/hcp-recommendations.html & https://www.acmg.net/docs/pp-g-ASD-schaffer-aop-gim201332a.pdf.*

Acute and Chronic Illness

Case Vignette 2.4 Katie is a 17-year-old girl who has complex psychiatric and other medical comorbidities, who takes multiple medications and who requires close follow-up. Katie was diagnosed with DiGeorge syndrome, schizophrenia, and congenital heart disease (Tetralogy of Fallot, status post-surgical repair). Her diagnosis was confirmed with genetic testing for the 22q11.2 deletion, and she has a full team of medical, educational, and social work professionals working with her and her family to meet her needs. She has an IEP, does well at school in an intensive learning center (ILC) setting, and has a skills trainer at home. Her nuclear family is supported by the extended family, friends, and twice monthly respite care. She is being treated with olanzapine for psychotic symptoms and aggressive behavior and has had a positive response. She also takes polyethylene glycol 3350 for chronic constipation, cetirizine for allergic rhinitis, fluticasone and albuterol for moderate asthma, and iron supplements for iron-deficiency anemia.

At her monthly follow-up appointment, Katie's parents report that she has had progressively worsening aggressive behaviors over the past three to 4 weeks. She is more often non-compliant and will yell when her parents insist that she do something that she is refusing. Additionally, she has been hitting herself in the head and is very difficult to redirect. Sleep, which has been a chronic struggle, has become even more problematic over the past couple of weeks. There have not been any overt signs of psychosis observed, but determining whether Katie is experiencing any psychotic symptoms is challenging because she is mostly nonverbal. Her parents admit that she misses taking her medications once or twice a week, but this pattern is no different than in the past. You inquire about any recent changes to the patient's schedule, school, or home life. The family shares that they adopted two kittens. The pet adoption has been a positive experience for the whole family, and the patient enjoys playing with them. The family notes that there have been no changes to Katie's activities, schedule, or providers both at home and school. As you think through the differential for this worsening behavior and the possible adjustments to Katie's medications, you conduct a general review of systems and learn that Katie has had continual nasal congestion and cough, with intermittent fever, for the past 4 weeks. In fact, you now recall that the whole family has been ill over the last several months. "We just keep passing these colds around," says Katie's father. They share that the illness appears to have triggered Katie's asthma, and they have been giving her albuterol twice per day over the past few weeks with some temporary improvement in her respiratory symptoms and acetaminophen as needed for fever. As you think about the possibilities and wonder why the patient has been sick for so long with a common cold, Katie begins to hit herself in the head. You are concerned that the patient has been ill for such a long period of time, and you recommend that Katie be evaluated by her pediatrician. You wonder if there is a medical problem causing an increase in her behavioral symptoms, and you wonder what the best approach would be to address them. After discussing the available options with the family, they agree to take Katie to her pediatrician as soon as possible and to subsequently follow up with you to evaluate the need for medication adjustments.

Later that week, you receive a note from Katie's pediatrician, Dr. Ray. He has diagnosed her with acute otitis media in both ears and an asthma exacerbation, secondary to an upper respiratory tract infection, further complicated by allergic rhinitis and conjunctivitis. It seems that on top of the infections, the family's newly adopted kittens are also triggering the patient's asthma and allergy symptoms. Dr. Ray prescribed a seven-day course of amoxicillin/clavulanate for the patient's ear infection, acetaminophen and ibuprofen as needed for fever or pain, and albuterol four times daily (delivered via spacer and mask, because of refusal of the nebulizer) for the asthma exacerbation. Dr. Ray has placed non-compliance on the patient's problem list, specifically with the fluticasone and cetirizine, and recommends their regular use to decrease overall atopy symptoms. Dr. Ray also recommends getting rid of the cats, or at least not allowing them in the patient's bedroom. Pediatrics follow-up has been scheduled in 1 week to reevaluate the patient.

You call Katie's mother and learn that the patient seems to be slowly improving since starting the medication regimen a few days ago. Katie is breathing more comfortably and is more compliant with requests compared to in prior weeks. She still hits herself in the head, but the frequency is decreasing, and overall, her parents feel that the medical interventions are working. Together, you decide to schedule the patient's next appointment after her medical treatment and pediatric follow-up, to reassess the patient's behavioral issues.

What medical ailments can masquerade as behavioral health problems?

The general challenge of other common medical considerations for behavioral symptoms is discussed in Chap. 9. In the context of developmental disability, medical problems can present as worsening behavioral or emotional symptoms. Time course and symptom type can be helpful to determine or localize the source of an illness. Rapid changes suggest an acute process such as development of acute otitis media or urinary tract infection. Symptoms such as increased self-harm may indicate pain, and consultation with a pediatrician is highly recommended in patients with limited communication to rule out other medical causes for psychiatric decompensation. Other potential causes of behavioral symptoms include painful menstrual cycles in female patients, exacerbations of chronic medical problems such as allergies, or medical interventions including invasive procedures. Chronic conditions can also cause or contribute to psychiatric symptoms: obstructive sleep apnea or hypothyroidism may mimic depression, or Graves' disease may be incorrectly diagnosed as generalized anxiety or panic disorder Seizures, encephalitis, and other neurologic disorders can masquerade as primary psychiatric disorders.

How do pediatricians approach management of chronic illness?

Pediatricians typically emphasize the family's role and the developmental impact of chronic illness more often than their adult medicine counterparts. The medical home model, held as the ideal for pediatric care, establishes a primary care physician as the central hub for coordinating a patient's care. This is an especially important concept for children with special healthcare needs who see multiple specialists.

Case 2.4 (continued) You receive a call from the pediatric hospitalist, informing you that Katie has been admitted for complications secondary to her congenital heart defect. You learn that, despite the surgical repair done early in her life, Katie has developed pulmonary backflow requiring another surgical correction. You provide consultation to the inpatient pediatric team regarding her psychiatric medications and provide suggestions to minimize agitation in the immediate postoperative period and while recovering in the hospital. Katie's surgery goes well, and with the coordinated efforts of the medical team, child life unit, her family, and yourself, her hospital stay is relatively uneventful. On the day Katie is to be transferred from the pediatric intensive care unit to the regular pediatric floor, her mother stops you and shares that she is very anxious to get home to the rest of her children. "She's doing so great, when do you think they will discharge her?" You admit to yourself that you were wondering the same thing, and tell the mother honestly that while you do not know the answer, you will work to find out and get back to her as soon as possible.

What are general criteria for pediatric hospital admission and discharge?

Knowledge of the pediatric thought process regarding hospital admission and discharge can provide valuable information for a consulting psychiatrist and can increase empathy with children receiving inpatient care and their families. Although admission and discharge decisions are always evaluated in the context of each individual patient and family, there are overarching principles and practices that apply more generally. In practice, there are several triggers for pediatric admission that differ substantially from those for adults. General criteria for hospitalization include lower thresholds for admission in younger patients, such as infants with fever or a toddler with a limp, who are admitted not only on basis of the clinical picture and physiologic increased risk for negative outcomes but also, in part, because of their developmentally limited capacity for accurate communication of history. An adolescent or adult with average communication skills is assumed to be able to communicate with the medical provider regarding the development of their symptoms. These skills are not automatically assumed to be present for younger children. This assumption relates to many aspects of a medical history, such as a child's communication of their pain level, localization of symptoms, and description or timing of symptom development. Even simple, concrete communication of circumstances, such as a child reporting (or denying) that he put an object in his ear, is checked with a physical examination and not necessarily accepted as fact. Additionally, histories are often provided by caregivers, who are one layer removed from the patient and not necessarily optimally reliable.

In terms of practical considerations, for children with respiratory conditions, respiratory effort is an important indicator for admission, as is lowered oxygen concentration. Oxygen saturation of <90% alone is criteria for admission in many pediatric centers. For children with infectious conditions, important indicators for admission and intravenous antibiotics include current level of infection and potential for complications or further progression (e.g., sepsis or infection of adjacent vital organ). In general, the risk for a potentially negative impact on a child's development or outcome is also considered, especially when the exact cause is not known (e.g., for a brief unresponsive episode in an infant). Although the social environment affects treatment outcomes for patients of all ages, medical problems are always evaluated within a child's social context. This approach highlights one overarching principle of balancing autonomy and beneficence. Autonomy is often given more weight in adult cases compared to pediatric patients. In contrast, pediatrics often places more weight on the potential risk to the child. An example would be a patient with an infection, thought to be treatable with oral antibiotics and outpatient follow-up if good compliance could be guaranteed; in many settings, admission would likely be recommended more often for a homeless child as compared to a homeless adult. Admissions such as these are sometimes referred to as "social admissions," as they are not based purely on clinical assessment of illness severity, but in part on the physicians' assessment of the level of risk posed by the patient's social environment. In the United States, an extreme example of the differing balance between autonomy and beneficence would be the ability for adults to decline, based on their religious beliefs, a life-saving blood transfusion for themselves, but not for their dependent children. Similarly, a discharge from the hospital or emergency department to the street would rarely if ever be considered acceptable for a minor patient, while a competent adult may readily choose to decline shelter placement or other offers of assistance despite a medical provider's evaluation of potential negative impact on medical outcomes.

Regarding discharge, hospitals will usually require documentation and demonstration that caregivers have the necessary skills and means to provide for appropriate follow-up care post-discharge and will arrange for help if difficulties are foreseen. In adult patients, although post-discharge needs are also assessed, the assumption of competence after instruction is the default. Postoperative patients such as in case vignette 2.4 are assessed for level of recovery, risk of complications, post-discharge needs, and potential comorbidities. For example, if a patient such as Katie has severe behavioral difficulties, limited cognition, or significant aggressive/self-harming behaviors, precautions would need to be taken to ensure that complications could be prevented or minimized (e.g., by removing stitches and IV lines) and to confirm that the patient's needs can be met in the outpatient setting. Following cardiac or other complicated surgery, pediatric patients will most often be "stepped down" from intensive care to a regular ward for observation prior to discharge. As previously mentioned, public health nurses or care coordinators are often utilized for children with special healthcare needs or complicated social situations, to prevent negative developmental impact/outcomes, reduce readmission rates, and improve follow-up care.

References

Almandil, N., et al. (2013). Weight gain and other metabolic adverse effects associated with atypical antipsychotic treatment of children and adolescents: A systematic review and meta-analysis. *Paediatric Drugs, 15*(2), 139–150. https://doi.org/10.1007/s40272-013-0016-6.

American Diabetes Association. (2016). Standards of medical care in diabetes—2016. *Diabetes Care, 39*(suppl 1), S1–S106.

Care for transgender adolescents. (2017). Committee opinion no. 685. American College of Obstetricians and Gynecologists. *Obstetrics and Gynecology, 129*, e11–e16.

Correll, C., & Carlson, H. (2006). Endocrine and metabolic adverse effects of psychotropic medications in children and adolescents. *Journal of the American Academy of Child and Adolescent Psychiatry, 45*, 771–791.

Correll, C. U., et al. (2009). Cardiometabolic risk of second-generation antipsychotic medications during first-time use in children and adolescents. *Journal of the American Medical Association, 302*(16), 1765–1773.

Dietary Guidelines for Americans. (2005). http://www.healthierus.gov/dietaryguidelines
Dori, N. & Green, T. (2011, October). The metabolic syndrome and antipsychotics in children and adolescents. *Harefuah, 150*(10), 791–796, 814, 813.
Falkner, B. (2010). Hypertension in children and adolescents: Epidemiology and natural history. *Pediatric Nephrology, 25*(7), 1219–1224.
George, M. et al. (2014). Hypertension screening in children and adolescents – National Ambulatory Medical Care Survey, National Hospital Ambulatory Medical Care Survey, and Medical Expenditure Panel Survey, United States, 2007–2010. MMWR Supplements September 12, 2014/*63*(02), 47–53.
Goeb, J. L., et al. (2010). Metabolic side effects of risperidone in early onset schizophrenia. *Encephale, 36*(3), 242–252. Epub 2009 Dec 1.
Hembree, W., et al. (2017). Endocrine treatment of gender-dysphoric/gender-incongruent persons: An endocrine society clinical practice guideline. *The Journal of Clinical Endocrinology & Metabolism, 102*(11), 3869–3903. https://doi.org/10.1210/jc.2017-01658.
Human Rights Campaign, AAP. (2017). *Supporting and caring for transgender children*. September 2016. https://www.aap.org/en-us/Documents/solgbt_resource_transgenderchildren.pdf
Loy, J. H., et al. (2017). Atypical antipsychotics for disruptive behaviour disorders in children and youths. *Cochrane Database of Systematic Reviews, 8*, CD008559. Epub 2017 Aug 9.
Overbeek, W. A., et al. (2010). Antipsychotics and metabolic abnormalities in children and adolescents: A review of the literature and some recommendations. *Tijdschrift voor Psychiatrie, 52*(5), 311–320.
Strickland, B. B., et al. (2004). Access to the medical home: Results of the national survey of children with special healthcare needs. *Pediatrics, 113*, 1485–1492. https://doi.org/10.1542/peds.113.5.S1.1485.
Uddin, S. et al. (2016, May). *Physician office visits by children for well and problem-focused care: United States, 2012*. CDC NCHS Data Brief No. 248.
Wilmot, E., & Idris, I. (2014). Early onset type 2 diabetes: Risk factors, clinical impact and management. *Therapeutic Advances in Chronic Disease., 5*(6), 234–244. https://doi.org/10.1177/2040622314548679.

Chapter 3
Essential Child and Adolescent Psychiatry and Substance Use Disorders for the Nonpsychiatrist

Bernhard Weidle

Introduction

The time from first appearance of mild psychological stress to the development of a serious child and adolescent psychiatric condition varies, but sometimes it might be short. Usually, a family's search for help will involve a meeting with primary pediatric healthcare services before they are referred for specialized psychiatric healthcare.

Psychiatric and primary healthcare providers will need common approaches and baseline knowledge to optimally help children and families. This chapter aims to describe systems for the description and classification of disorders as tools to understand symptoms, to communicate about them, to relate them to our established base of knowledge, and to thereby form grounds for the evaluation and treatment of the symptoms and provides an overview of the most common disorders in the specialty of child and adolescent psychiatry.

1. The multiaxial classification in the ICD (International Classification of Diseases), introduced by the World Health Organization (WHO 1996), is currently in its 10th edition (ICD 10) and contains all conditions, psychiatric and medical, based on symptom descriptions. A revised version (ICD 11) is planned to be published by 2018.
2. The DSM system (Diagnostic and Statistical Manual of Mental Disorders), developed by the American Psychiatric Association, is currently in its 5th edition (DSM-5), published in 2013 (APA 2013).

B. Weidle (✉)
Department of Mental Health, Norwegian University of Science and Technology (NTNU), Regional Centre for Child and Youth Mental Health and Child Welfare, Trondheim, Norway
e-mail: b-weidle@online.no

A. P. S. Guerrero et al. (eds.), *Pediatric Consultation-Liaison Psychiatry*,
https://doi.org/10.1007/978-3-319-89488-1_3

3. The ICPC (International Classification of Primary Care) system, owned by the World Organization of Family Doctors (WONCA 1972), is a third classification system, widely used by general practitioners.

Our diagnostic systems are categorical, i.e., based on the assumption that an individual can be defined as either healthy or ill, based on certain criteria. However, there is little evidence that one can establish a sharp delineation for when a psychiatric condition is normal or pathologic (Angold and Costello 2009; Kendell and Jablensky 2003). Therefore, psychiatric conditions such as anxiety or depression may be better described as dimensional phenomena, with several symptoms lacking a clear threshold between disorder and not disorder. This principle is illustrated in a study (Fergusson et al. 2005) exploring the continuity of depressive symptoms between youth and adulthood. The extent of depression – whether meeting the threshold for the diagnosis of a major depressive disorder or not – at ages 17–18 years was associated with future depression and suicidal behavior. While both patient and provider at one point have to think categorically to start or to decline treatment based on a diagnosis, they should also think dimensionally when evaluating the effect of a treatment intervention or prioritizing the role of more intensive monitoring and prevention. As Pickles and Angold (2003) put it, "the central question is not 'is psychopathology scalar or categorical,' but 'under what circumstances does it make sense to regard psychopathology as being scalar and under what circumstances does it make sense to treat psychopathology as being categorical.'"

The following vignettes review the most common and important psychiatric disorders in childhood and adolescence that are not reviewed more in depth in the subsequent chapters of this book. The examples in the specific vignettes were chosen based on prevalence and significance of the symptoms to illustrate somewhat "typical" cases. The vignettes do not attempt to cover the diagnosis and treatment of *all* psychiatric disorders, and for less common disorders that nevertheless occur in childhood and adolescence, the reader is referred to general textbooks of child and adolescent psychiatry.

Common Psychiatric Disorders

Attention-Deficit Hyperactivity Disorder (ADHD)

Vignette 3.1

Brian is a 6-year-old boy brought for evaluation by his mother, who lived alone with him. She was concerned about his symptoms of restlessness, high activity most of the day, and his angry outbursts, in spite of a charming personality. The mother seems to underreport his symptoms. Brian attends the last year of kindergarten. The staff describes a full crisis: His restlessness causes significant difficulties for him, the other children, and the staff. Brian himself commented, "none of the adults can handle me." He did not seem to listen to messages directed to the whole class, and he did not seem to listen to direct messages to him unless an adult provided frequent reminders. He exhibited significant problems in transitional situations. He could play with other children only for a short time, and he would easily lose his patience and run into conflicts with other children and staff members. His rage outbursts resulted in both physical and verbal attacks. The mother admitted a sense of insufficiency because of the high levels of conflicts at home. A visit at the supermarket usually ended with him yelling at her to buy unhealthy food or expensive toys and leaving her in the untenable situation of having to either accept his demands or argue in front of waiting customers. Visits to friends' households always became a challenge because of his impulsivity and tendency to explore the surroundings in high speed, often breaking items in his way. Because of these challenges, the mother eventually avoided all shopping and other outings except for visits to very close family.

Worldwide, possible ADHD is one of the most frequent reasons for referral to child and adolescent psychiatric services. The prevalence rate of this disorder is approximately 5% depending on study methods (Polanczyk et al. 2014). The case above illustrates a variety of ambiguous symptoms leading to one pathway of referral. At this stage, the differential diagnosis is broad and includes both psychiatric and other medical disorders, family dysfunction, trauma, abuse, and neglect. A diagnosis of ADHD is based on characteristic behavior over time in different settings, e.g., home, school/preschool, or leisure activities. Primary healthcare providers should be able to recognize possible ADHD and refer the child for further assessment as clinically appropriate. The history should include specific symptoms and their onset, duration, and severity; degree of functional impairment; symptoms suggestive of other differential diagnoses and comorbidities (including depressive, anxiety, specific learning, and substance use disorders); family and developmental history; and information from school/preschool. Comprehensive assessment should also include ADHD-specific parent and teacher questionnaires (DuPaul et al. 2016). A physical examination, including evaluation of vision and hearing, should rule out other medical conditions (e.g., anemia, diabetes, thyroid disorders) that could explain the symptoms.

Specialized healthcare services will often add a structured interview and psychoeducational and IQ testing to establish a comprehensive diagnostic conclusion.

Initial therapeutic interventions include psychoeducation of the child, parents, and teachers and home and classroom accommodations (structure, predictability, minimization of distractions) to compensate for lacking executive functions. If these interventions are not satisfactory, additional treatment should be offered, and the treatments best supported by the evidence base are behavioral modification therapies at school and home, stimulant medication, or a combination of the two. Some families will be in need of additional social support.

Conduct Disorder

Vignette 3.2

Andrew was 15 years old when he was brought for a pediatric examination. He had been caught in the act of committing car theft and ruthless vandalism, and he sustained some minor injuries while he tried to escape. Despite his young age, he was frequently out from home at night. If mother asked where he was she just got an angry answer: "with my friends of course!" When he was referred to you for a medical assessment, it turned out that both he and some of his friends were old acquaintances of the police. Andrews's father did not live together with the family, and Andrew had almost no contact with him. During the assessment, the mother complained about never having gotten help from public healthcare services despite her difficult situation. She reported that Andrews's misbehavior started in kindergarten, where the other children avoided or openly rejected him. He was an unruly boy, and he could destroy both toys and the games children played. The mother remembered one episode when a new nursery school worker became interested in Andrew. They played together most of the day. Later, she discovered that he had lifted her wallet from her pocket. The next day, when she tried to talk about the incident, he seemed completely untouched, and he denied all wrongdoing and asked her when they could play again.

Irritability, temper tantrums, rage outbursts, oppositional behavior, and aggression are common symptoms occurring in many psychiatric and other medical conditions. In addition, the presence of one or more other disorders may aggravate behavioral and conduct problems. Therefore, when conduct disorder is suspected, assessment of potential comorbid or differential diagnostic conditions is mandatory. The diagnosis is based on characteristic patterns of behavior observed over time and in different settings. The history should include specific symptoms, including duration, extent, and onset; psychomotor development; family medical and psychiatric history; family function and interaction; parenting style; and child's areas of interest and strength. Both screening forms such as the *Strength and Difficulty Questionnaire (SDQ)* and specific parent questionnaires such as the *Eyberg Child Behavior Inventory* (Eyberg and Ross 1978) might be helpful for primary healthcare services in assessing the degree of severity and potential need to refer for specialized healthcare services.

Specialized healthcare services may add a systematic child psychiatric interview, e.g., *Schedule for Affective Disorders and Schizophrenia* (*Kiddie-SADS*), which also contains a diagnostic supplement for further assessment of behavioral disorders. In the presence of personality traits with limited prosocial emotions and lack of remorse or guilt, callous lack of empathy and disregard about the feelings of others, no concern about poor/problematic performance at school or in other important activities, and shallow or deficient affects, the *Inventory of Callous-Unemotional Traits (ICU)* (Kimonis et al. 2008) could be helpful. To rule out comorbid intellectual developmental and specific learning disorders, psychoeducational and IQ testing may be necessary.

Guidelines, such as those issued by the National Institute for Health and Clinical Excellence in the UK (NICE 2013), for the assessment and treatment of behavioral disorders, underline the need for identification and treatment of comorbid conditions and for multimodal treatment interventions to reduce antisocial behavior.

As illustrated by the vignette above, frequently a variety of factors contribute to the development of behavioral disorders. Treatment of these disorders is challenging, and the patients find themselves easily involved in vicious, inescapable cycles. Because of the less-than-optimal prognosis, interventions will often need to be intensive, comprehensive, and multidisciplinary, involving medical and social services.

Many developmentally tailored, cognitive-behavioral therapy-based intervention programs have been shown to limit or reduce severe aggression. *Parent Management Training – Oregon Model (PMTO) (Patterson and Stouthamer-Loeber* 1984) and *The Incredible Years* (IY) program *(Webster-Stratton et al.* 2008*)* are examples for treatment interventions for families with younger children (3–12 years of age) with serious behavioral problems, while multisystemic therapy (MST) programs are developed to address adolescent criminal behavior (Henggeler 2011).

Mood Disorders, Depression, and Bipolar Disorders

Vignette 3.3
Mary was 15 years of age when she was brought to you for a medical evaluation. She has always been mild-mannered and reserved. During the last few months, the parents observed her to be increasingly withdrawn and isolative. Previously she liked to play guitar, but now she felt it was just boring, and she told her mom that she couldn't bear it any more. Going to school (only a few blocks away) had become such a demanding task for her that her parents had to drive her several days a week. She told her parents that it made no sense for her to go to school, as she had no energy and was not able to concentrate on lessons anyway. She was full of regret and remorse, and she had decreased self-confidence. During a long conversation with mother, Mary admitted to feeling sad nearly every day. She implied that life was too difficult for her to manage, but when asked directly, she denied any thoughts about taking her life. She mentioned that she had quarrels with some of the other girls in her grade but denied that there have been any serious incidents for her to feel bad about. After having been passive and lacking energy for more than 2 months, a physical examination and blood test to screen for other medical disorders were obtained but showed no abnormality. Mother was particularly concerned about Mary's condition because she remembered Mary experiencing a similar episode 2 years ago. Fortunately, the symptoms resolved completely after a few months. In addition, family history revealed that Mary's grandfather also had recurrent episodes, where he lay in bed for several days.

Sad feelings are a part of all people's daily life, and children need to be comforted in sad situations.

However, when the sadness is associated with depressed mood; tiredness; lack of energy, initiative, and interest in previously enjoyed activities; and persistence of symptoms even with comforting, a diagnosis of major depression should be ruled out. Additional symptoms include guilty feelings, low self-confidence, self-accusation, suicidal ideation, concentration problems, sleep pattern changes, and appetite changes. Also in depression, comorbid conditions are frequent (Angold et al. 1999), and the former and the latter often influence each other.

Assessment involves gathering information from all available sources, as children with depression might find it difficult to describe their symptoms. The main symptoms that are required to make the diagnosis are those listed above: four to five symptoms may indicate a mild depressive episode, six to seven symptoms a moderate one, and eight to ten a severe one. There are many questionnaires for children, parents, and professionals, such as the Mood and Feelings Questionnaire (Angold et al. 1995) or the Beck Depression Inventory (Bennett et al. 1997). The diagnosis cannot be based solely on the use of such questionnaires, but they can be used as a starting point to introduce the subject or as an interviewing tool to systemize information. Suicidal risk and other medical conditions causing low energy must be ruled out during the assessment.

The clinician should assess for potential psychosocial stressors and concomitant problems such as lack of social network, bullying, parent conflicts, and substance use. These concerns are unfortunately common triggers of depression (Goodyer et al. 2000). The UK-based National Institute for Health and Clinical Excellence (NICE) guidelines outline best practices for assessment and treatment (NICE 2005).

The clinician should assess for periods of unusual elated mood, especially if the child has experienced recurrent depressive episodes. In DSM-5, a manic episode is characterized by three (or more) of the following symptoms: inflated self-esteem or grandiosity; decreased need for sleep; tendency to keep talking; flight of ideas; easy distractibility and drawing of attention to unimportant or irrelevant items; psychomotor agitation or increased activity either socially, at work or school, or sexually; or excessive involvement in pleasurable activities that have a high potential for painful consequences. Irritability is common in all phases of mania. According to the DSM-5, bipolar I is characterized by changes between manic and depressive episodes and the presence of at least one manic episode, while bipolar II means the presence of depressive episodes but only hypomanic episodes. Hypomanic episodes have the same symptoms as manic episodes, but mood elation is less severe and occurs over a shorter time span (4 days are enough), and psychotic features are never present.

Evidence-based efficient treatments for depression include cognitive behavior therapy (CBT), interpersonal therapy, and pharmacotherapy, predominantly with selective serotonin reuptake inhibitors (SSRIs). CBT has the strongest evidence base (Webb et al. 2012; Weersing and Brent 2006), but interpersonal therapy (IPT) also has documented effectiveness (Brunstein-Klomek et al. 2007). Psychoeducation with family involvement and supportive psychotherapy can be sufficient in milder cases (Birmaher et al. 2007). Untreated, a depressive episode usually lasts between 3 and 8 months. However, relapse is frequent, and within a time frame of 5 years, 70% experience a new depressive episode (Birmaher et al. 2007). Among children with early-onset depression, about 20–40% may develop bipolar disorder. Therefore, particularly if this disorder occurs in the family, or if psychomotor retardation is a salient symptom, this possibility must carefully be ruled out. There is some evidence that lithium and lamotrigine may be effective for bipolar depression in children. It is not clear whether SSRIs are effective for bipolar depression, and they may increase the risk for development of manic symptoms. The main principle is not to use antidepressive medication without concomitant use of mood stabilizers in bipolar disorders. Despite a lifelong vulnerability for new manic and depressive episodes, many individuals with this diagnosis – treated appropriately – have a good life with long symptom-free periods. Good premorbid function and high IQ seem to improve prognosis.

Close to a fifth of patients with bipolar disorder end their life in suicide, which occurs most frequently in males, during adolescence, and during a depressive phase (McClellan et al. 2007). Suicide prevention tasks, including psychoeducation and close follow-up, are therefore extremely important.

Anxiety Disorders and Obsessive-Compulsive Disorder

Vignette 3.4

Jane has always been a cautious child. From the age of 12 years on, she became gradually more anxious and worried about new things and situations that seemed unfamiliar to her. Parents had tried to soothe and reassure her that her worries were without foundation. This reassurance made her feel better for a little while, but soon her anxious thoughts and feelings came back. She could be worried about everything, from being unable to answer a teacher's question to being kidnapped on her way to the neighborhood store. In addition, she became more and more irritable and inattentive in class. Jane's preoccupations persisted despite reassurances from her parents, who sometimes lost their patience, demanding that she just leave these unreasonable and unfounded concerns and not waste so much time worrying. Sometimes her anxious thoughts about dangers on her way to school prevented her from going to school, and father had to bring her by car. When her grades went down, her teacher and the parents agreed on the need for medical assessment. During the consultation, Jane was reluctant to talk about her problems even when her parents waited outside. When the doctor told her about other patients feeling this way, she revealed piece by piece her exaggerated concerns and worries, which were worsened by her perception that nobody took her seriously.

Anxiety disorders are one of the most common childhood problems, with prevalence rates ranging (depending on study methods) from 5 to 20%. Nearly 60% of adolescents with anxiety disorders have further episodes in adulthood. In addition, childhood anxiety disorders often precede adolescent and adult depression (Essau 2008; Patton et al. 2014). Therefore, therapeutic interventions that shorten the duration of anxiety episodes are important as they could prevent much morbidity later in life (Patton et al. 2014).

Typical sources of anxiety differ, depending on developmental stage: Babies and toddlers experience anxiety when exposed to sensory stimuli such as high noise, physical restriction, or fast-moving objects. One-year-olds commonly experience separation and stranger anxiety. Preschool children are often afraid of animals, darkness, and fantasy figures. School-aged children commonly fear injuries and other physical threats and experience achievement anxiety, while adolescents commonly experience anxiety around body image, medical symptoms, sexuality, social acceptance, and major threats such as death and catastrophes. The feeling of anxiety is commonly regarded as protection against danger and as a regulator of social relations, improving survival and reproduction. In pathologic anxiety, the same themes may be present, but the feelings are either without foundation, grossly exaggerated, or age and developmental stage-inappropriate. For example, while stranger anxiety is normal in toddlers, separation anxiety persisting beyond 3 years of age is regarded as pathologic. Anxiety reactions should be considered as a disorder if they are either developmentally inappropriate or cause troublesome avoiding behavior and impairment of daily functioning. Panic attacks, characterized by an abrupt and intense fear of losing control or dying, and usually accompanied by other medical symptoms, such as shortness of breath, palpitations, sweating, shaking, and light-headedness, are more frequent in adolescents and adults than in children of younger age.

As always, assessment starts with a careful history from both child and parents: symptoms, including onset, development (including provoking factors), severity, and impact on the family; family's effort to solve the problems; and family history of other psychiatric problems. Questionnaires might be helpful to map anxiety disorders in general, e.g., *Screen for Child Anxiety Related Emotional Disorders (SCARED)* (Muris et al. 2004), or specific anxiety symptoms (e.g., the *Spider Phobia Questionnaire*). Once the diagnosis is established, psychoeducation is important. While many families may believe that they ought to protect their child from anxiety-provoking situations, cognitive-behavioral therapy (CBT) with exposure to the anxiety-provoking situation has the best documented effect. CBT is a highly structured treatment with testing of hypotheses; correcting of automatic thoughts, misconceptions, and underlying false beliefs related to symptoms; and exposure exercises with application of anxiety management strategies. In children, it is always important to include parents or the whole family in therapy to change their patterns of cooperation. Psychoeducation for parents is necessary, especially if they are themselves anxious and overprotecting. For isolated phobias, brief treatment formats are available, for example, a single exposure session with booster sessions if needed (Ost 1989). Medication is not recommended as first-line treatment but could be helpful for nonresponders following an adequate trial of CBT or in combination with CBT.

School refusal is a symptom rather than a specific disorder. Defined as a determined refusal to leave home for school or increasing anxiety as school is approached, school refusal may present acutely or insidiously, often triggered by a specific event and accompanied by physical symptoms (poor appetite, headaches, nausea, vomiting, abdominal pain, diarrhea). Phobic anxiety of school is one of a variety of reasons that may account for the refusal, and these reasons may include separation anxiety, family dysfunction, bullying, poor peer relationships, academic underachievement, vulnerable identity, weak self-confidence, and other psychiatric conditions, mainly depression (Egger et al. 2003). To ascertain and resolve these underlying problems, parental counseling, school liaison, and CBT are tools to help the child to expeditiously return to school.

Obsessive-compulsive disorder (OCD) affects about 1% of the childhood population and, untreated, leads to a chronic course in about 40–60% of those affected (Stewart et al. 2004). In DSM-5, OCD was moved to a category that is discrete from the anxiety disorders and inclusive of hair pulling and hoarding disorder, which share common features such as obsessive thoughts and repetitive behaviors. In common with the anxiety disorders, OCD involves physiological arousal, wherein certain thoughts or obsessions, for example, about contamination, cause anxiety and trigger behaviors or compulsions determined to reduce the anxiety, for example, extensive handwashing rituals. Individuals with a non-OCD anxiety disorder do not engage in ritual behaviors (other than avoiding the feared situation) that they believe will relieve their symptoms. Also, the contents of anxiety-provoking thoughts and concerns are slightly different: in anxiety disorders, the concerns involve real-life situations, even though these concerns are exaggerated and out of context, while in OCD, the fears are more unrealistic, such as contamination via impossible or highly unlikely transmission routes. In OCD, both assessment and treatment closely follow anxiety management principles.

Interestingly the history of OCD illustrates the evolution of psychiatric treatments. Not more than 30–40 years ago, OCD was considered to be a serious psychiatric condition with a very poor prognosis. In the 1970s, medication first became available, followed by a treatment method now known as exposure and response prevention (ERP) (Rachman et al. 1971). Today, prognosis is considered as good, with a treatment response rate of about 70% (Torp et al. 2014).

Tic Disorders

Vignette 3.5
Parents consulted you, as their primary care physician, to discuss concerns about their son Scott, who was 6 years old and had normal development during the first 5 years of his life. Last year, Scott developed an "annoying habit" with repeated eye blinks and "weird" deviations of his mouth. During the last few months, he had started to shake his head from side to side, to shrug his right shoulder, and to jerk his arms. Parents have noticed frequent short hard coughs and throat cleaning. These movements and sounds wax and wane and may nearly disappear for a few days. Scott experienced these symptoms as very unpleasant and developed a tendency to avoid social gatherings except for school and contact with his old friends. His father remembered, from his own childhood, that he had frequent eye blinking and facial grimacing. Both parents were very worried about these symptoms, especially because they seemed to impair Scott's social life.

About 20% of all children might experience transient tics during normal development. Tourette's disorder, which involves a combination of motor tics and at least one vocal or phonic tic, occurs in about 1% of a childhood population (M.M. Robertson 2008). Tics are seldom the child's single or biggest problem (Khalifa and von Knorring 2006). Since the associated comorbidities often are more impairing than the tics, emphasis should be directed toward assessing the former. The conditions most frequently associated with Tourette's disorder are ADHD and OCD (Robertson 2000). Approximately 20–40% of children referred for Tourette's disorder report behavioral problems such as unpredictable rage outbursts, irritability, and aggression (Wright et al. 2012). Also, internalizing disorders such as depression, anxiety, and self-harm and certain personality disorders are common (Robertson 2000). Other medical conditions such as epilepsy, tardive dyskinesia, Sydenham's chorea, or other sequelae of streptococcal infections, dystonia, blepharospasm, Wilson's disease, neuroacanthocytosis, and medication side effects may cause tics and should be ruled out.

Reliable information, from both the child and parents' perspective, about symptom development is crucial. Structured interviews and comprehensive questionnaires, such as the Yale Global Tics Severity Scale (Leckman et al. 1989), may be helpful. In uncomplicated cases, accurate diagnosis and psychoeducation about nature and expected course are the most important measures and may constitute the only intervention needed. Usually, tics reach their peak intensity at 10–14 years of age and gradually diminish between 15 and 18 years. In adulthood, 25% of those with childhood tics will be without tics, 50% will be clearly improved, while 25% will have unchanged or worsening tics.

While tics are unintentional, they can be triggered by various environmental factors. Both positive and negative feedback regarding the tics may increase them, while a neutral environment typically will not. If tics cause functional impairment, pain, or social stigma, behavioral interventions (Frank and Cavanna 2013) such as habit reversal training are recommended as the first choice of treatment (Verdellen et al. 2011). If these treatments are not sufficient or not available, medication should be considered. As mentioned initially, comorbid conditions, especially ADHD, should be ruled out because they might cause more impairment than tics and because their treatment may improve the tics as well.

Autism Spectrum Disorders

Vignette 3.6

The parents brought Kevin, age 12 years, for a pediatric assessment. They had always cherished his high intelligence, but during the last 3 years in school, they have become increasingly worried about his behavior. A week ago, he had a serious temper tantrum, provoked by the mother cleaning his room and moving one of his collector's items to a slightly different location. This was "the final straw that broke the camel's back" and the reason to make an urgent appointment. Previously, they whisked away their concerns with the thought that nothing could possibly be wrong in a boy with such superior skills.

He talked endlessly about reptiles. By the fourth grade, he had surpassed his teacher in knowledge about these animals. For many of these creatures, he knew the scientific names, even when they were complicated and difficult for others to remember. Often, conversation with him would become conversation about reptiles. Despite his memory skills, he had surprising problems in many academic subjects. His teacher believed that his poor performance in language and social studies was because of lack of interest. While he partly mastered the math curriculum and could perform basic arithmetic operations without problems, it was difficult for him to solve math word problems. After school, during leisure time, he preferred to use his computer to read more about his favorite subjects or to play games. Kevin's movements were somewhat stiff, and he rarely joined his classmates for soccer. When his mother would try to motivate him to play outside with others, he would become very angry. No one in the family could disturb his activities or change his plans. Parents remembered that he was quite "a loner" as far back as in kindergarten. When picking him up, quite often they found him on his own in bushes or trees or in the fringe of the playground. He had only a few friends, and all of them were much younger than he. Mostly, they would come to play computer games, and he is popular in this group because of his computer skills.

The term autism spectrum disorder (ASD) covers a wide range of symptoms and clinical presentations (varying by intellectual ability and degree of functional impairment) with a common denominator of basic deficits in social communication and restricted interests and repetitive behaviors.

Primary care providers should be able to recognize ASD symptoms and refer, where appropriate, for comprehensive assessment and specialized services. A careful history from the child, the parents, and others who know the child well is essential. Assessment of hearing and language development is also essential, as lack of skills in these domains may look like ASD. Usually, kindergarten teachers and staff will become concerned when a child avoids contact or uses unusual ways to make contact with other children or adults, plays in a stereotyped manner, or presents a deviant language development. The *M-CHAT (Modified CHecklist for Autism in Toddlers*) (Kleinman et al. 2008) is a screening instrument that is easy to administer (available on http://www.firstsigns.org/downloads/m-chat.PDF) and helpful in ruling out a suspicion of autism. For older children (4–11 years), screening questionnaires like *the Childhood Autism Spectrum Test* (CAST) (Williams et al. 2006) or *the high-functioning Autism Spectrum Screening Questionnaire (ASSQ)* (Ehlers et al. 1999) for children and adolescents 6–17 years of age can be helpful in determining the need for further referral.

Comprehensive evaluations in specialized healthcare services will include assessments of cognitive and language development; observations of play, behavior, and social abilities; assessments of adaptive functioning; and possibly specific questionnaires and structured observations of communication and social situations via the *Autism Diagnostic Interview-Revised, (ADI-R)* (Lord et al. 1994) and the *Autism Diagnostic Observation Schedule* (*ADOS*), regarded as a gold standard (Lord et al. 1989). Medical conditions associated with autism are frequent. Therefore, the following investigations are recommended: chromosomal analysis, EEG, and brain MRI (to evaluate conditions like XYY, deletions, fragile X, epilepsy, migration disorders, tuberous sclerosis, neurofibromatosis, corpus callosum agenesis) as well as ophthalmology evaluation and hearing assessment.

Children with ASD and their families need comprehensive, sustained support and psychoeducation about the condition. Treatment goals include fostering social development and learning without overtaxing the child. Education needs to involve structured and predictable routines and schedules, motivation via special interests, help with interpretation of common social rules, feedback and support in case of inappropriate emotional responses, and eventual career counseling with the goals of as much autonomy and quality of life as possible.

There exist a variety of behavioral modification programs. *Early intensive behavioral intervention* (*EIBI)* is based on intensive home coaching of the child and the parents and is currently one of the most studied treatment programs (Dawson and Burner 2011). The program is highly resource-demanding, involving 20 or more weekly hours of intervention over 2 or more years (Vismara and Rogers 2010).

Children with higher functioning may benefit from cognitive-behavioral therapy (Wood et al. 2014) which is indicated in the presence of comorbid OCD or anxiety disorders (Russell et al. 2013; Sukhodolsky et al. 2013). While there is no specific medication for autism, pharmacologic treatment can be helpful for symptoms such as frequent severe rage attacks or extreme rigidity (McPheeters et al. 2011; Sharma and Shaw 2012) and for treatment of comorbid conditions. ADHD is comorbid in approximately 60–85% of children with ASD and may improve with stimulants or atomoxetine (Harfterkamp et al. 2013) albeit with a lower overall response rate (50%) and more frequent side effects, in comparison with children with only ADHD (Mahajan et al. 2012).

Schizophrenia and Other Psychotic Disorders

Vignette 3.7

David was referred for a pediatric evaluation at the age of 15 years because his parents became more and more concerned about a change in his usual behavior. The teacher had informed the parents that he was often absent during the last months of school. At home, the mother noticed that he often went to his room for reading, and he withdrew from family chores. David had always been a bright boy. His teacher described him as being a bit introverted, but he achieved good grades and played keyboard in a band founded by him and some friends. At the time of evaluation, he took seldom the initiative to go out with his friends. Even the playing sessions with the band became less frequent, as he produced excuses as to why he was not able to join. When mother asked for his view about these behavior changes, he mentioned that it was more important for him to read about philosophy and religion and that he could follow up his school lessons even when he was absent. Sometimes he would talk extensively about the deeper meaning behind a picture or something he had read in a book in a way parents did not understand at all. Parents reported one incident where he had attacked his father with a fork during a minor dispute, without being able to explain or apologize for his behavior. On assessment, when asked about unusual auditory or visual experiences, he explained that sometimes he heard annoying voices criticizing him or telling him to perform a certain action.

Heading

The general symptoms of a psychotic condition are confusion, characterized by an inability to distinguish between what is real and what is not and difficulties with the regulation of thoughts, feelings, and behavior. DSM-5 lists the five key symptoms of psychotic disorders: (1) delusions, (2) hallucinations, (3) disorganized speech, (4) disorganized or catatonic behavior, and (5) negative symptoms. To make a diagnosis of schizophrenia, two of these five symptoms, with at least one among the first three in the list, are required. Disorganized behavior implies confused, disordered, and/or illogical thinking and sometimes bizarre behavior. Catatonia includes muscular rigidity, fixed posturing, persistent speechlessness, repetitive behaviors, and insensitivity to pain. Negative symptoms include affective flattening (e.g., decrease in the ability to express emotions), poverty of speech (e.g., brief or empty replies), and inability to initiate and persist in goal-directed activities (e.g., little interest in daily activities, such as personal hygiene, school, or pleasurable activities). The onset of psychosis leads usually to functional impairment, which can sometimes be subtle or gradual.

It can be difficult to discern delusions in children, as their perception of reality depends on developmental stage. Before the age of 4 or 5 years, children may not be able to differentiate between imagination and reality. Even older children might have such confusion in stressful situations or during play, without being psychotic. Psychotic symptoms occur in many conditions such as borderline personality disorder, severe depression, bipolar disorder, or following severe trauma. The most common types of psychoses in children are schizophrenia and bipolar disorder with psychotic features. The latter is classified as a mood disorder , but in young people, bipolar disorder often has its onset with psychotic symptoms. The prevalence of schizophrenia in the general population is about 1%, but the disorder is rarely diagnosed in children or adolescents, as symptoms usually first appear in early adulthood. However, the frequency increases with age, and a premorbid condition characterized by nonspecific psychiatric symptoms, for example, problems in relationships, school performance, social functioning, and motivation, may be present long before onset of the disorder. Early diagnosis is crucial, as early treatment may improve the prognosis.

In rare cases, for example, following extremely difficult life experiences, a child may develop a psychotic condition over a short period of time. "Brief psychotic disorder" is defined in the DSM-5 (APA 2013) as the presence of one or more psychotic symptoms with a sudden onset, absence of a mood or substance-induced disorder, and remission within 1 month. The prognosis for this type of psychosis is better than for the schizophrenia spectrum disorders (Remberk et al. 2014).

First-line healthcare services should be able to recognize symptoms suspicious of psychosis and to refer for specialized healthcare services without delay. A careful history, including family history, is the most important assessment tool, along with questionnaires like the *Positive and Negative Syndrome Scale (PANSS)* (Kay et al. 1987) or the *Brief Psychiatric Rating Scale (BPRS)* (Overall and Pfefferbaum 1982) which may be helpful in unclear cases. Other serious medical conditions such as metabolic disorders, intoxications, tumors, infections, or other central nervous system injuries should be ruled out prior to a diagnosis of primary psychosis.

Treatment involves a combination of psychosocial and pharmacological interventions. Psychoeducation is obligatory, and CBT might be helpful to reduce psychotic symptoms (Browning et al. 2013). Treatment with antipsychotic medication should start early in order to reduce the development of motor, speech, social, and cognitive problems (Kranzler and Cohen 2013). Side effects often include obesity and metabolic syndrome. Therefore, the advantages of medications should be carefully and individually weighed against the potential side effects. While the long-term prognosis of the disorder is variable, a recent meta-analysis of schizophrenia outcome in all ages showed recovery in one in seven (Jaaskelainen et al. 2013).

Substance Use Disorders

Vignette 3.8

Three years later, you see David (from Vignette 3.7) in follow-up. He is doing better on antipsychotic medications and has entered a liberal arts program at a junior college. In response to your usual screening questions, he endorses that he uses marijuana "around two or three times per month," though denies any other substance use, including cigarettes and alcohol. He reports that the few friends that he has made "sometimes use it to calm their nerves," and he wonders if it is okay for him.

CNS-active drug use to alter consciousness is probably as old as mankind itself. In most human cultures (and even in some animal cultures), individuals have developed an amazing ingenuity to discover and to alter natural substances for this purpose. Mainly, this search seems to be motivated by religious or spiritual needs, but other incentives may include a desire to escape reality, to show one's belonging to a subculture, or to experience pleasure. In religious practices, the relation between reality and hallucinations might even be reversed: Indigenous Jivaro people from the Ecuadorian Amazon traditionally believed that the normal waking life is simply an illusion, while the true reality and the forces that determine daily events are supernatural and can only be seen and manipulated with the aid of hallucinogenic drugs (Harner 1973). Differentiation between use and misuse is not always easy and must be done in the context of religious and cultural values, traditions, and beliefs. Misuse involves excessive use leading to substantial harm and an inability to refrain from the drug because of craving, even when the user understands that the use causes damages. A common denominator for substance-related disorders is a compromised reward system: overactivated brain stress systems and compromised orbitofrontal/prefrontal cortex function, leading to intense activation of the brain reward system by drugs that are taken so excessively that normal activities are neglected (Koob 2006).

DSM-5 (APA 2013) distinguishes between substance-induced intoxication, withdrawal, and other disorders induced by substances. In addition, it identifies ten drug classes: alcohol; caffeine; cannabis; hallucinogens; inhalants; opioids; sedatives, hypnotics, and anxiolytics; stimulants (e.g., amphetamine-type substances, cocaine); tobacco; and other or unknown substances. However, substance use disorder does not yet specifically apply to caffeine, as it is not clear whether excessive caffeine use is a clinically significant disorder, and it is included only to encourage further research. The diagnosis of a substance use disorder – which would be important to assess for in the case above – is based upon four criteria related to the use of one or more of the listed substances: (1) impaired control, e.g., spending excessive time on substance use or using larger amounts than intended and being unable to reduce the use because of intense cravings that make it difficult to think about anything else; (2) social impairment including work or school absences, poor school performance, and interpersonal problems leading to loss of contact with family members or important friends; (3) risky use, including use in dangerous situations such as while operating machinery or driving a car; and (4) pharmacological symptoms such as tolerance (need to increase the amount to achieve the same effect) and withdrawal symptoms after abrupt cessation. To make a diagnosis of substance use disorder, at least two of these criteria must be present. The DSM-5 chapter of substance use-related disorders also includes gambling disorder, reflecting the similarities between these disorders in terms of clinical symptoms, involvement of the brain's reward system, comorbidity, and treatment.

Most of the psychiatric disorders discussed in this chapter (with the exception of autism) occur frequently together with substance use disorders, leading to so-called dual diagnosis, which implies a mutual influencing relationship: the psychiatric condition can often lead to substance use problems and conversely, using substances can trigger or worsen a psychiatric condition. Most studies on dual diagnoses are predominantly on adults. One exception is a study from Norway showing that frequent alcohol intoxications in 13–19-year-old youth were associated with anxiety and depressive symptoms among girls and with attention and conduct problems in both genders (Strandheim et al. 2009).

Clinicians should always consider and screen for the possibility of substance use disorder. Screening tools like the easy-to-administer six-item questionnaire *CRAFFT (Knight et al.* 2002*)* might help to nonjudgmentally introduce the topic. Treatment usually needs to broadly address all factors involved and include the family (Stanton and Shadish 1997). During the last decades, empirically supported treatments for adolescent substance use disorders have been developed. Family therapy is the treatment with the strongest evidence for effectiveness, although most types of treatment appear to be beneficial in helping adolescents to reduce their substance use (Tanner-Smith et al. 2013). However, long-term outcome is hampered by the high frequency of relapse, which may be, in part, driven by high rates of comorbidity with other psychiatric disorders (Hulvershorn et al. 2015).

Conclusion

Using illustrative case vignettes, this chapter provides an overview of common child and adolescent psychiatric disorders from the perspective of general pediatric practice. The chapter underlines the role of pediatric psychosomatic medicine as a mediator between psychiatric, medical, and psychosocial disorders and comorbidities that have an impact on healthcare outcomes, not only during childhood and adolescence but also throughout the lifespan.

References

Angold, A., & Costello, E. J. (2009). Nosology and measurement in child and adolescent psychiatry. *Journal of Child Psychology and Psychiatry, and Allied Disciplines, 50*(1–2), 9–15. https://doi.org/10.1111/j.1469-7610.2008.01981.x.

Angold, A., Costello, E. J., Messer, S. C., Pickles, A., Winder, F., & Silver, D. (1995). Development of a short questionnaire for use in epidemiological studies of depression in children and adolescents. *International Journal of Methods in Psychiatric Research, 5*, 237–249.

Angold, A., Costello, E. J., & Erkanli, A. (1999). Comorbidity. *Journal of Child Psychology and Psychiatry, 40*(1), 57–87.

APA. (2013). *Diagnostic and statistical manual of mental disorders (DSM-5)*. Washington, DC: American Psychiatric Association.

Bennett, D. S., Ambrosini, P. J., Bianchi, M., Barnett, D., Metz, C., & Rabinovich, H. (1997). Relationship of Beck depression inventory factors to depression among adolescents. *Journal of Affective Disorders, 45*(3), 127–134.

Birmaher, B., Brent, D., Bernet, W., Bukstein, O., Walter, H., Benson, R. S., et al. (2007). Practice parameter for the assessment and treatment of children and adolescents with depressive disorders. *Journal of the American Academy of Child and Adolescent Psychiatry, 46*(11), 1503–1526.

Browning, S., Corrigall, R., Garety, P., Emsley, R., & Jolley, S. (2013). Psychological interventions for adolescent psychosis: A pilot controlled trial in routine care. *European Psychiatry, 28*(7), 423–426. https://doi.org/10.1016/j.eurpsy.2013.05.008.

Brunstein-Klomek, A., Zalsman, G., & Mufson, L. (2007). Interpersonal psychotherapy for depressed adolescents (IPT-A). *Israel Journal of Psychiatry and Related Sciences, 44*(1), 40–46.

Dawson, G., & Burner, K. (2011). Behavioral interventions in children and adolescents with autism spectrum disorder: A review of recent findings. *Current Opinion in Pediatrics, 23*(6), 616–620. https://doi.org/10.1097/MOP.0b013e32834cf082.

DuPaul, G. J., Reid, R., Anastopoulos, A. D., Lambert, M. C., Watkins, M. W., & Power, T. J. (2016). Parent and teacher ratings of attention-deficit/hyperactivity disorder symptoms: Factor structure and normative data. *Psychological Assessment, 28*(2), 214–225. https://doi.org/10.1037/pas0000166.

Egger, H. L., Costello, E. J., & Angold, A. (2003). School refusal and psychiatric disorders: A community study. *Journal of the American Academy of Child and Adolescent Psychiatry, 42*(7), 797–807.

Ehlers, S., Gillberg, C., & Wing, L. (1999). A screening questionnaire for Asperger syndrome and other high-functioning autism spectrum disorders in school age children. *Journal of Autism and Developmental Disorders, 29*(2), 129–141.

Essau, C. A. (2008). Comorbidity of depressive disorders among adolescents in community and clinical settings. *Psychiatry Research, 158*(1), 35–42. https://doi.org/10.1016/j.psychres.2007.09.007.

Eyberg, S. M., & Ross, A. W. (1978). Assessment of child behavior problems: The validation of a new inventory. *Journal of Clinical Child Psychology, 7*(2), 113–116.

Fergusson, D. M., Horwood, L. J., Ridder, E. M., & Beautrais, A. L. (2005). Subthreshold depression in adolescence and mental health outcomes in adulthood. *Archives of General Psychiatry, 62*(1), 66–72. https://doi.org/10.1001/archpsyc.62.1.66.

Frank, M., & Cavanna, A. E. (2013). Behavioural treatments for Tourette syndrome: An evidence-based review. *Behavioural Neurology, 27*(1), 105–117. https://doi.org/10.3233/ben-120309.

Goodyer, I. M., Tamplin, A., Herbert, J., & Altham, P. M. (2000). Recent life events, cortisol, dehydroepiandrosterone and the onset of major depression in high-risk adolescents. *The British Journal of Psychiatry, 177*(6), 499–504.

Harfterkamp, M., Buitelaar, J. K., Minderaa, R. B., van de Loo-Neus, G., van der Gaag, R. J., & Hoekstra, P. J. (2013). Long-term treatment with atomoxetine for attention-deficit/hyperactivity disorder symptoms in children and adolescents with autism spectrum disorder: An

open-label extension study. *Journal of Child and Adolescent Psychopharmacology, 23*(3), 194–199. https://doi.org/10.1089/cap.2012.0012.
Harner, M. J. (1973). The sound of rushing water. In M. J. Harner (Ed.), *Hallucinogens and shamanism* (pp. 15–27). New York: Oxford University Press.
Henggeler, S. W. (2011). Efficacy studies to large-scale transport: The development and validation of multisystemic therapy programs. *Annual Review of Clinical Psychology, 7*, 351–381. https://doi.org/10.1146/annurev-clinpsy-032210-104615.
Hulvershorn, L. A., Quinn, P. D., & Scott, E. L. (2015). Treatment of adolescent substance use disorders and co-occurring internalizing disorders: A critical review and proposed model. *Current Drug Abuse Reviews, 8*(1), 41–49.
Jaaskelainen, E., Juola, P., Hirvonen, N., McGrath, J. J., Saha, S., Isohanni, M., & Miettunen, J. (2013). A systematic review and meta-analysis of recovery in schizophrenia. *Schizophrenia Bulletin, 39*(6), 1296–1306. https://doi.org/10.1093/schbul/sbs130.
Kay, S. R., Fiszbein, A., & Opler, L. A. (1987). The positive and negative syndrome scale (PANSS) for schizophrenia. *Schizophrenia Bulletin, 13*(2), 261–276.
Kendell, R., & Jablensky, A. (2003). Distinguishing between the validity and utility of psychiatric diagnoses. *The American Journal of Psychiatry, 160*(1), 4–12.
Khalifa, N., & von Knorring, A. L. (2006). Psychopathology in a Swedish population of school children with tic disorders. *Journal of the American Academy of Child and Adolescent Psychiatry, 45*(11), 1346–1353. https://doi.org/10.1097/01.chi.0000251210.98749.83.
Kimonis, E. R., Frick, P. J., Skeem, J. L., Marsee, M. A., Cruise, K., Munoz, L. C., & Morris, A. S. (2008). Assessing callous-unemotional traits in adolescent offenders: Validation of the inventory of callous-unemotional traits. *International Journal of Law and Psychiatry, 31*(3), 241–252. https://doi.org/10.1016/j.ijlp.2008.04.002.
Kleinman, J. M., Robins, D. L., Ventola, P. E., Pandey, J., Boorstein, H. C., Esser, E. L., et al. (2008). The modified checklist for autism in toddlers: A follow-up study investigating the early detection of autism spectrum disorders. *Journal of Autism and Developmental Disorders, 38*(5), 827–839. https://doi.org/10.1007/s10803-007-0450-9.
Knight, J. R., Sherritt, L., Shrier, L. A., Harris, S. K., & Chang, G. (2002). Validity of the CRAFFT substance abuse screening test among adolescent clinic patients. *Archives of Pediatrics and Adolescent Medicine, 156*(6), 607–614.
Koob, G. F. (2006). The neurobiology of addiction: A neuroadaptational view relevant for diagnosis. *Addiction, 101*(Suppl 1), 23–30. https://doi.org/10.1111/j.1360-0443.2006.01586.x.
Kranzler, H. N., & Cohen, S. D. (2013). Psychopharmacologic treatment of psychosis in children and adolescents: Efficacy and management. *Child and Adolescent Psychiatric Clinics of North America, 22*(4), 727–744. https://doi.org/10.1016/j.chc.2013.06.002.
Leckman, J. F., Riddle, M. A., Hardin, M. T., Ort, S. I., Swartz, K. L., Stevenson, J., & Cohen, D. J. (1989). The Yale global tic severity scale: Initial testing of a clinician-rated scale of tic severity. *Journal of the American Academy of Child and Adolescent Psychiatry, 28*(4), 566–573. https://doi.org/10.1097/00004583-198907000-00015.
Lord, C., Rutter, M., Goode, S., Heemsbergen, J., Jordan, H., Mawhood, L., & Schopler, E. (1989). Autism diagnostic observation schedule: A standardized observation of communicative and social behavior. *Journal of Autism and Developmental Disorders, 19*(2), 185–212.
Lord, C., Rutter, M., & Le Couteur, A. (1994). Autism diagnostic interview-revised: A revised version of a diagnostic interview for caregivers of individuals with possible pervasive developmental disorders. *Journal of Autism and Developmental Disorders, 24*(5), 659–685.
Mahajan, R., Bernal, M. P., Panzer, R., Whitaker, A., Roberts, W., Handen, B., & Veenstra-VanderWeele, J. (2012). Clinical practice pathways for evaluation and medication choice for attention-deficit/hyperactivity disorder symptoms in autism spectrum disorders. *Pediatrics, 130*(Suppl 2), S125–S138. https://doi.org/10.1542/peds.2012-0900J.
McClellan, J., Kowatch, R., & Findling, R. L. (2007). Practice parameter for the assessment and treatment of children and adolescents with bipolar disorder. *Journal of the American Academy of Child and Adolescent Psychiatry, 46*(1), 107–125.

McPheeters, M. L., Warren, Z., Sathe, N., Bruzek, J. L., Krishnaswami, S., Jerome, R. N., & Veenstra-Vanderweele, J. (2011). A systematic review of medical treatments for children with autism spectrum disorders. *Pediatrics, 127*(5), e1312–e1321. https://doi.org/10.1542/peds.2011-0427.

Muris, P., Dreessen, L., Bogels, S., Weckx, M., & van Melick, M. (2004). A questionnaire for screening a broad range of DSM-defined anxiety disorder symptoms in clinically referred children and adolescents. *Journal of Child Psychology and Psychiatry, and Allied Disciplines, 45*(4), 813–820. https://doi.org/10.1111/j.1469-7610.2004.00274.x.

NICE. (2005). *Depression in children and young people: Identification and management (Last update 2015)*. Retrieved from London https://www.nice.org.uk/guidance/cg28

NICE. (2013). *Antisocial behaviour and conduct disorders in children and young people: Recognition, intervention and management*. Retrieved from http://www.guideline.gov/content.aspx?id=44087

Ost, L. G. (1989). One-session treatment for specific phobias. *Behaviour Research and Therapy, 27*(1), 1–7.

Overall, J. E., & Pfefferbaum, B. (1982). The brief psychiatric rating scale for children. *Psychopharmacology Bulletin, 18*(2), 10–16.

Patterson, G. R., & Stouthamer-Loeber, M. (1984). The correlation of family management practices and delinquency. *Child Development, 55*(4), 1299–1307.

Patton, G. C., Coffey, C., Romaniuk, H., Mackinnon, A., Carlin, J. B., Degenhardt, L.,. .. Moran, P. (2014). The prognosis of common mental disorders in adolescents: A 14-year prospective cohort study. Lancet, 383(9926), 1404–1411. doi:https://doi.org/10.1016/s0140-6736(13)62116-9.

Pickles, A., & Angold, A. (2003). Natural categories or fundamental dimensions: On carving nature at the joints and the rearticulation of psychopathology. *Development and Psychopathology, 15*(3), 529–551.

Polanczyk, G. V., Willcutt, E. G., Salum, G. A., Kieling, C., & Rohde, L. A. (2014). ADHD prevalence estimates across three decades: An updated systematic review and meta-regression analysis. *International Journal of Epidemiology, 43*(2), 434–442. https://doi.org/10.1093/ije/dyt261.

Rachman, S., Hodgson, R., & Marks, I. M. (1971). The treatment of chronic obsessive-compulsive neurosis. *Behaviour Research and Therapy, 9*(3), 237–247.

Remberk, B., Bazynska, A. K., Krempa-Kowalewska, A., & Rybakowski, F. (2014). Adolescent insanity revisited: Course and outcome in early-onset schizophrenia spectrum psychoses in an 8-year follow-up study. *Comprehensive Psychiatry, 55*(5), 1174–1181. https://doi.org/10.1016/j.comppsych.2014.03.013.

Robertson, M. M. (2000). Tourette syndrome, associated conditions and the complexities of treatment. *Brain, 123*(Pt 3), 425–462.

Robertson, M. M. (2008). The prevalence and epidemiology of Gilles de la Tourette syndrome. Part 2: Tentative explanations for differing prevalence figures in GTS, including the possible effects of psychopathology, aetiology, cultural differences, and differing phenotypes. *Journal of Psychosomatic Research, 65*(5), 473–486.

Russell, A. J., Jassi, A., Fullana, M. A., Mack, H., Johnston, K., Heyman, I.,. .. Mataix-Cols, D. (2013). Cognitive behavior therapy for comorbid obsessive-compulsive disorder in high-functioning autism spectrum disorders: A randomized controlled trial. Depression and Anxiety, 30(8), 697–708. doi:https://doi.org/10.1002/da.22053.

Sharma, A., & Shaw, S. R. (2012). Efficacy of risperidone in managing maladaptive behaviors for children with autistic spectrum disorder: A meta-analysis. *Journal of Pediatric Health Care, 26*(4), 291–299. https://doi.org/10.1016/j.pedhc.2011.02.008.

Stanton, M. D., & Shadish, W. R. (1997). Outcome, attrition, and family-couples treatment for drug abuse: A meta-analysis and review of the controlled, comparative studies. *Psychological Bulletin, 122*(2), 170–191.

Stewart, S. E., Geller, D. A., Jenike, M., Pauls, D., Shaw, D., Mullin, B., & Faraone, S. V. (2004). Long-term outcome of pediatric obsessive-compulsive disorder: A meta-analysis and qualitative review of the literature. *Acta Psychiatrica Scandinavica, 110*(1), 4–13. https://doi.org/10.1111/j.1600-0447.2004.00302.x.

Strandheim, A., Holmen, T. L., Coombes, L., & Bentzen, N. (2009). Alcohol intoxication and mental health among adolescents--a population review of 8983 young people, 13-19 years in North-Trondelag, Norway: The Young-HUNT Study. *Child Adolesc Psychiatry Ment Health, 3*(1), 18. https://doi.org/10.1186/1753-2000-3-18.

Sukhodolsky, D. G., Bloch, M. H., Panza, K. E., & Reichow, B. (2013). Cognitive-behavioral therapy for anxiety in children with high-functioning autism: A meta-analysis. *Pediatrics, 132*(5), e1341–e1350. https://doi.org/10.1542/peds.2013-1193.

Tanner-Smith, E. E., Wilson, S. J., & Lipsey, M. W. (2013). The comparative effectiveness of outpatient treatment for adolescent substance abuse: A meta-analysis. *Journal of Substance Abuse Treatment, 44*(2), 145–158. https://doi.org/10.1016/j.jsat.2012.05.006.

Torp, N. C., Dahl, K., Skarphedinsson, G., Thomsen, P. H., Valderhaug, R., Weidle, B.,. .. Ivarsson, T. (2014). Effectiveness of cognitive behavior treatment for pediatric obsessive-compulsive disorder: Acute outcomes from the Nordic Long-term OCD Treatment Study (NordLOTS). Behaviour Research and Therapy, 64, 15–23. doi:https://doi.org/10.1016/j.brat.2014.11.005.

Verdellen, C., van de Griendt, J., Hartmann, A., & Murphy, T. (2011). European clinical guidelines for Tourette syndrome and other tic disorders. Part III: Behavioural and psychosocial interventions. *European Child & Adolescent Psychiatry, 20*(4), 197–207. https://doi.org/10.1007/s00787-011-0167-3.

Vismara, L. A., & Rogers, S. J. (2010). Behavioral treatments in autism spectrum disorder: What do we know? *Annual Review of Clinical Psychology, 6*, 447–468. https://doi.org/10.1146/annurev.clinpsy.121208.131151.

Webb, C. A., Auerbach, R. P., & Derubeis, R. J. (2012). Processes of change in CBT of adolescent depression: Review and recommendations. *Journal of clinical child and adolescent psychology: The official journal for the Society of Clinical Child and Adolescent Psychology, American Psychological Association, Division, 41*(5), 654–665. https://doi.org/10.1080/15374416.2012.704842.

Webster-Stratton, C., Jamila Reid, M., & Stoolmiller, M. (2008). Preventing conduct problems and improving school readiness: Evaluation of the incredible years teacher and child training programs in high-risk schools. *Journal of Child Psychology and Psychiatry, and Allied Disciplines, 49*(5), 471–488. https://doi.org/10.1111/j.1469-7610.2007.01861.x.

Weersing, V. R., & Brent, D. A. (2006). Cognitive behavioral therapy for depression in youth. *Child and Adolescent Psychiatric Clinics of North America, 15*(4), 939–957. ix.

WHO. (1996). *Multiaxial classification of child and adolescent psychiatric disorders. The ICD-10 classification of mental and behavioural disorders in children and adolescents*. Cambridge: Cambridge University Press.

Williams, J., Allison, C., Scott, F., Stott, C., Bolton, P., Baron-Cohen, S., & Brayne, C. (2006). The childhood Asperger syndrome test (CAST): Test-retest reliability. *Autism: The International Journal of Research and Practice, 10*(4), 415–427. https://doi.org/10.1177/1362361306066612.

WONCA. (1972). World Organization of National Colleges, Academies and Academic Associations of General Practitioners/Family Physicians. http://www.globalfamilydoctor.com/

Wood, J. J., Fujii, C., Renno, P., & Van Dyke, M. (2014). Impact of cognitive behavioral therapy on observed autism symptom severity during school recess: A preliminary randomized, controlled trial. *Journal of Autism and Developmental Disorders*. https://doi.org/10.1007/s10803-014-2097-7.

Wright, A., Rickards, H., & Cavanna, A. E. (2012). Impulse-control disorders in gilles de la tourette syndrome. *The Journal of Neuropsychiatry and Clinical Neurosciences, 24*(1), 16–27. https://doi.org/10.1176/appi.neuropsych.10010013.

Chapter 4
Psychopharmacological Principles

Susan Solimine and Anthony P. S. Guerrero

General Principles

It is important to understand that the use of psychopharmacology in the pediatric population is not necessarily the same as in adults. Child and adolescent psychiatrists will often say that children are "not just small adults," and therefore the treatment choices and dosages may be similar or different to those used in adults. Additionally, we must acknowledge that data on the usage of psychotropic medications in children is limited, and many commonly used agents are not necessarily approved by national regulatory organizations for use in this population. Providers may, at times, use psychotropic medications "off-label" to target specific treatment needs of the patient while maintaining the standard of care.

This chapter will review the complexity of psychopharmacology in youth with medical or other conditions. Additionally, it is important to consider when it may or may not be appropriate to begin psychotropic medications in youth. This chapter will focus on high-yield topics of mood, anxiety, and delirium which can be experienced in medically ill pediatric patients.

S. Solimine (✉)
Department of Psychiatry, Tripler Army Medical Center, CAFBHS, Honolulu, HI, USA
e-mail: Susan.Solimine.Civ@mail.mil

A. P. S. Guerrero
Department of Psychiatry, University of Hawai'i John A. Burns School of Medicine, Honolulu, HI, USA
e-mail: GuerreroA@dop.hawaii.edu

A. P. S. Guerrero et al. (eds.), *Pediatric Consultation-Liaison Psychiatry*,
https://doi.org/10.1007/978-3-319-89488-1_4

Case Vignette 4.1: Depression and Drug-Drug Interactions

Joshua is a 13-year-old male who was diagnosed with leukemia 18 months ago. He has had multiple inpatient medical hospitalizations for multiple infections as well as multiple hospital days spent receiving chemotherapy. Joshua is currently admitted to the medical floor because of severe gastrointestinal side effects from one of his medications. He was overheard mumbling to himself, and when the nurse asked him what was wrong, he stated, "I am done with this, I give up, I am tired of it all." Joshua discusses his frustration with the frequent blood draws and other procedures he has undergone, as well as the multitude of different medications with which he has been treated, ultimately resulting in adverse effects. He also mentions believing that he is a burden on his family. He is no longer able to enjoy any pleasurable activities, including time with family. He has a very poor appetite, isn't sleeping well, and describes his mood as "miserable." Joshua has been in therapy throughout his treatment because he was developing anxiety related to procedures and fear of having to be hospitalized for an infection. The medical team has now consulted the psychiatry team to further assist with the treatment of this patient.

As the consultant, you find that Joshua has been experiencing severe nausea and vomiting resulting in dehydration, and he is now receiving intravenous fluids. A review of his records also shows a significant amount of weight loss over the past 18 months. His cancer treatments have indeed been complicated by the adverse effects of multiple medications. In addition to his persistent anxiety, Joshua is now experiencing depressive symptoms.

When considering psychotropic options, one must be mindful of possible drug-drug interactions (DDIs), especially when antineoplastic (AN) agents are already being prescribed. The reader is referred to readings on psychopharmacology in the general child and adolescent population and to readily available (and often updated) references on DDIs. Particularly for the consultation-liaison patient population, it is important to recall that pharmacokinetic interactions mainly occur through cytochrome P450 isoenzymes, while pharmacodynamic interactions can result in alterations to therapeutic index which can be additive, synergistic, or antagonistic (Oliveira and Santos 2015).

Antidepressants can be used to target mood symptoms associated with cancer illness. They can also help those whom have experienced pain, gastrointestinal distress, wasting/cachexia, fatigue, and cognitive impairment associated with cancer. Among the antidepressants used in cancer patients, sertraline is most often described in the literature (Pao et al. 2006; Oliveira and Santos 2015). However, other literature advises caution when using selective serotonin reuptake inhibitors (SSRIs) such as sertraline, fluoxetine, paroxetine, and fluvoxamine due to the possibility of pharmacokinetic DDIs particularly associated with the cytochrome P450 isoenzymes (Oliveira and Santos 2015). For example, fluvoxamine is a strong CYP3A4 inhibitor with many DDIs. The use of escitalopram, citalopram, venlafaxine, and mirtazapine appears to be safer in cancer patients due to their minimal potential for impact on the CYP P450 system (Oliveira and Santos 2015).

The psychiatric symptoms most commonly reported by oncology patients include depressive symptoms (not necessarily meeting criteria for a full major depressive episode), anxiety, and insomnia. In these cases, mirtazapine, due to its antihistaminic activity at lower doses, has shown to be useful in targeting symptoms of sleep disturbance and anorexia (Oliveira and Santos 2015).

Tricyclic antidepressants (TCAs) are used much less often in the general pediatric population due to risks in overdose, higher side effect profile, and more drug-drug interactions. However, in the cancer population, they have been used to target insomnia and pain associated with pediatric cancers (Pao et al. 2006).

Mood stabilizers have also been used in pediatric cancer patients, particularly in those who experience seizures, pain, and peripheral neuropathy. The more commonly used mood stabilizers, such as valproic acid and carbamazepine, are less clinically useful in medically ill patients due to their delayed onset of action and potential for DDIs and hepatic, hematologic, and metabolic toxicities (Pao et al. 2006). Gabapentin, however, has been used in pediatric cancer to target peripheral neuropathy and pain and has been well tolerated in those with epilepsy (Pao et al. 2006).

Psychostimulants may also have a role in the treatment of symptoms in pediatric cancer patients. They can target the fatigue and poor concentration associated with some chemotherapy agents. They can also help to counter opiate-induced sedation (Pao et al. 2006).

The use of psychopharmacology in patients undergoing cancer treatments has been shown to have a positive impact on quality of life, particularly in those with depressive symptoms.

Take-Home Points from Vignette 4.1

- The use of antidepressants to treat cancer-associated depression and anxiety has been shown to improve quality of life.
- Although sertraline may be a commonly prescribed antidepressant, escitalopram, citalopram, venlafaxine, and mirtazapine have been shown to be safe and effective with the least DDIs.
- Gabapentin may help with mood stabilization as well as other cancer-related symptoms, such as peripheral neuropathy and pain.
- While TCAs have been used in the pediatric population to target pain and depression, significant caution must be exercised in the CL population because of these medications' greater side effect profiles, potential DDIs, and risk of death in overdose.

Case Vignette 4.2: Anxiety and Medication Side Effects

Emily is an 8-year-old girl who suffered from respiratory syncytial virus as an infant and now has severe asthma. She has had multiple inpatient medical hospitalizations due to asthma exacerbations that have required intubation. She has since developed some panic and depressive symptoms and is now endorsing symptoms of post-traumatic stress disorder from her frequent hospitalizations and has fear of being intubated again.

Psychiatric disorders are common in patients with pulmonary disease, particularly anxiety and depression. Asthma is reported to affect 5–7% of the US population, and up to 33% of these children and adolescents also meet criteria for an anxiety disorder (Levenson 2007).

Medications that are often used to treat respiratory diseases such as asthma can precipitate or exacerbate symptoms of anxiety. For example, theophylline and beta-adrenergic bronchodilators can result in anxiety, tremor, and tachycardia. There are also nonprescription asthma preparations that contain sympathomimetics, which can also cause symptoms of anxiety (Levenson 2007).

Overall, the SSRIs (except fluvoxamine) have been reported to be well tolerated in those with pulmonary disease.

The antituberculosis medication rifampin is a powerful CYP3A4 inducer with the potential for significant interactions with some antidepressants. The combined use of rifampin with TCAs, bupropion, or trazodone may lead to lower antidepressant blood levels. This would possibly result in the need to titrate antidepressant dosages while on rifampin to maintain adequate control of depression and anxiety symptoms (Levenson 2007).

For those patients with pulmonary disease who are also treated with lithium, theophylline can lower lithium levels.

Beta-blockers are sometimes prescribed for anxiety disorders, but they should be avoided in patients with reactive airway diseases because of the risk for bronchoconstriction.

Take-Home Points for Case Vignette 4.2

- Medications commonly prescribed to treat pulmonary diseases can result in anxiety symptoms; anxiety is commonly diagnosed in patients with pulmonary disease.
- Theophylline is often prescribed to treat pulmonary diseases but has multiple DDIs (e.g., with fluvoxamine, a significant CYP 1A2 inhibitor), so checking for interactions is important.
- Exercise caution in the use of beta-blockers in patients with reactive airway disease and anxiety.
- Most SSRIs are well tolerated in those with pulmonary diseases.

Case Vignette 4.3: Delirium and Antipsychotic Medications

Jason is a 14-year-old male who was recently seen by his pediatrician for flu-like symptoms. He was diagnosed with a viral illness and sent home. Overnight, Jason developed a very high fever and was noted to have changes in his mental status. Jason is usually calm, but he has been more irritable, and he seems to stare into space when others are speaking to him. His father brought him to the emergency room for an evaluation as he was concerned that there may be a more serious problem.

Although delirium's core features of disturbances in attention and cognition are seen throughout the lifespan, its presentation may differ in the pediatric population due to developmental factors. Children may present with abrupt developmental regression or loss of previously acquired skills. Examples include an acute decrease in eye contact, or parents suddenly being unable to console their child. Other prominent symptoms may include irritability, affective lability, agitation, sleep-wake disturbances, and fluctuations in alertness (Thom 2017).

The first step in treatment is to perform a thorough assessment to identify the underlying cause of delirium. Common causes include infection, medication-related factors, and autoimmune-related factors (Thom 2017). Chapter 8, "Acute Mental Status Change," provides additional information on pediatric delirium.

The use of benzodiazepines, opioids, and anticholinergic agents in medically ill patients can result in a delirium. Tapering or immediately discontinuing agents that may be contributing to the presentation is recommended whenever possible. Pharmacologic intervention is generally recommended when the symptoms impose a safety concern, if they impede advancement of medical care, if they are bothersome to the patient, or if the contributing agent (s) must be continued for the appropriate management of a co-occurring medical condition.

In general, the atypical antipsychotics are preferred over the typical antipsychotics for children and adolescents due to their lower side effect profile and tolerability.

In a retrospective study of children ages 1–18 who were diagnosed with delirium, olanzapine and risperidone were shown to be safe and effective in decreasing symptoms (Turkel et al. 2012; Thom 2017).

In a separate retrospective study, 23% of children who received intravenous haloperidol experienced adverse reactions including dystonia and hyperpyrexia (Thom 2017). Lowering the dosage or tapering with discontinuation often resulted in resolution of side effects. However, both typical and atypical antipsychotics are commonly used to treat pediatric delirium. The following table presents the usual dose ranges and important considerations when prescribing antipsychotics for the treatment of delirium.

Antipsychotic medications in pediatric CL psychiatry

Medication name	Initial dosing	Maximum dosing	Miscellaneous
Olanzapine	5–10 mg at bedtime	20 mg/day	Lower dose and titration
			Associated with lower risk of developing side effects
Risperidone	0.25–0.5 mg at bedtime	6 mg/day	Titration of dosage every 3–7 days; may initiate dosing at 0.5–1 mg/day
			For youth >16 years old
Quetiapine	25 mg BID	800 mg/day[a]	Slower titration leads to less side effects, especially in terms of sedation
Ziprasidone	20 mg BID	40–160 mg/day[a]	A detailed cardiac history is recommended due to risk of QTc prolongation; recommend baseline and follow-up ECG; must be taken with food
Aripiprazole	Weight based	30 mg/day	<25kg, start 1mg/day and for >25kg, start 2mg/day.
Haloperidol (13)	(For delirium) Oral: 0.01–0.1 mg/kg q12 h	Should not exceed 0.15 mg/kg/day	Need to monitor for extrapyramidal symptoms (rigidity, tremor, other involuntary movements, etc.), especially for children
	IV: 0.005–0.07 mg/kg every 30 min; once stable, use ½ of needed dose divided q12 h		Consider baseline and follow-up electrocardiogram to evaluate QTc interval

[a]divided dosing

Take-Home Points for Vignette 4.3

- Delirium may present somewhat differently in children than in adults.
- Treatment recommendations begin with finding and addressing the underlying cause, including stopping any agents that may be contributing to the presentation if possible.
- Haloperidol is still widely used in treatment, likely due to its effectiveness and availability in oral, intramuscular, and intravenous forms, despite its potential side effects.
- The atypical antipsychotics have been shown to be effective in treating pediatric delirium and are associated with a lower side effect profile.

General Considerations

The child and adolescent psychiatry practice parameters recommend the following standards of care whenever considering the use of psychotropic medications. Prior to pharmacotherapy initiation:

1. Perform a complete psychiatric evaluation.

2. Perform a complete medical history.
3. Ensure that a comprehensive medical examination and any indicated diagnostic studies have been completed and any identified medical conditions potentially contributing to the problem addressed.
4. Obtain collateral information from parents, school, or any others that will be involved in the youth's care.

The next recommendations are regarding the actual treatment plan:

1. The consultant will collaborate with the family and members of the treatment team to develop a psychopharmacologic and psychosocial approach to treatment "based on the best available evidence."
2. The consultant will set clear recommendations to monitor the patient's response to current methods of treatment.

Both the patient and legal guardians should be actively involved in the informed assent and consent process throughout the course of assessment and treatment. The discussion should include the potential risks, benefits, and alternatives to the recommended treatment. All questions should be answered by the provider prior to initiation of treatment including the anticipated duration and expectations of treatment. It is important to also address the possibility of treatment failure and what steps could be taken if this were to occur. This process should be documented in the patient medical record prior to the initiation of psychopharmacologic medications.

Especially in pediatric CL settings, it is of utmost importance for psychiatrists to refer to reasonably updated references in general pediatric psychopharmacology (Vitiello 2012) and to engage in other aspects of solid psychopharmacological practice, which includes clearly defining and monitoring target symptoms (and utilizing collateral information where appropriate); determining and considering the patient and family members' previous responses to medications; "starting low and going slow" in initiating and titrating the medication; continuing to raise the dose until one has either satisfactorily treated all symptoms, reached the recommended upper dose limit of the medication, encountered side effects that make further titration intolerable, or reached a plateau in improvement or worsening of symptoms with an increase in dose; following recommended guidelines in monitoring vital signs, other physical parameters, and laboratory values; and recognizing medically ill patients' potential sensitivity to medication side effects (Vitiello 2012), especially in the context of situations – including renal or hepatic insufficiency – that could affect drug metabolism and that require consultation with official prescribing guidelines and up-to-date references. Also, the consultant should make sure to consider the possibility of current or future pregnancy and lactation in adolescent females.

Often, medications must be given for urgent situations, and it is especially important to follow the latest evidence, to utilize protocols where available, and to consider locally available options. Chapter 5 in this textbook provides up-to-date recommendations on psychopharmacological management of aggression.

In keeping up to date on approved medications, we recommend consultations with the websites of relevant agencies (e.g., the US Food and Drug Administration at https://www.fda.gov/default.htm). At the time of this writing, there are also internet references (Guerrero and Matsu 2007) that summarize lists of psychotropic medications used in children and the status of FDA approval.

Furthermore, and as illustrated in the above vignettes, because of the likelihood that patients in pediatric consultation-liaison settings will have medical comorbidities and may be on other medications, it is especially important to consult with updated references on DDIs (http://www.ohiomindsmatter.org/documents/Psychotropic%20Medication%20List.pdf, n.d.). Chapter 9, on other medical presentations and considerations in pediatric consultation-liaison psychiatry, provides examples of medication side effects severe enough to warrant pediatric hospitalization.

In summary, the authors recommend the following "rules" for pediatric psychopharmacology, especially in consultation-liaison settings (Vitiello 2012):

1. Very carefully consider evidence for safety and efficacy in children and adolescents, specifically.
2. (Generally) the fewer the medications, the better.
3. Although official approval is not necessarily everything, pay attention to the various categories of medications:

    (A) Approved for treating children/adolescents with the condition for which the medication is being used (e.g., stimulants for attention-deficit hyperactivity disorder, fluoxetine for major depressive disorder)
    (B) Approved for treating adults with the condition but also approved for treating children/adolescents with a different condition (e.g., sertraline for major depression rather than obsessive-compulsive disorder)
    (C) Approved for treating adults with the condition and with some evidence for safety/efficacy for children/adolescents with the condition (e.g., certain atypical antipsychotics for pediatric psychotic disorders)
    (D) Not approved either for the condition being treated or for children/adolescents for any indication

4. When multiple conditions amenable to psychopharmacological treatment are possibly present and there is a need to be conservative in medication choices, consider a rough (and potentially modifiable, depending on new evidence) hierarchy of evidence for safety and efficacy:

$$\text{Stimulants} > \text{serotonin-selective reuptake inhibitors} > \text{antipsychotics} > \text{mood stabilizers}$$

5. Finally, it is important to realize that good psychopharmacology depends upon various other components, illustrated in the form of a pyramid in the figure below. Many of this textbook's chapters will emphasize that, particularly in pediatric settings, where a complex network of people surrounds the patient, teamwork with the patient, the family, and the healthcare providers is foundational in optimizing the assessment and overall care. Chapter 3, covering essential aspects

of child and adolescent psychiatric disorders, provides a basis for accurate diagnosis, while Chap. 10, covering formulation, insures that all biopsychosocial factors are considered in treatment, whether inclusive of medications or otherwise. Indeed, good psychopharmacology "is more than just medications" particularly in pediatric CL psychiatry.

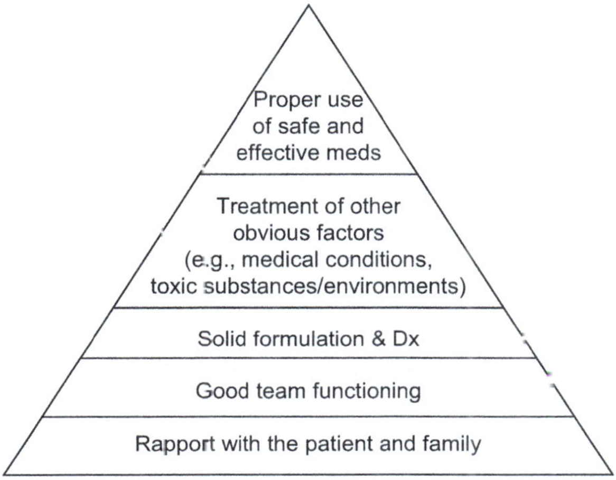

References

Guerrero, A. P. S., & Matsu, C. R. (2007). Chapter 24: Children and adolescents. In H. Leigh & J. Streltzer (Eds.), *Handbook of consultation-liaison psychiatry* (pp. 316–340). New York: Springer.

Indiana University School of Medicine Department of Medicine Clinical Pharmacology. *P450 Interaction Table*. http://medicine.iupui.edu/clinpharm/ddis/main-table. Accessed 1 Jan 2018.

Levenson, J. L. (2007). Psychiatric issues in pulmonary disease. *Primary Psychiatry, 14*(3), 25–28.

Minds Matter Ohio Psychotropic Medical Quality Improvement Collaborative. *Psychotropic medication list*. http://www.ohiomindsmatter.org/documents/Psychotropic%20Medication%20List.pdf. Accessed 1 Jan 2018.

Oliveira, L., & Santos, Z. (2015). Uses of psychotropics and drug-drug interactions in oncology: Reflections from a study in a Portuguese psycho-oncology unit. *Advances in Pharmacoepidemiology and Drug Safety, 4*(5), 194.

Pao, M., et al. (2006). Psychotropic medication use in pediatric patients with cancer. *Archives of Pediatrics & Adolescent Medicine, 160*(August), 818–824.

Thom, R. P. (2017). Pediatric delirium. *American Journal of Psychiatry, Residents Journal, 12*(2), 6–8.

Turkel, S. B., Jacobson, J., Munzig, E., et al. (2012). Atypical antipsychotic medications to control symptoms of delirium in children and adolescents. *Journal of Child and Adolescent Psychopharmacology, 22*(2), 126–130.

Vitiello B. (2012). Principles in using psychotropic medication in children and adolescents. In J. M. Rey (Ed.), *IACAPAP e-textbook of child and adolescent mental health*. Geneva: International Association for Child and Adolescent Psychiatry and Allied Professions http://iacapap.org/iacapap-textbook-of-child-and-adolescent-mental-health. Accessed 1 Jan 2018.

Further Readings

Birmaher, B., & Brent, D. (2007). Practice parameter for the assessment and treatment of children and adolescents with depressive disorders. *Journal of the American Academy of Child & Adolescent Psychiatry, 46*(11, , November), 1503–1526.

Bursch, B., & Forgey, M. (2013). Psychopharmacology for medically ill adolescents. *Current Psychiatry Reports, 15*, 395.

Chadwick, B., et al. (2005). Potentially hazardous drug interactions with psychotropics. *Advances in Psychiatric Treatment, 11*, 440–449.

Connolly, S. D., & Bernstein, G. A. (2007). Practice parameter for the assessment and treatment of child and adolescents with anxiety disorders. *Journal of the American Academy of Child & Adolescent Psychiatry, 46*(2, February), 267–283.

Connor, D. F., & Meltzer, B. M. (2006). *Pediatric psychopharmacology: Fast facts*. New York: W. W. Norton.

Findling, R. L., Drury, S. S., Jensen, P. S., & Rapoport, J. (2011). *Practice parameter for the use of atypical antipsychotic medications in children and adolescents*. Not yet published in *Journal of the American Academy of Child & Adolescent Psychiatry*, updated in 2011.

Lavid, N., & Budner, L. J. (2000). Review of the pharmacological treatment of delirium in the pediatric population with accompanying protocol. *Jefferson Journal of Psychiatry, 15*, 25–33.14.

Schieveld, J. N., et al. (2007). Pediatric delirium in critical illness: Phenomenology, clinical correlates and treatment response in 40 cases in the pediatric intensive care unit. *Intensive Care Medicine, 33*(6), 1033–1040.

Walkup, J. (2009, September). Practice parameter on the use of psychotropic medication in children and adolescents. *Journal of the American Academy of Child & Adolescent Psychiatry, 48*(9), 961.

Part II
Common Scenarios and Concerns in Traditional Inpatient Pediatric Consultation-Liaison Psychiatry

Chapter 5
Safety Issues in a General Medical Facility Setting

Say How Ong and Vicknesan J. Marimuttu

Society and the media have become increasingly concerned about self-harm and suicide in young people. This concern has led to an increasing worldwide focus on prevention and intervention. Young people who self-harm often present to hospitals via the emergency room (ER). The consultation-liaison team is often responsible to provide appropriate psychiatric assessment and management. This chapter will look to discuss self-harm, suicide, and dangerousness in young people in a general hospital setting.

Case Study: Suicide and Self-Harm

Agnes is a 16-year-old girl with a history of sexual abuse by her stepfather since she was 10 years old. She was fearful of speaking out for herself in the beginning, but at age 12 years, when she told her mother, her mother did not believe her and felt Agnes was scheming to get her stepfather out of the house. It was not until when Agnes told her school counselor that this matter was raised to the police who in turn alerted child protection services. Agnes was subsequently admitted into a juvenile residential facility under a child protection order due to the alleged abuse and her emerging conduct problems such as running away from home, smoking and drinking, and putting herself up with male acquaintances while she was on the run. She had also stopped going to school since entering the residential program, as she needs to be assessed for stability before resuming school.

In the residential home, Agnes' behavior had been particularly challenging. Her mood was perpetually angry and would "act out" or cut herself using any sharp items that she could find if she perceived that she had been treated unfairly by her

S. H. Ong (✉)
Department of Developmental Psychiatry, Institute of Mental Health, Singapore, Singapore
e-mail: say_how_ong@imh.com.sg

V. J. Marimuttu
Department of Psychological Medicine, KK Women's and Children's Hospital, Singapore, Singapore
e-mail: vicknesan.jeyan.marimuttu@singhealth.com.sg

A. P. S. Guerrero et al. (eds.), *Pediatric Consultation-Liaison Psychiatry*,
https://doi.org/10.1007/978-3-319-89488-1_5

peers or staff personnel. Agnes felt victimized after being sent to a residential program even though her stepfather had been imprisoned for the abuse.

Being in the residential home meant she had to stop going to her regular school and not meet with her peers. She admitted that they had been negative influences on her, teaching her to play truant, smoke, drink, and be introduced to other men or boys who were only slightly older than her. She regretted her actions and pleaded for a release. But as her mother now had to be the sole breadwinner, she was unable to closely supervise Agnes and do what was necessary to protect her.

Agnes became depressed 6 months into her residential program. She was unable to trust anyone and kept mostly to herself. She was preoccupied with negative thoughts and feelings and soon began to feel helpless and hopeless. She tried to kill herself several times in the home, but, due to the close surveillance, it was difficult for her to do so. This time, she could get another resident to smuggle in a razor blade for her. She hid herself in the washroom, drank a cup full of shampoo, and proceeded to cut herself. She did not tell anyone about this act and had planned it for weeks. She left a suicide note stating how sorry she had felt and how suicide was a solution for her to get away from her pain.

Agnes was found unconscious by one of the home staff during routine checks that night and was sent to the nearby pediatric hospital, where she was admitted for treatment of her wounds and ingestion of toxic substance.

A study by Sheridan et al. (2015) demonstrating a sizable prevalence of acute psychiatric conditions and substance use needing restraints or psychiatric admission among patients presenting to the pediatric ER highlights the importance of equipping general hospitals with the necessary resources and manpower in managing pediatric psychiatric consultations and admissions.

There are several aspects of safety and security challenges in general hospital setting. They can be categorized as follows:

Relational security
Risk of absconsion with multiple exit options and ward doors that are not locked
Easy access to surrounding sharps and medication for use in self-harm or suicide attempt
Ligature points in toilets/shower facilities
Risk of jumping from height with windows that can open out
Areas of hospital ward which are hidden from sight and where observation can be difficult (e.g., private rooms situated further from nursing station, toilets/shower areas, ward lounge area, etc.)
Lack of doors that open both outward and inward to allow staff to exit more easily when faced with an aggressive patient
Medical and nursing staffing concerns
Inadequate training of staff on issues regarding self-harm and suicide risk
Inadequate training on managing (e.g., via de-escalation or proper restraints) aggressive and violent behavior
Busy or inadequate number staff on the ward
Inaccurate risk assessment (e.g., admission of a highly suicidal patient to a bed further away from nursing station)

Insufficient observation and vigilance levels (e.g., not assigning one-to-one observation levels for a young person who is highly suicidal)
Lack of processes and protocols
Lack of ward-level nursing protocols for young people admitted following self-harm and suicide attempt (e.g., observation levels, need to check patient's belongings for sharps)
Lack of protocols on the medical management of distressed or aggressive patients (e.g., no clear protocols on the use of psychotropic medications in rapid tranquilization)
Lack of policy on the involvement of hospital security and the role they can play in supporting medical and nursing staff on the ward
Unavailability of policy for allowing patients to leave the ward
Unavailability of policy on the use of physical restraints
Unavailability of policy on when the hospital may seek support from the police

Suicidal attempts and ideations constitute a leading cause of psychiatric ER visits in youth (Grudnikoff et al. 2015). From time to time, suicidal patients have been admitted into general hospitals for concurrent medical or surgical conditions, especially if they had just overdosed on drugs or cut themselves. While it is not advisable to admit highly suicidal adolescents into a medical hospital due to limited resources and facility setup, health-care personnel are still required to attend to the patients' injuries and treat any acute or life-threatening physical conditions before transfers are made to a psychiatric facility. This situation poses medical dilemmas especially when both medical and psychiatric conditions are equally unstable or life-threatening. Unless there are existing safety protocols in place and the ward staff trained in some form of psychiatric nursing care, patients admitted for suicide risk can pose safety risks to themselves in hospital, leading to serious reportable incidents.

Though medical students and residents are trained in performing suicide risk assessments, not all feel confident or competent in doing so. Studies have also shown that suicidal behavior appears to generate, among ER staff, negative feelings and transferences, which in turn were largely due to societal attitudes, personal beliefs and biases, and lack of direction and support in managing suicidal behavior (Stefan 2006; Rossberg and Frills 2003). Only a minority of staff in general hospital ERs receiving pediatric patients with acute psychiatric crisis have received training in treating psychiatric patients (Santucci et al. 2003). ER doctors might not always be sufficiently trained to decide on the need for hospitalization or outpatient referral. Some studies (e.g., Case et al. 2011; Bridge et al. 2012) have shown that only one-third of adolescents who presented to the ER with mental health issues including self-harm or suicide attempt received a referral for psychiatric follow-up. Such knowledge gaps can only be rectified by ongoing education and active training for rotating as well as permanent doctors and nursing staff so that they can identify patients appropriately by their presenting issues and safety risk levels.

Suicide Attempts and Self-Harm

A suicide attempt can be defined as a self-destructive behavior performed with the intent to end one's life independent of the resulting damage (O'Carroll 1996). The term deliberate self-harm (DSH) (Madge et al. 2008) is frequently employed as a more encompassing term for all self-injurious behaviors with *and* without suicidal intent that have nonfatal outcomes. This term tends to be used predominantly within European countries and in Australia. In contrast, many studies published by researchers within Canada and the United States have employed the term non-suicidal self-injury (NSSI). More recently, the *Diagnostic and Statistical Manual of Mental Disorders (DSM-5)* has included NSSI in its fifth edition (American Psychiatric Association 2013).

NSSI is a subcategory of DSH and is defined as the deliberate, direct destruction or alteration of body tissue without conscious suicidal intent but resulting in injury severe enough for tissue damage (e.g., scarring) to occur (Favazza 1998). A key difference between DSH and a suicide attempt is the intent to end one's life. Individuals who engage in NSSI do not have intent to die, or they do not believe they will die from the NSSI behavior (Nock 2010). By contrast, suicidal self-harm is often characterized by high-lethality, low-frequency behavior, while NSSI is characterized by typically low-lethality, high-frequency, repetitive self-injurious behavior (Andover and Gibb 2010).

Epidemiology: Prevalence, Gender Differences, and Methods

Self-Harm

In exploring prevalence rates found in individual studies, Taliaferro et al. (2012) reported a 12-month prevalence estimate of 7.3% for NSSI. This study is one of the largest epidemiological studies of adolescents to date in the United States ($n = 61{,}767$). In a comparable epidemiological study of adolescents known as the Child and Adolescent Self-harm in Europe (CASE) study, Madge et al. (2008) found an average lifetime prevalence estimate of 17.8% and a 12-month prevalence of 11.5% for DSH. This was a large multicenter study conducted since 2005 and spans in seven countries (Australia, England, Ireland, Hungary, Belgium, the Netherlands, and Norway). It included 30,000 adolescents who were mainly 15- to 16-year-olds.

In terms of gender differences, female adolescents have a higher rate of self-harm when compared to male adolescents. The study by Evans et al. (2005) found the mean lifetime prevalence of self-harm to be 13.5% in females and 4.3% in males. 8.9% of females and 2.6% of males reported a self-harm episode in the previous year. A recent meta-analysis (Bresin and Schoenleber 2015) found that NSSI was 1.5 times more prevalent in females than in males.

Suicide and Attempted Suicide

The exploration of the prevalence of suicide is complicated by the way in which suicides are recorded by authorities responsible for death verdicts. Possible suicides are often given undetermined or accidental death verdicts (Gosney and Hawton 2007). Globally, suicide is the second leading cause of death in young people age 15–19 years old (WHO 2014). It is the third most common cause of death in male adolescents (after road-traffic accidents and violence) and the most common cause of death in female adolescents aged 15–19 years old (Patton et al. 2009). According to the World Health Organization (WHO), it is estimated that there were 804,000 suicides in 2012. The suicide rate for male adolescents is higher by 2.6 times than female counterparts (Wasserman et al. 2005). Suicide rates are lowest for those under 15 years old. It was previously reported (Bertolote and Fleischmann 2002) that there are 1.2 deaths per 100,000 boys aged 5–14 years, and this number increases to 19.2 deaths per 100,000 male adolescents aged 15–24 years. A comprehensive review of self-harm and suicidal behavior was published in 2005 (Evans et al. 2005). It included 513,188 adolescents in 128 studies. In the review, 9.7% of adolescents reported having attempted suicide in their lifetime, of which 6.4% occurred in the previous year. 29.9% of adolescents reported that they had suicidal thoughts at some point in their lives. The review reported higher prevalence of both suicidal thoughts and behaviors in females as compared to males.

Reported suicide rates vary widely between countries. Hawton et al. (2012) have summarized the suicide rates of individuals aged 15–24 years in several countries. The highest rates are reported in eastern European countries like Russia (43.7 per 100,000 males and 7.4 per 100,000 females; 2006), Lithuania (41.3 per 100,000 males and 6.3 per 100,000 females; 2009), and Ukraine (26.5 per 100,000 males and 4.5 per 100,000 females; 2009). Scandinavian countries like Finland (26.4 per 100,000 males and 8.7 per 100,000; 2009) and Norway also report higher rates. In Asia, Japan (20.4 per 100,000 males and 9.8 per 100,000 females; 2009) has reported higher suicide rates when compared to Hong Kong (11 per 100,000 males and 5.8 per 100,000 females; 2009) and China. In China, the rates of suicide in rural adolescent (8 per 100,000 males and 12.9 per 100,000 females; 1999) populations are higher than their urban (3 per 100,000 males and 4.1 per 100,000 females; 1999) counterparts. This difference may be due to ready availability of pesticides. The variations found among the different countries may be influenced by various factors. These include variations among countries in terms of socioeconomic status, geography and climate (e.g., light exposure and depression), access to lethal means (e.g., poisons or firearms), use of alcohol and drugs, and religious beliefs.

Method of Self-Harm and Suicide Attempts

Self-harm may involve self-cutting, self-poisoning with household cleaning products or over-the-counter or prescription medications, self-battery, or jumping from heights. The most common method used in self-harm in community samples is self-cutting (Madge et al. 2008). Among young people who self-harm and present to the hospital, self-poisoning is the most common method (Olfson et al. 2005). Paracetamol is often taken in self-poisoning (Hawton et al. 2003).

The case vignette examined common reasons. The most common reason for self-harm is "to get relief from a terrible state of mind," and the second most common reason is "to die." It is also common to report multiple reasons for self-harm. There is some relationship between the method used in the self-harm and the reason for self-harming. Repetition among young people has been noted to be high. In the same study, 55% of female adolescents and 53% of male adolescents reported multiple self-harm events. Repetition is more likely with self-cutting than with self-poisoning (Hawton et al. 2010). Some of the predictors of repeated self-harm include having depression, history of sexual abuse, exposure to self-harm among peers, and having concerns about one's own sexual orientation (O'Connor et al. 2009a, b).

Hospital Presentations

The lifetime prevalence of self-harm in psychiatrically hospitalized adolescents has been reported as high as 82% (Muehlenkamp et al. 2012). In the United States, the National Center for Injury Prevention and Control as part of the Centers for Disease Control and Prevention (CDC) records all self-harm presentations to emergency departments in hospitals across the country. The centers' definition of self-harm does not differentiate between NSSI and suicide attempts. It found that the self-harm presentations in those under 18 years old increased significantly from 89.21 per 100,000 in 2001 to 138.22 per 100,000 in 2013 (CDC 2013). The data also showed that females are 2–3 more likely to present to hospitals with self-harm every year.

Associated Factors in Self-Harm and Suicide

Genetics

A systematic review and meta-analysis (Geulayov et al. 2012) determined that offspring of parents who died of suicide were almost twice as likely to die of suicide themselves relative to control offspring of two living parents. The study noted a similarly increased risk of suicide attempts was noted for children of parents who attempted suicide.

A meta-analysis and systematic review of twin studies investigating the genetics of suicide found that the concordance for completed suicide was much higher in monozygotic twin pairs versus dizygotic twin pairs. The review estimated that the heritability of suicidality (including ideation, plans, and attempts) is in the range of 30–55% and that the heritability is largely independent of that of psychiatric disorders (Voracek and Loibl 2007).

Biological Factors

The serotonergic system has an important role in impulse control. Abnormalties in this system have been associated with suicidal behavior and have been extensively studied in adult samples. Low CSF 5-hydroxyindoleacetic acid (5-HIAA), which is a metabolite of serotonin, has been associated with impulsive aggression and suicidal behavior in adults (Mann 1998). Tryptophan hydroxylase is an important rate-limiting enzyme involved in serotonin biosynthesis. In adults, tryptophan hydroxylase gene polymorphisms (TPH1 and TPH2) have been linked to suicidality in Caucasians (Bellivier et al. 2004; Li and He 2006 and González-Castro et al. 2014).

There is a lack of studies exploring the role of serotonergic systems in younger samples. In a study of 15 teenage suicide victims, Pandey et al. (2002) found evidence indicating higher levels of 5-HT2A receptor, protein, and mRNA expression in the prefrontal cortex and hippocampus.

In terms of structural brain factors, a smaller anterior cingulate gray matter and white matter volume associated with increased suicidality have been observed in adolescents with borderline personality disorder and comorbid major depression. This is similar to findings found in adults with similar diagnoses (Goodman et al. 2011).

Additional brain changes include the appearance of white matter hyperintensities. White matter hyperintensities appear as hyperintense signals on T2-weighted magnetic resonance images (MRI). These can appear in the deep white matter or periventricular area. A higher prevalence of white matter hyperintensities was reported to be significantly linked to past suicide attempts in children and adolescents with major depressive disorder (Ehrlich et al. 2004). This mirrors the findings found in adults (Ahearn et al. 2001).

Family and Environmental Factors

Adversity in the family can have a significant impact on the development of children and adolescents. Disruptions to the family system in the form of parental separation, divorce, and parental loss through the death of a parent have been associated with the risk of self-harm (O'Connor et al. 2009a, b; Fergusson and Lynskey 1995; Johnson et al. 2002). Stressful life experiences including interpersonal difficulties during adolescence have been found to be independent predictors of suicide attempts in late adolescence and early adulthood (Johnson et al. 2002). Such interpersonal difficulties include difficulty making new friends, loneliness, and frequent arguments with adults in positions of authority and peers. Other forms of interpersonal stressors like bullying have also been associated with self-harm in cross-sectional school-based studies (Hawton et al. 2002). More serious traumatic childhood experiences in the form of physical and sexual abuse are also associated with self-harm during adolescence (Madge et al. 2008; O'Connor et al. 2009a, b). Young people who have lesbian, gay, bisexual, or transgender (LGBT) sexual orientation have been found to have six times higher risk of attempted suicide when compared to young people with a heterosexual orientation (Fergusson et al. 1999).

Psychiatric Comorbidity

In terms of psychiatric disorders, depression and anxiety disorders have been found most commonly in young people who present with self-harm. One study showed that 87% (Manor et al. 2010) of young people who present to hospital with self-harm have some form of psychiatric disorder. Self-harm is commonly associated with young people who have received an early diagnosis of personality disorder (Nock et al. 2006).

Alcohol misuse has been found to be a risk factor for adolescents who self-harm. One study found that binge drinking is associated with self-harm and that this link is most pronounced for young people aged 13 years or younger (Aseltine et al. 2009). It is currently unclear if lifestyle factors like smoking, binge drinking, or substance misuse are directly linked to self-harm or are forms of coping with underlying emotional distress.

Previous suicide attempts are an important risk factor for future repeated attempts as well as completed suicide. The risk of completed suicide is 20 times higher for individuals who have attempted suicide versus those who have not (Spirito and Esposito-Smythers 2006). Self-harm is another major risk factor and increases the risk of subsequent completed suicide by tenfold (Hawton and Harriss 2007). It is estimated that 1 in 25 patients who present to hospital following an episode of self-harm will die of suicide in the following 5 years (Carroll et al. 2014). With such an elevated risk for completed suicide, appropriate and timely management of patients referred to the ER may mitigate the psychosocial risk factors that often lead patients to end their lives.

Assessment of Suicide Risk

Suicide Risk

Suicidal and self-harming adolescents contribute to a significant number of ER visits (Ting et al. 2012) and are often accompanied by their parents or school counselors and sometimes escorted by police officers who responded to public calls for help. These adolescents are often uncooperative and not forthcoming with information. Doctors practicing in pediatric ERs are often pressured to admit them for observation instead of referring them directly to a psychiatric facility even if there were no medical or surgical indications for admission. Admission into a psychiatric facility can be extremely stigmatizing, and the idea is often rejected by patients and parents. This rejection can pose a challenge if there are no child psychiatric services or secured wards in the hospital. Early or urgent psychiatric consultations may not be possible in some countries, especially after office hours. Hence, in some states in the United States, inpatient or outpatient crisis units are being embedded within the medical ERs, e.g., the Comprehensive Psychiatric Emergency Program model. In pediatric hospitals without consultation-liaison child psychiatrists after office hours, telepsychiatry and phone consultations can help determine whether the youth requires admission into the medical ward or to a psychiatric facility or can be adequately managed in the community. Parker et al. (2003) found that a rapid response urgent consultation model reduced admission rates to the psychiatric inpatient ward from 22% to 2% in 1 year. Latimer et al. (2014) studied a rapid response team (RTT) intervention model and found it to be cost-effective compared to usual care for suicidal youth presenting at the ER.

Basic skills in suicide assessment and profiling of high-risk patients should be taught not just in pediatric ERs but also in the general medical and surgical wards. Patients and parents should be interviewed separately first and then together to address any uncertainty about symptoms and issues and to help them understand reasons for suicide attempts, their medical consequences, and legal implications. Based on the suicide risk ladder from the predicament model of suicide (Pridmore and Jamil 2009), an individual's suicide risk is influenced by complex and unique interactions of individual baseline suicidality factors, stress impact, and momentary position which represents the suicide risk of the individual at a particular moment. Suicide in several countries is still considered illegal and reportable by law. Asking about suicide does not increase risk of suicide, contrary to what many used to believe. By talking directly about suicide, patients often feel relieved that this topic was brought up and they no longer have to keep it a secret. This directness could encourage a more open and honest conversation between patients and health-care staff.

Even in high-income countries, patients with suicide-related behavioral presentations in the hospital may not always receive specialist psychosocial assessments (Kapur and associates 2008). Because of the high prevalence of psychiatric, family, school, and social problems among medically hospitalized youth who have attempted suicide (Gasquet and Choquet 1994), clinical histories should elicit depression, mania, psychosis, anxiety, substance use, past suicide attempt and self-harm, impulsivity, aggression, and assess for family and social support. Several studies on suicide have shown that significant suicide triggers include family conflicts or disputes, breakups, bullying (including cyberbullying), academic problems or failures, and impending disciplinary or legal actions.

The Australian Triage Scale and the Canadian Emergency Department Triage system for psychiatric patients are tools commonly used at ER settings to determine

Table 5.1 HEADSS assessment tool

H – Home (consider living arrangements, transience, relationships with carers/significant others, community support, supervision, abuse, childhood experiences, cultural identity, and recent life events.)
E – Education, employment, eating, and exercise (consider school/work retention and relationships, bullying, study/career progress and goals, nutrition, vegetarianism, eating patterns, weight gain/loss, exercise, fitness, and energy.)
A – Activities, hobbies, and peer relationships (consider hobbies, belonging to peer group, peer activities and venues, lifestyle factors, risk-taking, injury avoidance, and sun protection.)
D – Drug use (consider alcohol, cigarettes, caffeine, prescription/illicit drugs and type, quantity, frequency, administration, interactions, access, recent increases/decreases, past treatments, education, and motivational interviewing.)
S – Sexual activity and sexuality (consider sexual activity, age onset, safe sex practices, same sex attraction, history pap smears/STI screening, sexual abuse, and pregnancy/children.)
S – Suicide, depression and mental health, and safety/risk (consider normal vs clinical depression, anxiety, reactions to stress, and if appropriate risk assessment.)

HEADSS mnemonic adapted from Goldenring and Cohen (1988)

priority of intervention based on behavioral presentation and time parameters (Downey et al. 2015). For example, the Australian Triage Scale (Smart et al. 1999) specifies a time frame in which treatment or intervention should be carried out based on triage category (emergency, urgent, semi-urgent, or urgent) with patient descriptors such as whether patient was violent, aggressive, or suicidal, was distressed or acutely psychotic, and was suffering from a long-standing mental health disorder and whether family support/escort was available.

Suicide assessment should be based on both dynamic and static risk factors as well as protective factors. Features that increase completed suicide risk are male gender, age 14–19 years, poor family and social support, highly lethal suicide means (e.g., hanging, drowning, jumping), premeditation, and concealment. Even if a failed suicide attempt was not the presenting issue, admitting and attending doctors should be trained to routinely assess the potentially triggering psychosocial circumstances of each adolescent.

Psychosocial factors can be elicited using the HEADSS assessment tool (Goldenring and Cohen 1988), an easy-to-perform face-to-face interview that could be performed by a junior doctor, a resident, an allied health staff, or a nurse and that can be used in both inpatient and ER (HEADS-ED, Cappelli et al. 2012) settings. See Table 5.1.

The Pediatric Symptom Checklist (PSC; Jellinek et al. 1988) may also improve the recognition and treatment of psychosocial problems in children (see Table 5.2, 17-item version; reproduced with permission).

Studies (e.g., Lopez-Castroman et al. 2016; O'Connor et al. 2012; Jobes 2006) have shown that a significant number of suicide victims felt ambivalent before the act itself. Many so-called suicidal acts were a call for help, and had there been a way to relieve emotional pain, the victims might have reconsidered suicide. A proportion of them also did not think through all their available options and may have had an existing impulsivity and a lack of foreplanning.

Table 5.2 Pediatric Symptom Checklist (PSC-17)

Please mark under the heading that best describes your child:				
	Never	Sometimes		Often
	(0)	(1)	(2)	
1. Feels sad, unhappy				
2. Feels hopeless				
3. Is down on self				
4. Worries a lot				
5. Seems to be having less fun				
6. Fidgety, unable to sit still				
7. Daydreams too much				
8. Distracted easily				
9. Has trouble concentrating				
10. Acts as if driven by a motor				
11. Fights with other children				
12. Does not listen to rules				
13. Does not understand other people's feelings				
14. Teases others				
15. Blames others for his/her troubles				
16. Refuses to share				
17. Takes things that do not belong to him/her				
Does your child have any emotional or behavioral problems for which she/he needs help?				
__No__Yes				

It is extremely important to differentiate genuine suicidal intent from a cry for help or means to achieve short-term relief through non-suicidal self-injury. Several pediatric survivors of potentially lethal ingestions had actually hoped to "sleep over it," to simply wanting to "forget problems," or to feel "alive" or to at least feel something even if pain. Admittedly, for some fatal drug overdoses, it is not possible to know whether the act was a suicide or accidental death, self-harm and NSSI

Like suicide attempts, NSSI contributes significantly toward health-care costs and workload in the pediatric ERs and inpatient setting. Many nonpsychiatric doctors may not know how to approach an adolescent patient with repeated self-harm behaviors. They might feel uncomfortable broaching the topic if at all, while others might have a strong countertransference. Many teens have disclosed to the psychiatrists and psychiatric case managers that ER staff often view them in a disapproving manner, pass sarcastic or judgmental remarks about their repeated ER attendances, and disregard their complaints.

While the majority of self-harm behavior assessments, such as the Self-Injury Inventory (SII; Zlotnick et al. 1995) and the Deliberate Self-Harm Inventory (DSHI; Gratz 2001), were developed for adults, these measures are examples of available brief tools specifically developed for adolescents.

Self-Report Measures

(i) The Functional Assessment of Self-Mutilation (FASM; Lloyd et al. 1997): self-report measure of the methods, frequency, and functions of self-mutilation behavior (SMB)
(ii) The Ottawa Self-Injury Inventory (OSI; Cloutier and Nixon 2003): 38-item self-report measure that offers a comprehensive assessment of NSSI, including both measurement of its functions and potential addictive features
(iii) Self-Harm Survey and Motivations Underlying Self-Harm Questionnaire (Laye-Gindhu and Schonert-Reichl 2005): 44-item component on six dimensions of self-injury and 29-item component on motivations, to explore frequency, context, and reasons for self-harm
(iv) Adolescent Risk Inventory (ARI; Lescano et al. 2007): 33-item, self-report inventory, with mostly yes/no response options, that explores high-risk behaviors and attitudes including six items exploring self-harm behavior including self-cutting and suicide attempts

Clinician-Rated Structured Measures

(i) Self-Injurious Behavior Questionnaire (SIB-Q; Gutierrez et al. 2001): 25-item scale with Likert-style response options that measures self-injurious behavior among those with developmental disabilities
(ii) Self-Injurious Thoughts and Behaviors Interview (SITBI; Nock et al. 2007): 169-item scale composing five modules evaluating presence, frequency, and characteristics of suicidal ideation, plans, gestures, attempts, and NSSI

There is no one perfect assessment tool, and the choice of tool used would be dependent on clinician experience, training, and comfort and simplicity of use in a busy pediatric unit.

NSSI is a form of maladaptive coping behavior often related to underlying psychopathology. To appropriately plan treatment, the clinician must screen for the following:

1. Depression
2. Borderline personality traits or disorder
3. Alexithymia
4. Chronic low self-esteem
5. Low tolerance to stress, frustration, and disappointments
6. Low propensity for self-soothing and emotional regulation
7. Psychotic or schizoaffective disorders

Case Study: Violence and Aggression

Ten-year-old Jimmy was admitted into a community hospital's pediatric ward following suspicions of non-accidental injury (NAI) by one of his biological parents. Jimmy became increasingly restless while waiting for his medical examination. By the next day, he was pacing about in the ward, interfering with the nurses doing their work, and arguing with other pediatric patients within his ward cubicle. When requested to return to his bed, Jimmy shouted that he wanted to go home, kicked the side table, and tried to attack his nurse. The ward milieu was interrupted, and the other patients were terrified of him. Four nursing staff, with security backup, restrained him in his bed. The child psychiatrist was called in to assess the patient's mental state. A review of his clinical notes suggested that he had earlier been diagnosed to have attention-deficit hyperactivity disorder (ADHD), which was not treated due to his social circumstances. The psychiatrist excused all the security officers and nursing staff as their presence appeared to be aggravating Jimmy's anger and frustration. He pleaded to be released from his 5-point restraint. The psychiatrist drew the curtain to keep Jimmy out of sight from the other patients. Speaking in a soft and calm voice, he spent the next hour talking to Jimmy in a reassuring manner and encouraged him to relax himself so that he could be released as soon as possible. There was no need for intramuscular or oral sedation as Jimmy could settle down eventually. His legal guardian was informed of his being physically restrained. A debrief was conducted with the ward nurses and manager. One of the recommendations was to assign a quiet room to allow agitated patients to calm themselves down without traumatizing other patients. A protocol describing de-escalation techniques and appropriate medication use was also incorporated into the hospital's patient care protocol.

Dangerousness includes violence and verbal and physical aggression that could place the safety of others at risk. Rarely seen in a pediatric setting, it can be easily overlooked especially in a crowded inpatient ward or ER.

Aggression is defined as any behavior that is intended to be destructive to self, others, or objects and property (Swann 2003). Aggression is typically considered as maladaptive and can be divided into premeditated, predatory aggression or reactive, affective aggression. McAneney and Shaw (1994) found that high-volume pediatric ERs, compared with low-volume ones, were at greater risk for verbal threats, physical attacks, and injury to staff, patients, and visitors, independent of whether there were 24-h security or locked doors. Connor et al. (2006) reported that clinically referred children and adolescents often exhibit aggression in the 6 months prior to child psychiatric referral, regardless of their diagnosis. Maladaptive aggression in clinical settings takes up a large quantity of resources and is a significant public health problem in the United States and other parts of the world.

Social factors causing aggression include substance use, alcoholism, poor and overcrowded neighborhoods such as ghettos with high crime rates, and easy access to fire weapons. Medical and psychiatric causes (Table 5.3) can also contribute to violence and aggression.

While some psychiatric or other medical causes of violence or aggression are readily treatable and reversible, others may take time to resolve. Although a challenge, it is essential to safely and appropriately provide nursing care within the pediatric ward, as safety events could happen during the least expected moments. In assessing violence risk, it is particularly helpful to note previous violent offenses, past admissions for agitation, and past violent episodes due to substance misuse.

The Structured Assessment of Violence Risk in Youth™ (SAVRY™) (Borum et al. 2002, 2006) can help to assess a youth's violence risk upon on admission. It includes twenty-four items in three risk domains (historical risk factors, social/con-

Table 5.3 Common medical and psychiatric causes that can cause safety concerns

Acute delirium (arising from, e.g., toxins, head injuries, illicit drugs, metabolic disorders, etc.)
Developmental delays and intellectual disability
Neurodevelopmental disorders (e.g., autism spectrum disorders, ADHD)
Conduct disorders
Acute psychotic disorders (typically with grossly disorganized behaviors, command hallucinations, and paranoia)
Bipolar mood disorders (especially during acute manic episodes)
High anxiety, fear, or frustration, which could arise from environment-related or post-trauma stress issues

textual risk factors, and individual/clinical factors), a three-level rating structure for each risk item, six protective factor items (either present or absent), emphasis on both reactive and proactive aggression subtypes, and consideration of dynamic factors that can be useful targets for intervention and prevention.

Other tools available for assessment of children and adolescents include the Behavioral Activity Rating Scale (BARS) (Swift et al. 2002) and the Modified Overt Aggression Scale (MOAS) (Kay et al. 1988). BARS is frequently used in nonmedical setting to determine whether a patient needs transfer to a higher level of care. MOAS is a four-part behavior rating scale designed to measure four types of aggressive behavior as witnessed in the past week – verbal aggression, aggression against property, autoaggression (aggression toward oneself), and physical aggression. Its use is recommended by the American Academy of Pediatrics.

Management and Interventions

Safety considerations, be it for patients, their family, or health-care staff, remain paramount when a child or adolescent patient is admitted into a general ward. The typical pediatric medical and surgical wards are not the best equipped to house patients with high risks for suicide, self-harm, or violence. First, the ward layouts do not always offer line of sight for nursing care. In some countries, the wards for non-paying/partial paying (subsidized) patients often house between four to six pediatric beds in a single large cubicle, possibly tucked far away from the nursing counter. The physical distance and lack of line of sight do not provide the much-needed close surveillance for at-risk patients.

Second, while nursing staff are generally proficient in responding to medical emergencies, the majority are not trained in psychiatric emergencies or "code gray" situations. Psychiatric knowledge and mental health literacy among health-care professionals can be surprisingly deficient, even among doctors, because of inadequate emphasis on psychiatry in undergraduate medical or nursing school. Lack of competency may further be perpetuated by negative countertransference toward patients with mental health issues.

Table 5.4 Helpful nursing interventions identified by parents and children

Intervention theme	Category of intervention	Example of actions
Caring for the child as a special person	1. Getting to know the child	Being warm, talking and listening to child
	2. Personalizing care	
	3. Being available	Attending and responding to each child's unique needs
	4. Communicating calmly	Being consistently present and available
Caring for the parents	1. Being available to parents	Explicitly making time for parents
	2. Reassuring parents through talking	Being present and attentive to their needs
		Sharing information and perspectives in a comforting way
Managing the child's illness	1. Including parents in the care team	Linking thoughts to feelings and physical symptoms
	2. Teaching coping behaviors	Sharing knowledge of mental health care with families
Creating a therapeutic environment	1. Managing physical spaces	Helping the child make personal choices and taking care of their immediate environment
	2. Managing the social environment	Fostering relationships between children within the unit
		Ensuring safety and well-being of children in critical situations

In a qualitative study of admitted patients, Montreuil et al. (2015) identified specific helpful nursing interventions (Table 5.4). These interventions should be regarded as basic communication and behavioral intervention tools to prevent safety risks posed by either patients or family members.

Ward Protocols for Patients at Risk for Suicide and Self-Harm

When the health-care staff or clinician strongly suspects that a patient is in imminent danger of harming self or others, caregivers and family members must be informed of the risk so that necessary precautions can be taken in accordance with the hospital's suicide and self-harm protocols. Table 5.5 shows a list of precautionary measures to be initiated as soon as the ward receives a patient with high risk.

Ward Protocols for Patients at Risk for Violence or Aggression

Aggressive or violent behavior is especially distressing in a pediatric hospital which is supposed to be a safe place for sick and recuperating patients.

Table 5.5 Suicide precautionary measures in the inpatient unit

Keep patient near to the central nursing station
Keep patient within line of sight of the nursing staff
Restrict patient from leaving his/her bed without accompanying staff or adult caregiver
Check and chart patient's status every half an hour
Keep curtains open except during medical examinations or procedures
Keep alcoholic hand-rub solutions or gels and any sharps away from the patient's bed
Inform child psychiatrist on duty whenever there is change in mental status
Keep multidisciplinary team updated after each psychiatric consultation
Take patient off suicide caution when instructed by child psychiatrist

Formulated from expert consensus and available evidence, Treatment Recommendations for the Use of Antipsychotics for Aggressive Youth (TRAAY; Pappadopulos et al. 2003) address severe impulsive aggression over four phases of care: evaluation, treatment, stabilization, and maintenance. Many recommendations continue to be relevant in current practice, including psychosocial crisis management before medication, atypical antipsychotics for aggression with comorbid psychiatric conditions, and sparing use of emergency or as-needed medications.

According to Best Practices in Evaluation and Treatment of Agitation (Project BETA; Consensus Statement of the American Association for Emergency Psychiatry 2012), when working with an aggressive or agitated patient, priorities include (1) ensuring the safety of patient, staff, and others in the area; (2) helping the patient manage his emotions and distress and maintain or regain control of his behavior; (3) avoiding the use of restraint when at all possible; and (4) avoiding coercive interventions that escalate agitation. Safety protocols are imperative for any inpatient unit. Periodic safety "walks" by senior management are often helpful in identifying gaps in preparedness to deal with an aggressive patient. Safety drills can be held regularly to keep all staff well prepared when such situations occur. Clinicians and nurses can be appointed as safety officers or "champions." Generally, for pediatric patients, physical restraints are discouraged as they might further aggravate the patient or cause unnecessary trauma. Worse, a staff or the patient might be injured during the process. Physical restraints are hence often a last resort after failing to manage the child's aggression through appropriate medication.

For nonmedical causes of aggression, the first of management is for the staff to talk calmly with the child and remove the child away from the provocative situation to a quieter and private part of the ward. This intervention often helps the child to no longer perceive himself as being threatened. See Table 5.6 for a list of de-escalation techniques. The second line of management includes seclusion and restraint. However, not all inpatient units have seclusion rooms that are specifically built for

Table 5.6 De-escalation techniques

Use a quiet, private, and calming space
Talk to the child and listen actively
Acknowledge feelings of anger, frustration, and disappointment
Motivate the child by encouraging the child to help himself or work together with you
Use relaxation techniques like deep breathing, muscle relaxation, and counting down
Distract the child to focus on something positive
Set reasonable limits for behaviors
Teach him what to say or do when he feels that way again

this purpose. Nurses should try not to handle an aggressive child alone and should always keep another nurse informed. Should the situation escalate, security backup may be needed. It can be extremely helpful for ward nurses and security personnel to be trained in crisis management techniques by certified trainers, who often work primarily in psychaitric inpatient or correctional facilties. However, not all hospital staff have access to such training. Aggression management (or "code gray") teams, comprising staff members from different disciplines and led by an emergency consultant and hospital administrator, may be helpful in responding to safety concerns unresponsive to verbal de-escalation (Hopper et al. 2012).

As the third line of management, the nurse can further offer the child a medication like lorazepam to manage agitation. The choice of medication should be based on the underlying cause or causes of acute agitation and after considerations of the balance of risks, benefits, and side effects (Sonnier and Barzman 2011). Table 5.7 describes suggested medications, dependent on availability. International guidelines on the use of seclusion, restraint, and medication include the AACAP Practice Parameter for the Prevention and Management of Aggressive Behavior in Child and Adolescent Psychiatric Institutions (with special reference to Seclusion and Restraint) (Masters et al. 2002), the National Institute for Health and Care Excellence (NICE) guidelines and algorithms (2013, 2014, 2015), and Project BETA (2012).

All patients should be given the choice whether to take the medication orally (TRAAY; Pappadopulos et al. 2003). By having a choice, patient can have a sense of personal control in their treatment and are made aware of the possible effect that accompanies the intake of the medication. Oral medications also prevent unnecessary exposure to trauma arising from an intramuscular injection (Currier and Medori 2006; Martin and Volkmar 2007). It is important to note that oversedation is not a goal of medication treatment, as it would prohibit further mental state examination and collaborative treatment planning (Zimbroff 2008).

Second-generation or atypical antipsychotic medications are generally preferred over first-generation or typical antipsychotics due to their shorter-term side effects and less propensity for serious side effects such as extrapyramidal symptoms, dyskinesia, and neuroleptic malignant syndrome. Among the typical antipsychotic

Table 5.7 Medications used in acute agitation

Suggested ORAL medications	Suggested intramuscular injections
Children 6–12 years old:	Children 6–12 years old:
Promethazine 0.5–1 mg/kg stat (max. 25 mg)	IM diphenhydramine 1 mg/kg/dose stat (max. 50 mg)
Hydroxyzine 0.6 mg/kg stat (max 25 mg)	IM lorazepam 0.02 mg/kg/dose–0.06 mg/kg/dose (max 1 mg)
Diazepam 0.2–0.3 mg/kg stat (max. 10 mg)	IM haloperidol 1–3 mg stat (max. 0.15 mg/kg/day)
Risperidone 0.25–0.5 mg/day (liquid or ODT[a])	IM olanzapine 2.5 mg stat
Olanzapine 2.5 mg stat (ODT[a])	
Above 12 years old:	Above 12 years old:
Oral promethazine 12.5–25 mg stat	IM diphenhydramine 50–100 mg stat
Oral hydroxyzine 12.5–25 mg stat	
Oral lorazepam 1–2 mg stat	IM lorazepam 0.5–1 mg stat
Risperidone 0.25–0.5 mg/day (liquid or ODT[a])	IM haloperidol 2–5 mg stat IM olanzapine 5–10 mg stat
Olanzapine 5–10 mg stat (ODT[a])	

References: 1. Pereira S, Gard D, Brandford D, CPD online (May 2009)
2. Adimando, A. J., Poncin, Y. B., Baum, C. R. (2010)
3. Sonnier, L., Barzman, D. (2011)
[a]ODT = oral disintegrating tablet

medications, haloperidol is of high potency, relatively well tolerated, and hence widely used in emergency settings. Risperidone and olanzapine, in the form of liquid or orodispersible/oral disintegrating tablets, are the more commonly used atypical antipsychotics currently.

Post-medication Monitoring

Especially in situations where medication use fits the definition of chemical restraint according to the Joint Commission International (JCI) definition, the youth must be closely monitored for paradoxical reactions, including hyperactive/aggressive behavior (as has been reported with benzodiazepines, particularly in children/adolescents and patients with developmental delay, intellectual disabilities, autism spectrum disorders, and neurologic disorders):

- Respiratory depression
- Anticholinergic toxic effects and reactive airway exacerbations from antihistamines, particularly in children with neurodevelopmental disorders
- Dystonic reactions, oculogyric crises, and akathisia particularly in antipsychotic-naïve children and adolescents' vital sign (blood pressure, pulse, respiratory rate, temperature, oxygen saturation) instability
- Circulatory compromise and injuries in the peripheral limbs

In managing aggression, patients and staff are potentially at risk for physical or emotional harm and possible legal action. Important follow-up steps include a discussion with the patient, to ensure an opportunity to express feedback; a discussion with the parents/guardians, to ensure that they are properly informed; and a root-cause analysis, to ensure that the health-care team has had an opportunity to debrief and identify areas of improvement. Patients subjected to restraint can become extremely terrified or traumatized after the incident if not handled appropriately. To ensure sound clinical justification and to manage medicolegal risk, the clinician must properly document indication (including less restrictive measures tried), explanation to patient and/or caregiver, and response to intervention. Training must highlight that any form of restraint is a matter of last resort, and close monitoring of restrained and sedated patients is critical to avoid adverse events (Dorfman 2000).

For patients with neurodevelopmental disorders, the causes for aggression can be very different from those without those conditions. Evaluation of the antecedent events, detection of communication difficulties, and assessment for any sensory issues or physical discomforts could help guide appropriate interventions. For children with autism spectrum disorders, it is necessary to consider transition planning in advance, to use alternative communication means (e.g., flashcards, computer, etc.), and to adjust environmental stimuli like noise and lighting, all of which could prevent aggression and meltdowns. Referral to an occupational therapist or applied behavioral psychologist might prove useful.

It is important not to disregard or minimise the psychological and emotional impact on health-care staff after an incident. Staff who have experienced or witnessed violence or aggression should be offered emotional support and counseling if needed. In the Child Guidance Clinic of Singapore, a peer support group called CHERISH (cherish to engage and renew in strength and hope) assists fellow colleagues who have received verbal or physical aggression from patients or visitors. This system allows timely response by peer volunteers who could empathize with their situations. The staff can be subsequently referred to specialist clinics for further interventions if necessary. These interventions are also intended to prevent staff burnout and loss of morale.

Outcomes and Level of Care

When a patient is deemed unstable and high risk for suicide or violence, the medical team should consider a transfer to a tertiary psychiatric facility or hospital with secured holding units. Depending on the country and state, there are relevant statutes or health acts that empower clinicians or allied health professionals such as medical social workers to admit the patient against his will in order to ensure safety. These are referred to as "formalized admissions" or "psychiatric holds." Depending on the local statutes and acts, patients could be held from as short as 48 hours to as long as 6 months.

Patients in pediatric ER who need acute psychiatric admission typically would be required to wait at the ER for transfer to another facility. For some, they may be admitted into the observation ward or a crisis unit while awaiting transfer. In a survey among 42 Californian counties, the average wait time for pediatric patients with a primary psychiatric diagnosis was 12.97 hours, usually because of lack of inpatient psychiatric beds (Stone et al. 2012). The ER is not ideal to hold psychiatric patients because of its environment and physical setup (Santiago et al. 2006), and may increase the likelihood for dangerous behaviors. During the hold, there must be adequate nursing resources to provide 1–1 supervision and monitoring of mental states and risk of violence or self-harm. Patients who can be discharged from medical wards should have received a psychiatric consult in hospital or at least an outpatient psychiatric referral. Safety plans should be discussed with caregivers and family members to prevent further suicide attempts or self-harm (Sher and LaBode 2011). Suicide risk is particularly high after discharge either because patients may feel more "energized" or have developed greater awareness of personal losses or failures after initiation of treatment. Impulsivity and lack of foreplanning are also factors likely to prompt adolescents to reattempt suicide upon facing subsequent emotional distress.

The safety plans include:

Supervision

(i) Mobilizing family and peer support network
(ii) Insuring close adult supervision
(iii) Limiting outings to only those with accompanying responsible adults
(iv) Looking out for warning signs and triggers of suicidal ideations

Means Restriction

(v) Keeping firearms (if applicable), sharps, and medications in locked cabinets
(vi) Randomly checking school bags, bedrooms, and bathrooms for pills, razor blades, and penknives
(vii) Keeping the bedroom door unlocked even if closed for privacy
(viii) For patients living in high-rise apartments, locking window grills especially if there had been incidents of climbing out of windows or threatening to jump

Coping Strategies

(ix) Engaging in healthy activities to provide distraction and increase sense of pleasure and mastery
(x) Adapting coping techniques to the home setting
(xi) Accessing resources as identified by the clinician (e.g., community mental health agencies, support groups, and crisis help lines)

Discharge Planning

Discharge planning is an important step to ensure continuity of care and maintenance of gains achieved during hospitalization. Used in both medical and psychiatric settings, discharge planning identifies the patient's needs and is done collaboratively with the patient, family, medical professionals, and community agencies or step-down care facilities. A dynamic process, discharge planning starts the moment a patient has been admitted to establish links between patient and these various resources. In addition to coordination of care and mobilization of necessary support, discharge planning also includes early intervention during crisis and relapse of illness and maintenance of optimal health and well-being (Babich and Brown 1991). Discharge of psychiatric patients should not be conducted prematurely or rushed under the pressures of inpatient bed shortages, depleted medical insurance coverage, or cost containment (Alghzawi 2012). Patient and family psychoeducation, post-discharge care management, community-based care, and home visits can prevent readmission and relapse and ensure a safer transition (Steffen et al. 2009; Vigod et al. 2013).

Poor adherence to follow-up after initial assessments for self-harm is a major barrier for adolescents to get the necessary help that they need (Granboulan et al. 2001) and confers a much less favorable psychosocial outcome (Pillay and Wassenaar 1995). Ougrin et al. (2010) studied 70 adolescents presenting to ER for self-harm and found that those who received therapeutic assessment (TA), a brief therapeutic intervention based on cognitive analytic therapy as compared to assessment as usual, were more likely to improve engagement with follow-up services 3 months after the initial assessment at ER. With the psychosocial factors behind self-harm and suicide attempts being potentially complex and overwhelming for the adolescents to overcome, active and early engagement with treatment is a necessary first step toward helping them achieve positive and realistic treatment goals.

Conclusion

Aggression and self-harm can be extremely challenging to manage in general medical hospital settings that have limited resources and access to psychiatric care. Collaboration between pediatric and psychiatric teams is the only way to ensure that children and adolescents presenting with these behaviors are effectively managed.

References

Adimando, A. J., Poncin, Y. B., & Baum, C. R. (2010). Pharmacological management of the agitated pediatric patient. *Pediatric Emergency Care, 26*(11), 856–860. https://doi.org/10.1097/PEC.0b013e3181f9dce4.

Ahearn, E. P., Jamison, K. R., Steffens, D. C., Cassidy, F., Provenzale, J. M., Lehman, A., et al. (2001). MRI correlates of suicide attempt history in unipolar depression. *Biological Psychiatry, 50*(4), 266–270.

Alghzawi, H. M. (2012). Psychiatric discharge process. *ISRN Psychiatry, 2012*, 1–7. https://doi.org/10.5402/2012/638943.

American Psychiatric Association. (2013). Nonsuicidal self-injury. In *Diagnostic and statistical manual of mental disorders* (5th ed.). Washington, DC: American Psychiatric Publishing.

Andover, M. S., & Gibb, B. E. (2010). Non-suicidal self-injury, attempted suicide, and suicidal intent among psychiatric inpatients. *Psychiatry Research, 178*, 101–105. https://doi.org/10.1016/j.psychres.2010.03.019.

Aseltine, R. H., Jr., Schilling, E. A., James, A., Glanovsky, J. L., & Jacobs, D. (2009). Age variability in the association between heavy episodic drinking and adolescent suicide attempts: Findings from a large-scale, school-based screening program. *Journal of the American Academy of Child and Adolescent Psychiatry, 48*, 262–270. https://doi.org/10.1097/CHI.0b013e318195bce8.

Babich, K. S., & Brown, L. (Eds.). (1991). *Discharge planning: A manual for psychiatric nurses*. Thorofare: Published by SLACK Incorporated.

Bellivier, F., Chaste, P., & Malafosse, A. (2004). Association between the TPH gene A218C polymorphism and suicidal behavior: A meta-analysis. *American Journal of Medical Genetics Part B, Neuropsychiatric Genetics, 124*(1), 87–91.

Bertolote, J. M., & Fleischmann, A. (2002). A global perspective in the epidemiology of suicide. *Suicidology, 7*(2), 6–8.

Borum, R., Bartel, P., & Forth, A. (2002). *Manual for the structured assessment for violence risk in youth (SAVRY)*. Tampa: University of South Florida.

Borum, R., Bartel, P., & Forth, A. (2006). *Manual for the structured assessment of violence risk in youth (SAVRY)*. Odessa: Psychological Assessment Resources.

Bresin, K., & Schoenleber, M. (2015). Gender differences in prevalence of nonsuicidal self-injury: A meta-analysis. *Clinical Psychology Review, 38*, 55–64. https://doi.org/10.1016/j.cpr.2015.02.009.

Bridge, J. A., Marcus, S. C., & Olfson, M. (2012). Outpatient care of young people after emergency treatment of deliberate self-harm. *Journal of the American Academy of Child and Adolescent Psychiatry, 51*(2), 213–222.e1. https://doi.org/10.1016/j.jaac.2011.11.002. Epub 2011 Dec 23.

Cappelli, M., Gray, C., Zemek, R., Cloutier, P., Kennedy, A., Glennie, E., Doucet, G., & Lyons, J. S. (2012). The HEADS-ED: A rapid mental health screening tool for pediatric patients in the emergency department. *Pediatric, 130*(2), e321–e327. https://doi.org/10.1542/peds.2011-3798.

Carroll, R., Metcalfe, C., & Gunnell, D. (2014). Hospital presenting self-harm and risk of fatal and non-fatal repetition: Systematic review and meta-analysis. *PLoS One, 9*(2), e89944. https://doi.org/10.1371/journal.pone.0089944.

Case, S. D., Case, B. G., Olfson, M., Linakis, J. G., & Laska, E. M. (2011). Length of stay of pediatric mental health emergency department visits in the United States. *Journal of the American Academy of Child and Adolescent Psychiatry, 50*(11), 1110–1119. https://doi.org/10.1016/j.jaac.2011.08.011. Epub 2011 Oct 2.

Centers for Disease Control and Prevention. (2013). *WISQARS nonfatal injury reports*. Retrieved from: http://webappa.cdc.gov/cgi-bin/broker.exe

Cloutier, P. F., & Nixon, M. K. (2003). The Ottawa self-injury inventory: A preliminary evaluation. Abstracts to the 12th international congress European society for child and adolescent psychiatry. *European Child & Adolescent Psychiatry, 12*(Suppl. 1), 1–94.

Connor, D. F., Carlson, G. A., Chang, K. D., et al. (2006). Juvenile maladaptive aggression: A review of prevention, treatment and service configuration and a proposed research agenda. *Journal of Clinical Psychiatry, 67*(5), 808–820.

Consensus Statement of the American Association for Emergency Psychiatry Project BETA Workgroup. (2012). Best practices in evaluation and treatment of agitation. *West J Emerg Med: Integrating Emergency Care with Population Health, 13*(1), 3–40.

Currier, G. W., & Medori, R. (2006). Orally versus intramuscularly administered antipsychotic drugs in psychiatric emergencies. *Journal of Psychiatric Practice, 12*(1), 30–40.

Dorfman, D. H. (2000). The use of physical and chemical restraints in the pediatric emergency department. *Pediatric Emergency Care, 16*, 355–360.

Downey, L. V., Zun, L. S., & Burke, T. (2015). Comparison of Canadian triage acuity scale to Australian emergency mental health scale triage system for psychiatric patients. *International Emergency Nursing, 23*(2), 138–143.

Ehrlich, S., Noam, G. G., Lyoo, I. K., Kwon, B. J., Clark, M. A., & Renshaw, P. F. (2004). White matter hyperintensities and their associations with suicidality in psychiatrically hospitalized children and adolescents. *Journal of the American Academy of Child and Adolescent Psychiatry, 43*(6), 770–776.

Evans, E., Hawton, K., Rodham, K., & Deeks, J. (2005). The prevalence of suicidal phenomenon in adolescents: A systematic review of population-based studies. *Suicide & Life-Threatening Behavior, 35*, 239–250.

Favazza, A. R. (1998). The coming of age of self-mutilation. *The Journal of Nervous and Mental Disease, 186*(5), 259–268.

Fergusson, D. M., & Lynskey, M. T. (1995). Childhood circumstances, adolescent adjustment and suicide attempts in a New Zealand birth cohort. *Journal of the American Academy of Child and Adolescent Psychiatry, 34*, 612–622.

Fergusson, D. M., Horwood, L. J., & Beautrais, A. L. (1999). Is sexual orientation related to mental health problems and sexuality in young people? *Archives of General Psychiatry, 56*, 876–880.

Gasquet, I., & Choquet, M. (1994). Hospitalization in a pediatric ward of adolescent suicide attempters admitted to general hospitals. *The Journal of Adolescent Health, 15*(5), 416–422.

Geulayov, G., Gunnell, D., Holmen, T. L., & Metcalfe, C. (2012). The association of parental fatal and non-fatal suicidal behaviour with offspring suicidal behaviour and depression: A systematic review and meta-analysis. *Psychological Medicine, 42*(8), 1567–1580.

Goldenring, J., & Cohen, E. (1988). Getting into adolescent heads. *Contemporary Pediatrics, 5*(7), 75.

González-Castro, T. B., Juárez-Rojop, I., López-Narváez, M. L., & Tovilla-Zárate, C. A. (2014). Association of TPH-1 and TPH-2 gene polymorphisms with suicidal behavior: A systematic review and meta-analysis. *BMC Psychiatry, 14*(1), 1.

Goodman, M., Hazlett, E. A., Avedon, J. B., Siever, D. R., Chu, K. W., & New, A. S. (2011). Anterior cingulate volume reduction in adolescents with borderline personality disorder and co-morbid major depression. *Journal of Psychiatric Research, 45*(6), 803–807.

Gosney, H., & Hawton, K. (2007). Inquest verdicts: Youth suicides lost. *Psychiatric Bulletin, 31*, 203–205.

Granboulan, V., Roudot-Thoraval, F., Lemerle, S., et al. (2001). Predictive factors of postdischarge follow-up care among adolescent suicide attempters. *Acta Psychiatrica Scandinavica, 104*, 31–36.

Gratz, K. L. (2001). Measurement of deliberate self-harm: Preliminary data on the deliberate self-harm inventory. *Journal of Psychopathology and Behavioral Assessment, 23*(4), 253–263. https://doi.org/10.1023/A:1012779403943.

Grudnikoff, E., Soto, E. C., Frederickson, A., Birnbaum, M. L., Saito, E., Dicker, R., Kane, J. M., & Correll, C. U. (2015). Suicidality and hospitalization as cause and outcome of pediatric psychiatric emergency room visits. *European Child & Adolescent Psychiatry, 24*(7), 797–814. https://doi.org/10.1007/s00787-014-0624-x.

Gutierrez, P. M., Osman, A., Barrios, F. X., & Kopper, B. A. (2001). Development and initial validation of the self-harm behavior questionnaire. *Journal of Personality Assessment, 77*, 475–490. https://doi.org/10.1207/S15327752JPA7703_08.

Hawton, K., & Harriss, L. (2007). Deliberate self-harm in young people: Characteristics and subsequent mortality in a 20-year cohort of patients presenting to hospital. *The Journal of Clinical Psychiatry, 68*(10), 1574–1583.

Hawton, K., Rodham, K., Evans, E., & Weatherall, R. (2002). Deliberate self-harm in adolescents: Self-report survey in schools in England. *British Medical Journal, 325*, 1207–1211.

Hawton, K., Hall, S., Simkin, S., Bale, L., Bond, A., Codd, S., & Stewart, A. (2003). Deliberate self-harm in adolescents: A study of characteristics and trends in Oxford, 1990–2000. *Journal of Child Psychology and Psychiatry, 44*(8), 1191–1198.

Hawton, K., Harriss, L., & Rodham, K. (2010). How adolescents who cut themselves differ from those who take overdoses. *European Child & Adolescent Psychiatry, 19*, 513–523.

Hawton, K., Saunders, K. E. A., & O'Connor, R. C. (2012). Self-harm and suicide in adolescents. *Lancet, 379*(9834), 2373–2382.

Hopper, S. M., Babl, F. E., Stewart, C. E., & Woo, J. W. (2012). Aggression management in a children's hospital setting. *The Medical Journal of Australia, 196*(3), 198–201.

Jellinek, M. S., Murphy, J. M., Robinson, J., Feins, A., Lamb, S., & Fenton, T. (1988). The pediatric symptom checklist: Screening school-age children for psychosocial dysfunction. *The Journal of Pediatrics, 112*, 201–209.

Jobes, D. A. (2006). *Managing suicidal risk: A collaborative approach*. New York: The Guilford Press.

Johnson, J. G., Cohen, P., Gould, M. S., Kasen, S., Brown, J., & Brook, J. S. (2002). Childhood adversities, interpersonal difficulties, and risk for suicide attempts during late adolescence and early adulthood. *Archives of General Psychiatry, 59*, 741–749.

Joint Commission International Accreditation Standards for Hospitals, 6th Edition. (2017). Assessed from http://www.jointcommissioninternational.org/

Kapur, N., Murphy, E., Jayne Cooper, J., et al. (2008). Psychosocial assessment following self-harm: Results from the multi-Centre monitoring of self-harm project. *Journal of Affective Disorders, 106*(3), 285–293.

Kay, S. R., Wolkenfelf, F., & Murrill, L. M. (1988). Profiles of aggression among psychiatric patients: I. Nature and prevalence. *The Journal of Nervous and Mental Disease, 176*, 539–546.

Latimer, E. A., Gariépy, G., & Greenfield, B. (2014). Cost-effectiveness of a rapid response team intervention for suicidal youth presenting at an emergency department. *Canadian Journal of Psychiatry, 59*(6), 310–318.

Laye-Gindhu, A., & Schonert-Reichl, K. A. (2005). Nonsuicidal self-harm among community adolescents: Understanding the "whats" and "whys" of self-harm. *Journal of Youth and Adolescence, 34*(5), 447–457. https://doi.org/10.1007/s10964-005-7262-z.

Lescano, C. M., Hadley, W. S., Beausoleil, N. I., et al. (2007). A brief screening measure of adolescent risk behavior. *Child Psychiatry and Human Development, 37*, 325–336. https://doi.org/10.1007/s10578-006-0037-2.

Li, D., & He, L. (2006). Further clarification of the contribution of the tryptophan hydroxylase (TPH) gene to suicidal behavior using systematic allelic and genotypic meta-analyses. *Human Genetics, 119*(3), 233–240.

Lloyd, E. E., Kelley, M. L., & Hope, T. (1997). *Self-mutilation in a community sample of adolescents: Descriptive characteristics and provisional prevalence rates*. Annual meeting of the Society for Behavioral Medicine, New Orleans, LA.

Lopez-Castroman, J., Nogue, E., Guillaume, S., Picot, M. C., & Courtet, P. (2016). Clustering suicide attempters: Impulsive-ambivalent, well-planned, or frequent. *Journal of Clinical Psychiatry, 77*(6), e711–e718. https://doi.org/10.4088/JCP.15m09882.

Madge, N., Hewitt, A., Hawton, K., Wilde, E. J., Corcoran, P., Fekete, S., Heeringen, K. B., De Leo, D., & Ystgaard, M. (2008). Deliberate self-harm within an international community sample of young people: Comparative findings from the child & adolescent self-harm in Europe (CASE) study. *Journal of Child Psychology and Psychiatry, 49*, 667–677. https://doi.org/10.1111/j.1469-7610.2008.01879.x.

Mann, J. J. (1998). The neurobiology of suicide. *Nature Medicine, 4*, 25–30.

Manor, I., Gutnik, I., Ben-Dor, D. H., et al. (2010). Possible association between attention deficit hyperactivity disorder and attempted suicide in adolescents – A pilot study. *European Psychiatry, 25*, 146–150.

Martin, A., & Volkmar, F. R. (Eds.). (2007). *Lewis' child and adolescent psychiatry: A comprehensive textbook* (4th ed.). Philadelphia: Lippincott Williams and Wilkins.

Masters, K. J., Bellonci, C., Bernet, W., Arnold, V., Beitchman, J., Benson, R. S., et al. (2002). Practice parameter for the prevention and management of aggressive behavior in child and adolescent psychiatric institutions, with special reference to seclusion and restraint. *Journal of the American Academy of Child and Adolescent Psychiatry, 41*(2 Suppl), 4S–25S. https://doi.org/10.1097/00004583-200202001-00002.

McAneney, C. M., & Shaw, K. N. (1994). Violence in the pediatric emergency department. *Annals of Emergency Medicine, 23*(6), 1248–1251.

Montreuil, M., Butler, K. J. D., Stachura, M., & Pugnaire Gros, C. (2015). Exploring helpful nursing care in pediatric mental health settings: The perceptions of children with suicide risk factors and their parents. *Mental Health Nursing, 36*(11), 849–859. https://doi.org/10.3109/01612840.2015.1075235.

Muehlenkamp, J. J., Claes, L., Havertape, L., & Plener, P. L. (2012). International prevalence of adolescent non-suicidal self-injury and deliberate self-harm. *Journal of Child and Adolescent Psychiatric and Mental Health Nursing, 6*, 10. https://doi.org/10.1186/1753-2000-6-10.

NICE Guideline. (2013). *Mental health crisis care: Physical restraint in crisis*. A report on physical restraint in hospital settings in England.

NICE Guideline. (2014). *Rapid tranquillisation in mental health settings: Promethazine hydrochloride*. Retrieved from: https://www.nice.org.uk/advice/esuom28/chapter/key-points-from-the-evidence

NICE Guideline. (2015). *Violence and aggression: Short-term management in mental health, health and community settings*. Retrieved from: https://www.nice.org.uk/guidance/ng10

Nock, M. K. (2010). Self-injury. *Annual Review of Clinical Psychology, 6*, 339–363. https://doi.org/10.1146/annurev.clinpsy.121208.131258.

Nock, M. K., Joiner, T. E., Jr., Gordon, K. H., Lloyd-Richardson, E., & Prinstein, M. J. (2006). Non-suicidal self-injury among adolescents: Diagnostic correlates and relation to suicide attempts. *Psychiatry Research, 144*, 65–72. https://doi.org/10.1016/j.psychres.2006.05.010.

Nock, M. K., Holmberg, E. B., Photos, V. I., & Michel, B. D. (2007). Self-injurious thoughts and behaviors interview: Development, reliability, and validity in an adolescent sample. *Psychological Assessment, 19*, 309–317. https://doi.org/10.1037/1040-3590.19.3.309.

O'Carroll, P. W. (1996). Beyond the tower of babel: A nomenclature for Suicidology. *Suicide & Life-Threatening Behavior, 26*(3), 237–252.

O'Connor, R. C., Rasmussen, S., Miles, J., & Hawton, K. (2009a). Self-harm in adolescents: Self-report survey in schools in Scotland. *The British Journal of Psychiatry, 194*, 68–72. https://doi.org/10.1192/bjp.bp.107.047704.

O'Connor, R. C., Rasmussen, S., & Hawton, K. (2009b). Predicting deliberate self-harm in adolescents: A six month prospective study. *Suicide & Life-Threatening Behavior, 39*, 364–375. https://doi.org/10.1521/suli.2009.39.4.364.

O'Connor, S. S., Jobes, D. A., Yeargin, M. K., FitzGerald, M. E., Rodríguez, V. M., Conrad, A. K., & Lineberry, T. W. (2012). A cross-sectional investigation of the suicidal spectrum: typologies of suicidality based on ambivalence about living and dying. *Comprehensive Psychiatry, 53*(5), 461–467. https://doi.org/10.1016/j.comppsych.2011.09.007.

Olfson, M., Gameroff, M. J., Marcus, S. C., Greenberg, T., & Shaffer, D. (2005). Emergency treatment of young people following deliberate self-harm. *Archives of General Psychiatry, 62*, 1122–1128. https://doi.org/10.1001/archpsyc.62.10.1122.

Ougrin, D., Zundel, T., Ng, A., Banarsee, R., Bottle, A., & Taylor, E. (2010). Trial of therapeutic assessment in London: Randomised controlled trial of therapeutic assessment versus standard psychosocial assessment in adolescents presenting with self-harm. *Archives of Disease in Childhood, 96*(2), 1–6. https://doi.org/10.1136/adc.2010.188755.

Pandey, G. N., Dwivedi, Y., Rizavi, H. S., Ren, X., Pandey, S. C., Pesold, C., Roberts, R. C., Conley, R. R., & Tamminga, C. A. (2002). Higher expression of serotonin 5-HT2A receptors in the postmortem brains of teenage suicide victims. *The American Journal of Psychiatry, 159*(3), 419–429.

Pappadopulos, E., Macintyre, J. C., Crismon, M. L., et al. (2003). Treatment recommendations for the use of antipsychotics for aggressive youth (TRAAY). Part II. *Journal of the American Academy of Child and Adolescent Psychiatry, 42*(2), 145–161.

Parker, K. C., Roberts, N., Williams, C., Benjamin, M., Cripps, L., & Woogh, C. (2003). Urgent adolescent psychiatric consultation: From the accident and emergency department to inpatient adolescent psychiatry. *Journal of Adolescence, 26*(3), 283–293.

Patton, G. C., Coffey, C., Sawyer, S. M., et al. (2009). Global patterns of mortality in young people: A systematic analysis of population health data. *Lancet, 374*, 881–892. https://doi.org/10.1016/S0140-6736(09)60741-8.

Pereira, S., Gard, D., & Brandford, D. (2009). *Rapid tranquilisation of acutely disturbed patient.* Royal College of Psychiatrists, CPD online www.rcpsych.ac.uk

Pillay, A. L., & Wassenaar, D. R. (1995). Psychological intervention, spontaneous remission, hopelessness, and psychiatric disturbance in adolescent parasuicides. *Suicide & Life-Threatening Behavior, 25*, 386–392.

Pridmore, S., & Jamil, M. Y. (2009). Two models of suicide. *Australasn Psychiatry, 17*(6), 466–471. https://doi.org/10.1080/10398560903281824.

Rossberg, J. I., & Frills, S. (2003). Staff members emotional reactions to aggressive and suicidal behavior of inpatients. *Psychiatric Services, 54*, 1388–1394.

Santiago, L. I., Tunik, M. G., Foltin, G. L., & Mojica, M. A. (2006). Children requiring psychiatric consultation in the pediatric emergency department: Epidemiology, resource utilization, and complications. *Pediatric Emergency Care, 22*(2), 85–89. https://doi.org/10.1097/01.pec.0000199568.94758.6e.

Santucci, K. A., Sather, J., & Baker, M. D. (2003). Emergency medicine training programs' educational requirements in the management of psychiatric emergencies: Current perspective. *Pediatric Emergency Care, 19*(3), 154–156. https://doi.org/10.1097/01.pec.0000081235.20228.7a.

Sher, L., & LaBode, V. (2011). Teaching health care professionals about suicide safety planning. *Psychiatria Danubina, 23*(4), 396–397.

Sheridan, D. C., Spiro, D. M., Fu, R., Johnson, K. P., Sheridan, J. S., Oue Alyssa, A., Wang, W., Van Nes, R., & Matthew, H. L. (2015). Mental health utilization in a pediatric emergency department. *Pediatric Emergency Care, 31*(8), 555–559. https://doi.org/10.1097/PEC.0000000000000343.

Smart, D., Pollard, C., & Walpole, B. (1999). Mental health triage in emergency medicine. *Australian and New Zealand Journal of Psychiatry, 33*, 57–66.

Sonnier, L., & Barzman, D. (2011). Pharmacologic management of acutely agitated pediatric patients. *Paediatric Drugs, 13*(1), 1–10. https://doi.org/10.2165/11538550-000000000-00000.

Spirito, A., & Esposito-Smythers, C. (2006). Attempted and completed suicide in adolescence. *Annual Review of Clinical Psychology, 2*, 237–266. https://doi.org/10.1146/annurev.clinpsy.2.022305.095323.

Stefan, S. (2006). *Emergency department treatment of the psychiatric patient: Policy issues and legal requirements* (1st ed.p. 232). Oxford: Oxford University Press.

Steffen, S., Kösters, M., Becker, T., & Puschner, B. (2009). Discharge planning in mental health care: A systematic review of the recent literature. *Acta Psychiatrica Scandinavica, 120*(1), 1–9. https://doi.org/10.1111/j.1600-0447.2009.01373.x.

Stone, A., Rogers, D., Kruckenberg, S., & Lieser, A. (2012). Impact of the mental health care delivery system on California emergency departments. *Western Jounal of Emergency Medicine: Integrating Emergency Care with Population Health, 13*(1), 51–56. https://doi.org/10.5811/westjem.2011.6.6732.

Swann, A. C. (2003). Neuroreceptor mechanisms of aggression and its treatment. *The Journal of Clinical Psychiatry, 64*(suppl 4), 26–35.

Swift, R. H., Harrigan, E. P., Cappelleri, J. C., Kramer, D., & Chandler, L. P. (2002). Validation of the behavioural activity rating scale (BARS): A novel measure of activity in agitated patients. *Journal of Psychiatric Research, 36*(2), 87–95.

Taliaferro, L. A., Muehlenkamp, J. J., Borowsky, I. W., McMorris, B. J., & Kugler, K. C. (2012). Factors distinguishing youth who report self-injurious behavior: A population-based sample. *of adolescents. Acad Pediatrics, 12*(3), 205–213.

Ting, S. A., Sullivan, A. F., Boudreaux, E. D., Miller, I., & Camargo, C. A., Jr. (2012). Trends in US emergency department visits for attempted suicide and self-inflicted injury, 1993–2008. *General Hospital Psychiatry, 34*(5), 557–565. https://doi.org/10.1016/j.genhosppsych.2012.03.020. Epub 2012 May 2.

Vigod, S. N., Kurdyak, P. A., Dennis, C. L., Leszcz, T., Taylor, V. H., Blumberger, D. M., & Seitz, D. P. (2013). Transitional interventions to reduce early psychiatric readmissions in adults: Systematic review. *The British Journal of Psychiatry, 202*(3), 187–194. https://doi.org/10.1192/bjp.bp.112.115030.

Voracek, M., & Loibl, L. M. (2007). Genetics of suicide: A systematic review of twin studies. *Wiener Klinische Wochenschrift, 119*(15–16), 463–475.

Wasserman, D., Cheng, Q., & Jiang, G. X. (2005). Global suicide rates among young people aged 15–19. *World Psychiatry, 4*, 114–120.

World Health Organization. (2014). *Preventing suicide: A global imperative*. Geneva: WHO.

Zimbroff, D. L. (2008). Pharmacological control of acute agitation: Focus on intramuscular preparations. *CNS Drugs, 22*(3), 199–212.

Zlotnick, C., Shea, T. M., Pearlstein, T., Simpson, E., Costello, E., & Begin, A. (1996). The relationship between dissociative symptoms, alexithymia, impulsivity, sexual abuse, and self-mutilation. *Comprehensive Psychiatry, 37*, 12–16.

Chapter 6
Eating and Feeding Disorders

Fiona McNicholas and Sara McDevitt

Introduction

Given the salient role that feeding (and eating) play in health and well-being, family functioning and relationship development, emotional regulation and the relatively frequent presentation of eating and feeding disorders, it is understandable that these difficulties are high priority in Pediatric Consultation-Liaison Psychiatry. Using case examples, this chapter reviews the clinical presentation of feeding and eating disorders throughout development, using DSM 5 diagnostic criteria, and suggests a potentially helpful assessment framework and a typical treatment plan.

Changes in the current DSM V diagnostic classification have (2014) included the addition of feeding disorders (FD), based on recognition that many individuals with eating disorders (ED) often had a previous history of childhood feeding difficulties (Uher and Rutter 2012) and that many mothers with either current or past ED have difficulty in feeding their infants (Agras et al. 1999), and the addition of binge eating disorder.

Feeding Disorders

DSM 5 lists three feeding disorders that, although typically presenting in childhood, can also present in adolescence or adulthood: (1) avoidant/restrictive food intake disorder, replacing DSM IV ‘feeding disorder of infancy or early childhood’, (2)

F. McNicholas (✉)
Child Psychiatry, University College Dublin, Dublin, Republic of Ireland
e-mail: Fiona.mcnicholas@ucd.ie

S. McDevitt
Child Psychiatry, HSE, Cork, Republic of Ireland
e-mail: sara.mcdevitt@hse.ie

A. P. S. Guerrero et al. (eds.), *Pediatric Consultation-Liaison Psychiatry*,
https://doi.org/10.1007/978-3-319-89488-1_6

Table 6.1 Classification of feeding disorders in infants and toddlers

Specific type	Typical age onset/ developmental phase	Main features
Feeding disorder of state regulation	Newborn period	Infant has difficulty regulating their arousal level to allow for effective feeding
Feeding disorder of reciprocity	2–6 months of age	Significant difficulties in social reciprocity and responsivity
Infantile anorexia	Often at transition to self-feeding	Lack of hunger or interest in food leading to inadequate food intake often accompanied by difficulties in infant-caregiver interactions
Sensory food aversions	Often at introduction of solid feeding	Avoidance often limited to specific food types, based on tastes, textures, appearance or smells. Normal ingestion of other foods
Feeding disorder associated with medical conditions	Can occur at any age	Concurrent medical condition often interfering with eating (cardiac) or leading to distress or pain (reflux)
Posttraumatic feeding disorder	Can occur at any age	Food refusal following traumatic medical (nasogastric [NG] feeding) or physiological (vomiting) events, leading to fear and avoidance

Chatoor (2002)

pica and (3) rumination disorder. This new classification shares many of the salient features present in the DSM IV criteria and also includes conditions proposed to occur at any age. Chatoor proposed several discrete syndromes, most occurring during infancy and childhood and associated with inadequate nutrition and growth failure (Chatoor 2002). Although these syndromes have not been universally accepted (Uher and Rutter 2012), elements are present in the current DSM V categories and highlight the interplay between infant and carer (Table 6.1). The salient role that feeding (and eating) plays in the development of interpersonal relationships and emotional regulation has been central to many of the proposed classifications, leading some researchers to conceptualise them fundamentally as a relational disorder and best termed 'Feeding Disorder Between Parent and Child' (Davies et al. 2006).

Case 6.1: Thomas

A 9-year-old boy, Thomas, was transferred from a local general hospital to a large paediatric hospital because of severe and rapid weight and an almost complete failure/refusal to eat. He was previously managed by his family doctor following a 1-week history of gastroenteritis with projectile vomiting and diarrhoea. He was slow to return to normal eating post recovery and remained fatigued and reluctant to attend school. After a 1-month period of failed treatment by his community primary care physician, he was admitted to his local hospital with continuing weight loss, increasing oppositionality around eating and increasing family discord. He accepted intravenous fluids but steadfastly refused to take any oral nutrition. After 2 weeks with further and significant weight loss, he was transferred to a paediatric hospital for the management of what was termed 'possible anorexia nervosa'.

You ponder how would you go about assessing this child?

'If-Me' Model of Assessment

For feeding disorders, it may be helpful to specifically assess (according to the If-Me or 'If it were Me going to a psychiatrist, what would I want in an assessment' mnemonic) individual, family, medical and environmental factors that contribute to the presenting complaint.

Assessment of Individual Symptoms The clinician needs to establish the child's food-related symptoms, their meaning, duration, development, associated impairment and other symptoms, including depression, anxiety or delusions.

Case 6.2

Thomas' food refusal was driven by an intense fear of vomiting rather than by fear of fatness, as would be typical in anorexia nervosa. Thomas described, because of the aversive experience of projectile vomiting while sick, an intense fear of vomiting that led to phobic avoidance of food, initially high-fat foods (which had been associated with most marked indigestion) but subsequently all foods other than clear fluids. His anxiety levels were pervasively high, and he dreaded the next attempt by family or medical staff to provide nutrition. This dread led to increasing bouts of oppositional behaviour, directed most prominently at his mother.

Assessing Family Factors and Parenting It is important to assess – general and especially more recent parenting styles – how parents have tried to intervene, how they generally relate to this child and their other children, membership of the family unit, family functioning and presence of any family psychopathology that might perpetuate the difficulty or interfere with treatment.

Case 6.3

In Thomas' case, a discussion about the family led the clinician to understand that the mother recently lost her father to pancreatic cancer 3 months prior to Thomas' gastroenteritis. Her father had many gastrointestinal symptoms, including vomiting, and she was aware of the salience of this symptom for Thomas. Mother was very close to her father and was bereft after his death. On reflection, she believes that Thomas's vomiting traumatised her by bringing flashbacks of her father's last weeks, and she opted out of her normal parenting role. Her husband, a successful but busy full-time farmer, was typically not involved in the homemaking or parenting and was unable to compensate for her withdrawal. Thomas' ongoing difficulty around eating, his reluctance to attend school, his demandingness on her time and the different parental perspectives on how best to manage these challenges led to significant inter-parental and family discord, which was uncharacteristic of the family functioning. Thomas' 15-year-old twin siblings, per mother's opinion, seemed relatively unaffected by the situation and had no history of mental health difficulties.

Studies of children with other feeding disorders have found certain caregiver risk characteristics, including tendencies of the mother to be more controlling and coercive in the feeding situation, to use physical punishment or force feeding and to be more angry and hostile in child interactions (Chatoor et al. 1998, Stice et al. 1999, Allen et al. 2014). In nonfeeding situations parents have also been observed to be less flexible, less affectionate and less attuned to emotional signals from the child, in turn more likely to appear withdrawn (Feldman et al. 2004). Parents with their own eating difficulties were found, in comparison to controls, to display more negativity and conflict during meal times and to have more negative infants (Stein et al. 1994). This interplay between parent and child has led some researchers to propose that feeding disorders should be conceptualised as 'relational disorders' (Davies et al. 2006). This interplay highlights the importance of conducting a good assessment of parenting, examining the relationship between parent and child and enquiring about the caregiver's mental health along with their relationship with food.

Assessing Medical Domain In Thomas' case, assessment of the medical domain includes assessment of immediate medical risk, along with medical developmental history. In general, a detailed dietary history must be collected, recording the exact amount and type of food being eaten, calculating the total daily calorie intake and estimating any deficits and duration of these deficits. Documenting a weight history by establishing the premorbid weight, recording actual weight loss and calculating the deviation from a mean body weight give an indication of the duration and severity of the nutritional deficit. Laboratory investigations will further refine the assessment of medical risk and will point to various interventions.

Case 6.4

Thomas presented after a 2-week period on predominantly IV dextrose, with fewer than 500 calories per day, placing him at a very high risk of refeeding. When Thomas was admitted, he weighed 55lbs (9th percentile), and his height was estimated at 4 feet 5 inches (37th percentile), giving him a current BMI (wt/ht2) of 13.8 (< 3rd percentile). A previous weight, 4 months prior to his illness, was 65lbs, (BMI 16.3, 50th percentile) representing a 15% drop in weight. Given that the mean male BMI at age 9 is 16.8, Thomas % mean BMW (also referred to as ideal body weight or IBW) was 82%, significantly lower. He appeared lethargic, had muscle wasting and hypotonia and had poor cardiac reserve with bradycardia (40 bpm), electrolyte disturbances (raised urea, low potassium and calcium) and hypothermia. Mother reported that Thomas met all his developmental milestones at the appropriate age and was medically well. He was perceived to be somewhat anxious, and 'measured', preferring familiarity to novelty and being slow to trying new foods and new activities. These traits had been accommodated by his family, and despite a somewhat selective diet and cautious personality, they were not viewed as impairing.

A clinical history is often enriched by observations of a feeding interaction, which might uncover developmental and medical factors and highlight any discordant relationships and coercive experiences. Clinical examination will assess general development, postural control, swallowing and sensory integration, which are all potential contributions to feeding disorders. The clinician may also wish to use a caregiver questionnaire to supplement clinical history and observations and to offer a more holistic and multi-rater perspective. The psychometric properties and clinical utility of several feeding questionnaires were reviewed by Sanchez et al. (2015), who recommended the Behavioural Paediatric Feeding Assessment Scale.

Assessing Environmental Domain This domain will typically encompass the young child's academic and behavioural progress at school along with their peer relationships. Additionally, it includes any psychosocial adversities in the home and neighbourhood. Even in affluent nations, poverty and lack of food continue to be a significant factor in feeding problems (Casey et al. 2001).

Case 6.5

An assessment of Thomas' environment suggested minimal stressors linked with academic or peer activities. He was perceived as an able and willing student, albeit somewhat perfectionistic and high achieving. He was likeable and had a small number of close friends. His only post-school activities were weekly attendance at chess club and scouts.

A diagnosis of avoidant/restrictive food intake disorder was made.

Avoidant/Restrictive Food Intake Disorder (ARFID)

The salient feature in this diagnostic category is difficulty or severe disinterest in eating (or, in an infant, being fed) leading to inadequate nutritional intake and weight loss (or, in growing children, failure to maintain weight trajectory). The reasons leading to such difficulties are many but do 'not' involve a prominent fear of weight gain or body image distortion, as would be typical in anorexia nervosa (Bryant Waugh 2013). Additionally, these difficulties may present at any age across the lifespan, not just during infancy or childhood. Although specific aetiologies are not assumed or required, examples of putative aetiological causes include, as in the case of Thomas, a reaction to a previous aversive experience, where choking or severe vomiting induces anticipatory anxiety upon eating, which is subsequently avoided. Other aetiologies include idiosyncratic preferences for various food textures, appearances, smells and tastes, often linked with other sensitivities. In ARFID, the eating disturbance must not be because of a concurrent medical or psychiatric condition, such as depression leading to a loss of appetite.

Prevalence of Feeding Problems Transient, non-impairing and self-limiting food restriction is common and occurs in up to 25% of children (Jacobi et al. 2008). If general feeding problems are considered, the prevalence in typically developing children increases to almost 1 in 2, linked with temporary weight or relationship difficulties that fall short of a more formal 'feeding disorder' (Linscheid et al. 2003). General feeding problems account for the commonest reason for primary caregiver consultations in the preschool age (Arvedson 2008). It is only when the difficulty persists, linked with weight percentile trajectory deviations, nutritional deficiency or significant interpersonal relationships, that it is considered pathological, with the child requiring additional high-calorie enteral nutritional supplements.

The prevalence of feeding problems is higher in children with developmental delay or attending specialists' clinics such as gastroenterology, speech and language or genetics clinics, where 8% met formal diagnostic criteria (Williams et al. 2009). When broader diagnostic criteria are applied, such as those suggested by Chatoor, up to 80% of children with developmental difficulties have feeding problems (1994). These may arise from structural or functional abnormalities, including oro-pharyngeal skills deficits, cleft lip or palate as may occur in 22q11 deletion syndrome or gastrointestinal reflux linking feeding and swallowing with pain and generating an aversive experience. Neurological issues such as cerebral palsy, leading to low muscle tone and dysphagia, may also be contributory and evident upon observation. Children with feeding problems also often have subclinical symptoms of obsessive-compulsive disorder, anxiety or autism (Schreck et al. 2004). Although some of these features were present in the case presented, as with many other cases, Thomas did not meet full diagnostic criteria for either autism or anxiety.

Additionally, aspects of the mother (carer)-child relationship may contribute, with suboptimal feeding experiences being linked with, for example, a mother being unaware of developmental stages or nutritional needs, unaware of child's inability to sit upright and self-feed or fearful of the infant choking, leading to delayed or shortened solid feeding and a transfer of anxiety to the infant. A mother with her own eating and body image-related concerns may control both food types and amounts offered to her child, along with meal time in general. Environmental factors, especially social adversity, poverty and lack of opportunity, may also play a part. The assessment of these difficulties requires a biopsychosocial approach, with an awareness of the often-combined contribution from several sources (Davies et al. 2006).

Treatment of Feeding Disorders

To date there are no evidenced-based guidelines for the treatment of ARFID, or indeed other feeding disorders, due to their recent conceptualisation. Given the differences in aetiological associations, it is likely that the treatment of feeding disorders, especially ARFID, will include cognitive, behavioural and psychological interventions and at times expert input from a multidisciplinary team, including mental health clinicians, paediatricians, dieticians and occupational and speech and language therapists. The body of evidence supporting the effectiveness of certain interventions appears to be growing, as indicated by publications in many varied journals (Strandjord et al. 2015).

The goal of treatment, based on a collaborative approach involving the young person, their family and the treating team, is to have the young person eating normally and adequately again. At a basic level, the focus is to have the child eat and subsequently to address other domains that may mediate or moderate their feeding problems. Once the medical risk has been stabilised, treatment typically commences by establishing the young person's motivation to engage and establish their position in the stages of change model (Prochaska et al. 2008). Clinicians need to enlist the support of their parent to a degree based on the child's maturity and ability to engage yet giving the responsibility for the feeding and treatment plan to parents. Information about what constitutes a healthy diet, the food pyramid and energy requirements and changes linked with puberty are all possible motivators in an otherwise disinterested or scared child.

A cBT (cognitive behavioural therapy) approach is used, with the small 'c' representing the degree of cognitive work that is commensurate with a child's developmental age and capacity to use metacognition, i.e. thinking about thinking. The plan includes behavioural experiments where new foods are added based on a hierarchy, beginning with foods deemed easiest or 'most wanted', i.e. foods that allow social reintegration, such as popcorn and pizza. The management of food-related anxiety is important, as oftentimes the food restriction is in response to some aversive experience, and sometimes even the thought or presentation of food is enough to re-traumatise the child. Anxiety symptoms may also be comorbid. Mindfulness allows for a more focused awareness of bodily sensations, including anxiety and autonomic instability with the approach of food or meal times. Practising relaxation, guided imagery and biofeedback may all be helpful. Family support is essential, as family may well have struggled heroically for long periods, particularly with AFRID, prior to seeking treatment (Forman et al. 2014). Parents may need help in reestablishing healthy meal time approaches and interactions with their child. They may need to examine their own prejudices regarding forbidden and unhealthy foods, and they may need to be reminded to separate their child from their illness through the process of externalisation (White and Epston 1990).

What factors do you think are relevant to target in Thomas' case?

Treatment of AFRID

Case 6.6

*Thomas was initially fed nasogastrically with small amounts of calories that were increased to his typical daily caloric intake by day 7. He was encouraged to take oral fluids in monitored amounts. The team used the 'IFME' framework. From individual assessment, there was no evidence that Thomas had any desire to be thin, there was no body image distortion and/or unwillingness to consider an appropriate range of calorie-dense foods. His current food preferences were not based on any sensory issues outside of the potential for a food item to get 'stuck in his throat' and to cause gagging and vomiting, his ultimate fear. He identified an acceptable range of 'less chokey foods'. The dietician introduced food items into his meal plan, starting with very small portions (*e.g. *one spoon of plain yoghurt, two spoons custard, one softened Weetabix) that were increased to more typical amounts with a corresponding reduction in the NG amounts. Thomas was coached in progressive muscle* *relaxation, deliberately starting with a focus on his feet, as far away from his mouth as possible. Guided mourning assisted the mother to overcome her grief and to be more available to the family unit. Family discussions led to a hierarchical shift, in which both parents were repositioned firmly at the top and in which siblings formed a supportive sibship group for Thomas. Attendance at hospital school allowed Thomas to experience social and academic engagement, which improved his mood. Consistent weight gain, normalisation of physical and laboratory tests and increasing food repertoire led Thomas to be more confident about trying increasing amounts of 'chokey' foods, and about trying these off the ward, starting with the hospital coffee shop and subsequently sites outside of the hospital. Following successful overnight leaves, Thomas was discharged from the hospital 4 weeks later with some food supplements. Thomas was followed up as an outpatient for ongoing review and growth monitoring, family-focussed work and individually focused cBT. His final review 18 months post-admission showed him to have regained his weight trajectory, with minimal residual anxiety symptoms and no food-related worries. His mother, who returned to work, reported more parenting competence and described a relaxed, happy household.*

Picky Eating

Picky eating refers to a child's tendency to eat a preferred but restrictive diet, to be avoidant of trying new foods (food neophobia), to exhibit strong likes and dislikes and to insist of food being prepared or served in certain ways, in the context of normal weight. Adherence to this repertoire may severely restrict nutritional intake (Carruth et al. 2004), may cause growth retardation (Dovey et al. 2008) and may contribute to family conflict (Mascola et al. 2010). A child's refusal to eat certain foods, or to insist that parents prepare separate meals, has been linked with other behavioural problems and may represent an effort of the child to exert their autonomy. Other behavioural problems, such as temper tantrums, sleeping problems or oppositional-defiant behaviour, may coexist and may need to be the focus of treatment, with the management of picky eating being secondary (Jacobi et al. 2008; Mascola et al. 2010; Rydell et al. 1995). Successful treatment of clinically significant picky eating involves careful assessment of not only the food consumed but also the feeding and general relationship of the child and caregiver. An integrated treatment approach is often required.

Previously and occasionally still referred to as selective eating, fussy or faddy eating, or food avoidance, picky eating is common (Cardona Cano et al. 2015; Timimi et al. 1997), with prevalence ranging between 14% and 50% in early childhood (Dubois et al. 2007; Carruth et al. 2004) and decreasing with age (Mascola et al. 2010). Usually short lived and resolving by middle childhood, many prospective longitudinal studies have shown that a significant minority persist into adulthood (Jacobi et al. 2008). Some cases have their onset in adolescence (Van Tine et al. 2017). Concerns about the pathologising of picky eating as a psychiatric disorder (Kirkey 2012) have been raised and in part reflect the lack of standardised definition and conflicting descriptions from studies that recruit different populations and that have heterogeneous samples (Norris et al. 2016). The inclusion of picky eating under the ED section might be understandable given the increased awareness, from several longitudinal studies, of the risk for subsequent disordered eating (Kotler et al. 2001, Van Tine et al. 2017, Mascola et al. 2010; Rydell et al. 1995). In the case presented above, although Thomas had many features of picky eating, i.e. preferred foods, his premorbid overall food intake was less restrictive, with severe selectivity being clearly linked with fear of choking or vomiting and resolving successfully following treatment.

Pica and Rumination Disorder

'Pica' refers to a 1 month or longer period of nonnutritive or non-food substance ingestion that is neither culturally sanctioned nor developmentally appropriate. This behaviour is also not part of another mental health disorder or, if so, is sufficiently severe to merit attention. Medical complications, such as bowel obstruction or infections, are more likely to uncover this behaviour than any nutrient or vitamin deficiency, as often there is adequate nutritional intake. Although there are no community studies on the prevalence, it is more common in children and individuals with autism or intellectual disability and can occur temporarily in pregnancy. Treatment, although not well studied, typically involves behavioural interventions and environmental manipulations.

Pica is distinguished from eating as part of culturally sanctioned or socially normative practices, i.e. ingestion of clay, mud or lime in India may be viewed to be spiritually desirable. As with most FD, the onset is usually but not exclusively in childhood. Pica may occur in pregnancy or as part of autism spectrum disorder, but for a diagnosis to be given, it should be severe enough to warrant independent clinical attention.

'Rumination disorder' refers to the regurgitation of previous chewing or swallowed food, in an effortless manner and without disgust or distress. Regurgitated food may be subsequently swallowed or spat out. As with pica, a minimum duration of 1 month is required, with behaviour occurring most often daily and not part of an eating or other mental health disorder. Unlike pica, rumination disorder is more often associated with failure to thrive, failure to gain weight or hunger states, especially in younger children if food is not re-swallowed. In older individuals, social etiquette may also lead to an avoidance of social eating resulting in weight loss. As with pica, it is more common in individuals with autism or intellectual disability, but exact prevalence rates are not available. Although generally assumed to be more common in early childhood, some studies have suggested a mean age of onset in young adolescence (Chial et al. 2003). Treatment is usually behavioural, but further study is necessary.

Table 6.2 DSM V criteria for eating disorders

	Anorexia nervosa (AN)	Bulimia nervosa (BN)	Binge eating disorder (BED)
Weight/BMI	Significantly underweight		
Fear of wt gain/ fatness	Intense		
Body image/shape disturbance	Significant		
Recognition of seriousness of weight loss	Absent		
Emotions			Disgust, depression, guilt and marked distress
Feeling of control		Lack of control	Lack of control
Restricted energy intake	Persistent		
Self-evaluation		Linked with shape/weight	Linked with shape/weight
Binging	Less likely	Significant amount 1/ week × 3/12 months	Significant amount 1/ week × 3/12 months
Purging (vomiting, laxatives)	Only if binge-purge subtype	1/week × 3/12 months	
Excessive exercising	Can occur	Can occur	
Subtypes	Restricting		
	Binge purging		
Notes		Not exclusively during AN	Not exclusively in AN/BN

Eating Disorders in Children and Adolescents

Anorexia Nervosa

Originally described in 1873 by Sir William Gull, anorexia nervosa (AN) is the most commonly presenting eating disorder in the acute hospital setting. DSM V made two key changes that enhance its applicability to the child and adolescent age group. Firstly, it removed the criteria of amenorrhoea, so it can now fully apply to prepubertal girls, girls with primary amenorrhoea and boys. Secondly, it did away with a strict weight guideline of less than 85% and specifically includes the concept of developmental trajectory. The diagnosis of an 'atypical anorexia' is considered when not all of the AN criteria are met (see Table 6.2), e.g. a child's weight is within the normal range, but their weight loss is very significant as the child was in the obese range to begin with. Atypical anorexia nervosa is classed as an 'other specified feeding or eating disorder (OSFED)' within DSM V.

Epidemiology

The lifetime community prevalence of anorexia nervosa in adolescents has been estimated at 0.3% (Swanson et al. 2011) and as high as 1% in other studies. An even higher proportion of adolescents report subthreshold symptoms of anorexia nervosa (McNicholas et al. 2010), while within the younger paediatric population group (8–15 years), eating disorders and anorexia are less common (0.1%). However, anorexia nervosa is the most common eating disorder diagnosed in the younger paediatric population, and its median age of onset in the paediatric population is 12.3 years (Swanson et al. 2011). The female/male gender ratio in childhood is much less pronounced at 2:1 (CDC 2013 accessed 2016), with female preponderance then developing during adolescence. A comprehensive study of primary care databases in the UK reported incidence rates of 13.1 per 100,000 in the 10–14-year-old group and 26.7 per 100,000 in the 15–19-year-old group (Micali et al. 2013). Incidence appears to be rising.

Aetiology

Anorexia nervosa has complex biopsychosocial origins that are not yet fully understood. Several twin, adoption and family studies indicate that genetic factors play a key role in determining vulnerability to developing anorexia, with heritability estimates of 50–60% most commonly reported (Trace et al. 2013). Heritability is likely to involve several additive genetic factors, including phenotypic variations of noradrenergic, serotonergic and dopaminergic systems; endocrine, leptin and appetite centres; and obesity receptors. Epigenetic factors that may then influence phenotypic expression of anorexia nervosa may include the phenotypic effects of feeding difficulties, starvation and puberty (Yilmaz et al. 2015, Zerwas and Bulik 2011).

Psychological Factors

Certain premorbid child and adolescent temperamental and personality traits have also been associated with a higher risk of developing anorexia nervosa and include perfectionism, obsessive-compulsive traits, anxious temperament, low self-esteem and harm avoidance (Anderluh et al. 2003; Jacobs et al. 2009; Gillberg et al. 2005; Fan et al. 2010). Premorbid body dissatisfaction has been noted in children as young as 8 years (Micali et al. 2015), who subsequently are more likely to overvalue their identity around appearance and control of food intake. Medical conditions such as diabetes mellitus and coeliac disease, where children have learned to count or restrict calories and avoid carbohydrates and other food types, and a high focus on athletic and gymnastic success also predispose genetically vulnerable children to developing an eating disorder, to manipulating their eating to cause weight change or to increase athletic performance (Bachle et al. 2016).

Social Influences

While social factors alone do not cause anorexia nervosa, they no doubt are associated with development and maintenance of AN particularly in adolescents. The socio-cultural pursuit of thinness, idealised by magazines, media and social media, has significantly contributed to body dissatisfaction in all ages, especially during the critical developmental stage of identity formation and socio-emotional growth (Harrison 2000, Goncalves et al. 2012). In a time of unparalleled access to social media in younger adolescents, this is important as both a risk and maintaining factor. Such influence may be mediated though the family's idealisation of thinness and attitudes towards eating, social interests and peer competition (Ferguson et al. 2012). Children and adolescents with anorexia nervosa often identify a precipitating critical life event, often bullying, peer conflict, family stressor, childhood trauma and abuse or negative change event. Such social factors may trigger a cycle of eating disorder behaviour and psychopathology that then becomes embedded. While much of the literature on anorexia nervosa is based in westernised cultures, this is an eating disorder that occurs globally, across culture, ethnicity and geographical boundaries.

Case 6.7: Amy

Amy is a 15-year-old teenager who sees her family doctor, Dr. Johnson, for a history, as reported by the mother, of noticeable weight loss (about 20 pounds) over the last 6 months. Previously of average weight and with good health, Amy has dropped three clothes sizes and has become irritable and tired. She has also withdrawn from family and friends. Amy announced 4 months ago that she had become vegan, and she is 'obsessed' with healthy eating magazines and Instagram pictures of models. She is a keen gymnast, but her mother is very concerned that her physical activity has become extreme. On two occasions recently, she became faint at school and was sent home, and her performance at gym has suffered. Amy is a bright student and has always pushed herself to do well, so this setback upset her greatly. She thinks she might need a multivitamin to help her concentrate and have more energy at school. Her mother thinks she may have an eating disorder: a few friends have had eating issues, as did an aunt.

How would you screen and assess Amy using the 'If-Me' framework, as described above?

Screening for Eating Disorders

Children and adolescents with eating disorders usually present initially to their family doctor, and so screening of Amy begins here with careful history taking and physical examination. The SCOFF screening tool (Morgan et al. 2000) is a useful framework for Dr. Johnson. He will also need to inquire about Amy's eating patterns, weight loss trajectory, exercise, physical symptoms and pubertal, growth and menstrual status. Amy will also require a physical examination with attention to height; weight; BMI and BMI percentile; sitting, lying, and standing pulse and blood pressure; temperature; any signs of starvation or medical instability; and an ECG

Case 6.8
Dr. Johnson concludes that Amy may have an eating disorder with significant risk: her heart rate is 50, she is losing 0.5 pounds per week, and she looks malnourished. He therefore refers her to the paediatric hospital and psychiatry team.

Assessment of Eating Disorders

When a patient presents to an eating disorder or child liaison team, she will meet with a child psychiatrist/paediatrician and therapist and will receive a full history, with a focus on thoughts and feelings about food, eating, weight and shape and a psychosocial history, mental status and physical examination and risk review.

Assessment of Individual Symptoms

Case 6.9
As well as school gymnastics practice, Amy disclosed that she participates in school gymnastics practice, goes to the gym three times per week for up to 2 hours at a time and runs each day to improve her performance and to be lean and 'healthy'. She checks her weight daily and skips breakfast and lunch on most days. While she plans to eat lunch at school, she tends to join friends in their decision to skip lunch. She admits to avoiding 'carbs'. She is upset that she tires easily and is moody. Amy is now very anxious and worried about missing school, and her doctor notes that she is irritated with her mother for making her go through an appointment. The doctors see that Amy's self-esteem is very low. She feels that the only thing that is going well for her is her eating plan, and she is worried that if she loses control of the situation, she will not reach her target of 100 pounds and will not make the gymnastics team. As Amy's insight seems to be poor, her doctor obtains collateral history from the parents and asks about symptoms of depression, suicidality, anxiety, obsessive-compulsive disorder, psychosis, autism as well as other medical disorders which might present similarly or complicate her treatment, e.g. *coeliac disease, diabetes, hyperthyroidism, other endocrine disorders,* etc. *The doctor also obtains a detailed medical and developmental history, including feeding history.*

Use of Supplementary Questionnaires

Especially when patients have difficulty discussing feelings about shape and weight, standardised questionnaires and instruments can supplement the clinical interview (Hay et al. 2014; Lock et al. 2015). For a 15-year-old patient like Amy, the children's eating attitudes questionnaire (ChEAT, Maloney et al. 1988) or the eating disorder examination-questionnaire (EDE-Q, Fairburn and Beglin 1994) are good options to explore thoughts, feelings and behaviours and to track progress during treatment.

Case 6.10
Amy finds the process of completing a questionnaire useful in helping her to realise how out of balance her life has become. She is now feeling scared and overwhelmed and recognises that she may need some help. Amy also completes a quality of life measure (the Clinical Impairment Questionnaire, Bohn et al. 2008*) and realises how her problem has taken over her friendships, family and activities. The doctor is hopeful that these insights might help with motivation and identification of recovery and treatment goals.*

Assessment of Family Factors

This step includes assessment of family composition, communication, relationships, major events, eating patterns, history of eating disorders or other mental health concerns and strengths and resilience factors. It also includes assessment of impact of eating disorder symptoms on the family.

Case 6.11
Amy lives with her mother; her father, who works long hours; and her sister, who is 11 years old and who has diabetes. Amy's close maternal aunt had an eating disorder when she was 19 years old. She is now recovered but, as a PE teacher, focuses significantly on fitness and shape. She spends a lot of time with Amy while the father is away at work. Amy's younger sister, Susan, spent two long periods in the hospital in the last 3 years. Susan is on insulin, monitors her blood sugars and follows a careful diet, which all the family are aware of. She and Amy are quite competitive. Amy has been frustrated at times when her sister has needed high levels of support and feels terribly guilty about being frustrated. The Parent Versus *Anorexia Scale (Rhodes et al.* 2005*) helps the team to recognise how un-empowered her parents feel they are in terms of helping Amy with her eating disorder on top of all the other stressors they face as a family.*

Assessment of Medical Factors

Case 6.12
The team reviews a 4-day eating diary and notes that there are long gaps of 6 hours between meals, and when Amy does eat, it is a mainly plant-based diet with little protein and no fat or complex carbohydrates. They estimate that she is eating 800 calories per day and using up 400 alone though exercise. They are relieved that there is no history of binging, purging or use of laxatives. They review the primary care physician's growth and weight charts and note that these were normal until

2 years ago. Amy met all her developmental milestones early and has no other significant medical history. Her history of fainting, occasional palpitations, skin deterioration and tiredness concern them.

Assessment of Environmental Factors

Case 6.13

Amy has been finding it hard to balance her school work with getting on the gym team, and this pressure has been building up now that exam time is approaching. There has also been a falling out among her group of friends in the last year, and Amy feels caught in the middle. She admits being an avid follower of two bloggers who have eating disorders. Academically, Amy has always achieved high grades and continues to do so with additional effort due to her fatigue.

At this point, construct a biopsychosocial formulation for Amy and include predisposing, precipitating, perpetuating and protective factors.

Physical Examination

The child psychiatrist and family doctor/paediatrician must collaboratively establish level of immediate physical risk. Unlike in adults, the healthy BMI range for children and adolescents varies over childhood, so it is essential that BMI is plotted onto an appropriate BMI percentile chart and that % BMI be calculated (RCPsych 2012). One study found that one-third of children under 13 years with early-onset eating disorders were medically unstable at presentation despite not being significantly underweight, and half of them required hospital admission (Hudson and Court 2012). Therefore, BMI % alone is inadequate in assessing risk, and a broad and systematised approach to physical risk assessment is required.

Case 6.14

Amy's doctors noted her cachectic appearance, lanugo (fine) hair on her face, dry skin, acrocyanosis in her fingers, brittle hair and cold intolerance. They reviewed the results of Dr. Johnson's investigations, with special attention to vital signs. Her height is 165 cm and her weight is 46 kg, giving her a BMI of 17 and a BMI % of 82.7. She is slightly dehydrated, but her heart rate is 55 with normal ECG, and there is no significant drop in postural systolic or diastolic blood pressure. She has proximal leg muscle wasting and scores a 2 on the sit up and squat test (SUSS) (RCPsych 2012*). In line with the history, there are no signs of self-induced vomiting: no enlarged parotid glands, Russell's sign (knuckle calluses) or eroded or loose dentition.*

Physical Investigation

Laboratory studies should screen for any nutritional deficiencies and the physiological impact of the eating disorder (Table 6.3). These will need to be repeated at regular intervals as part of regular risk monitoring.

Table 6.3 Physical investigations

Blood tests: Urea and electrolytes, calcium, liver function tests, coagulation, glucose, full blood count, white cell count differential, vitamin B-12, folate, vitamin D	Electrocardiogram
Endocrine thyroid function tests, follicle-stimulating hormone/luteinizing hormone/testosterone	Abdominal ultrasound (if no menstruation for >6/12 months)
Coeliac screen as history indicates	Dexa scan (if no menstruation for >6/12 months)

Case 6.15

The team concludes that Amy has anorexia nervosa, restricting subtype, and discusses the most appropriate treatment setting.

In which setting would you treat Amy?

What do you think that the key components of her treatment plan be?

Three principles to consider in the paediatric age group are that (1) early intervention is most effective (2). Psychosocial treatment involving families is most effective (3). Treatment begins with patient safety, and in AN refeeding is the most important first treatment.

Medical Admission

If physical risk assessment indicates physical instability or food intake less than 400 kcal per day, a paediatric inpatient medical admission is warranted to enable safe supervised refeeding and medical stabilisation. Two key frameworks that enable clinicians to take a systematic approach to decision-making are the Junior MARSIPAN guidelines, MARSIPAN checklist (RCPsych 2012, 2015) and Society of Adolescent Health and Medicine guidelines (2015). The goal is to minimise the risk of refeeding syndrome, a rare but potentially fatal consequence of the body's sudden shift from catabolic to anabolic state, which can result in electrolyte imbalance, multi-organ failure, seizures, coma and death (Mehanna 2008). Communication around eating disorders can be complex, as anorexia nervosa crosses the medical and mental health interface, and multiple clinicians and teams are involved. Suggestions to enhance communication, safety and care are included in Table 6.4. Patients may feel very anxious and angry at the idea of weight gain, which will need to be explained and enforced firmly, consistently and collaboratively by clinicians and parents, so that refeeding is effective and safe.

Outpatient Treatment

As soon as the patient is deemed medically stable, with improvement of the physical parameters that led to her hospitalisation (e.g. MARSIPAN checklist, RCPsych 2016 and a pattern of some restoration of her oral intake), she should be treated in an outpatient setting so that her family can become empowered quickly to manage

Table 6.4 Inpatient admission guidelines

Initiation of the refeeding plan immediately; food is the most important treatment
Formal weekly meeting of paediatrics, liaison psychiatry, nursing and dietary team
Collaborative written treatment plan by this multidisciplinary team
Clear communication, by a nominated person, of the plan, once formulated, with Amy and her family
Twice weekly weights (first thing in the morning while wearing hospital garments)
Daily physical and review of blood K, P, mg and white cell count for 5–7 days (highest refeeding risk)
ECG monitoring
Supervision of meals and use of toilets
Involvement of parents where possible early on to empower them (e.g during snack time)
Possible supplementation with thiamine and phosphate
Activities and activity level determined by psychiatry team consultation and advice
Goal of 0.5–1 kg weight gain per week in hospital
(Very rarely) bolus NG feeding may be needed as a short-term intervention
Admission of ED patients to the same ward to allow staff to build experience

the eating disorder (Lock 2013). In this age group, specialist outpatient eating disorder treatment is as effective as, and less costly than, specialist inpatient care (Gowers et al. 2010). For a small number of patients for whom outpatient care has failed or for whom parents are unable, a more structured programme of refeeding and psychological treatment may be needed, and an inpatient or day patient eating disorder programmes may be appropriate. A recent randomised open study comparing inpatient and day patient treatment in Germany for adolescents with moderate/severe anorexia following brief psychiatric admission found that day programmes were as effective as long-term inpatient admission for weight restoration, weight maintenance and safety and that they were less costly (Herpertz-Dahlmann et al. 2014). Adolescent day programmes in the UK such as multifamily therapy for anorexia nervosa are also options (Eisler et al. 2016).

Evidence-Based Psychosocial Treatment of Anorexia Nervosa

Families do not cause adolescent anorexia nervosa, but it is overwhelmingly clear from the literature that they are key to recovery and that systemic family therapy treatments are superior to individual therapy (Robin et al. 1994, Lock et al. 2010). Family-based treatment for anorexia nervosa (FBT) is the most systematically researched treatment to date and is regarded as the first-line treatment for adolescents with anorexia nervosa (Hay et al. 2014; Lock et al. 2015; Herpertz-Dahlman 2016).

Case 6.16

Amy's father will adjust his work to attend the family-based treatment sessions. The psychiatrist explains that this is a manualised treatment that lasts up 20 weeks and that will empower Amy's parents to take charge of refeeding, with weekly specialist support and monitoring of weight and physical parameters. They are told that this treatment is associated with BMI recovery rates of 40–50%, with a further 30% of adolescents having a partial recovery (Lock and Le Grange 2012*). They are encouraged to approach her illness as they would a serious, life-threatening medical condition requiring a programme of treatment. They are all clear that a goal of 0.2–0.5 kg weight gain per week is expected with outpatient treatment.*

If the patient were too obsessional, or if FBT were not possible for family reasons or otherwise ineffective, a broader systemic family therapy approach would be recommended (Lock et al. 2015). Second-line interventions include multifamily therapy for anorexia (Eisler et al. 2016), enhanced cognitive behavioural therapy for eating disorders (CBT-E) for older adolescents (Fairburn 2008) and day/inpatient programmes. To date, there is no evidence to suggest that psychopharmacological treatments are effective in treating Amy's anorexia nervosa, and so except for nutritional supplementation, medication would be used only for comorbidity (e.g. anxiety or depression) (Herpertz-Dahlman et al. 2015). Throughout her psychosocial treatment, Amy's psychiatrist/paediatrician will continue to monitor her physical parameters to ensure that her medical risk is monitored.

Prognosis of Paediatric Anorexia Nervosa

A recent meta-analysis of 35 studies found, for AN in the 15–19 age group, a 10% mortality rate, which is the highest for the mental disorders. Prompt engagement in treatment is therefore essential. For a significant subgroup, AN will become a chronic or life-limiting illness (Arcelus et al. 2011). On a positive note, adolescents appear to have a better prognosis than adults with anorexia nervosa, with one study reporting, for severe anorexia nervosa, a 75% full recovery rate at 10–15 years (Strober et al. 1997). Key to good outcomes is access to early specialist intervention and a focus on weight and behavioural outcomes.

Bulimia Nervosa

Epidemiology Bulimia nervosa (BN) is more common in childhood than anorexia nervosa, with a lifetime prevalence of 1–1.5% in paediatric community samples. Like with AN, a higher proportion of the paediatric population has subthreshold symptoms, but, in comparison to AN, BN presents less frequently to liaison services. There is a significant age effect, with an incidence of 2.9/100,000 in the 10–14-year-old group and 25.9/100,000 in the 15–19-year-old group. At 2–3:1, the female to male ratio for BN is lower than that for AN (Micali et al. 2013, Swanson et al. 2011).

Diagnostic Criteria

The main change in the DSM V for BN is that binging and purging cycles need only occur once weekly rather than twice as was the case in DSM IV-TR (Table 6.2).

Aetiology

The different eating disorders overlap substantially, and over time they can develop from one into the other. Indeed, a transdiagnostic approach to understanding and treating all eating disorders has been developed (Fairburn 2008).

Biological Factors Most twin and family studies estimate BN's heritability to be between 0.55 and 0.62 (Trace et al. 2013). Multiple candidate genes include those related to gender, obesity, weight and appetite and neurotransmitters such as serotonin and dopamine. Studies also indicate that early pubertal timing is a biological risk factor for the development of BN in girls (Klump 2013).

Psychological Adult studies associate BN with certain personality traits. A child or adolescent, who has difficulty in regulating their emotions, who is impulsive and who engages in risk behaviours such as substance misuse and self-harm, is more likely to develop BN (Fischer 2007; Pearson et al. 2015; Myers et al. 2006). The CBT-E formulation of BN identifies how low self-esteem leads to an overevaluation of shape and weight and subsequent dieting and compensatory behaviour. In a vulnerable adolescent, this process develops into binge behaviour and a cycle of escalation (Murphy et al. 2010).

Sociocultural Factors Adolescent social pressure around thinness and body dissatisfaction is associated with BN. Adolescents who want to become athletes, especially those interested in aesthetic sports (gymnastics, aerobics, dancing), modelling and bodybuilding (especially for males), are all at increased risk. With a 5–16% prevalence in such subgroups, BN is the most common eating disorder in athletes (Currie 2010; Joy et al. 2016). Other social risk factors for BN include a history of childhood trauma, abuse, poly trauma (Utzinger et al. 2016) and criticism.

Screening and Assessment of Bulimia Nervosa

Screening and assessment by the family doctor and specialist liaison or eating disorder team is identical to that described for Amy above. The EDE-Q can be particularly helpful for uncovering hidden bulimia-type behaviours such as laxative abuse and self-induced vomiting, which are often under-reported or not known to parents. Such diagnostic accuracy is particularly critical to decision-making around treatment.

Specifically, for BM, it is important to explore:

- Individual factors: comorbidity of depression, substance use, deliberate self-harm and suicidality.
- Family factors: adverse situations that may be a consequence to parental attempts to manage the ED and that may perpetuate the ED. Parental attitude to food, body shape and exercise are also important perpetuating factors that will need to be carefully reviewed.
- Medical factors: frequency of purging, which may lead to cardiac abnormalities, potassium depletion, metabolic alkalosis or acidosis, palpitations, fainting, breathlessness or haematemesis
- Environmental factors: such as reckless social behaviour and relationships, to ensure that safety is maintained.

Physical Examination and Investigation

In addition to following the same format as outlined for AN (Table 6.2), the examining doctor will look for signs of dehydration and purging (enlarged parotids, loose teeth), check urea and electrolytes and assess for hypokalaemia-induced cardiac changes on ECG patients with BN who are also at high risk of oesophageal tears or rupture. Dental referral may be required to identify and treat dental erosion and loose teeth. Even adolescents with bulimia who are not anaemic or underweight may be malnourished due to purging, and nutritional screening tests will also be needed.

Case 6.17

Michelle is a 15-year-old female with a % BMI of 105% who is referred by her family doctor for eating disorder assessment. In the last year, she describes having lost control of her eating, and she feels frustrated and hopeless. She makes herself sick 2 times per day on most days, particularly in the evenings after dinner when she feels at her lowest. She often skips breakfast and lunch, but then later in the day is overwhelmed by hunger and will eat anything she can find. Last night she had up to a loaf of bread, chips, a tub of ice cream as well as dinner and cookies. She finds it hard to remember what she eats or feels at the time. Afterwards however, she feels awful and usually makes herself sick. She has also cut her arms and thighs on several occasions. Michelle is frustrated as her weight is 68 kg, and she knows she is overweight, but she can't lose weight despite the purging and fasting. She goes to the gym in bouts of 2–3 h when she exhausts herself. She is then starving, irritable, 'all over the place' and angry. Her mother thinks that she is 'big' like her family and that Michelle is influenced by magazines and friends not realistic about how she can look.

What is your diagnosis and why?
Construct a formulation of Michelle.
Outline your physical and risk assessment of Michelle.
What investigations will you order?

Treatment of Bulimia Nervosa in Adolescents

Adolescents with BN rarely require medical admission unless they have hypokalaemia or ECG changes, in which case telemetry may be required, and so they are less likely to present to a paediatric liaison service. Once cardiac and gastroesophageal issues are resolved, treatment is generally on an outpatient basis. Hospital management principles are like those recommended for AN (Table 6.4), with individualised determination of weight goals and vitamin supplementation.

There is a very limited evidence base around the psychological treatment of adolescent BN. CBT-E has been recommended because of its evidence base in adults (Murphy et al. 2010; Lock et al. 2015). Like FBT, CBT-E is also a manualised treatment that is delivered by a skilled therapist and that involves a 20- or 40-session programme focused on normal eating pattern restoration through real-time recording, regular meal structure, weekly weights, psycho-education and formulation and eventually discussions of body shape evaluation, body checking and management of emotional triggers. It is adapted for adolescents and emphasises parents' important role in the treatment process. More recently, three randomised studies of older adolescents suggest that an adapted form of family-based therapy (FBT-BN) may be superior to individual therapy for BN (Le Grange et al. 2015). Guided self-help may also be considered for older adolescents. There is no evidence base around BN treatment in adolescent males. Outpatient psychosocial treatment is always complemented by regular meal planning, nutritional supplementation and physical monitoring.

As with adolescent AN, psychopharmacological treatment is reserved for comorbidity, and despite evidence of effectiveness for high doses of fluoxetine (60 mg) in adults with BN, there have been no robust trials in adolescents (Goldstein et al. 1995).

Prognosis Bulimia nervosa has a standardised mortality rate (SMR) of 2.22 based on 12 studies (Arcelus et al. 2011). Risk factors associated with poorer outcome in adolescents include family history of obesity, longer duration and poor early response to treatment. There is also a risk of developing AN.

Binge Eating Disorder

Binge eating disorder (BED) was previously classified as an atypical disorder under 'Eating Disorder Not Otherwise Specified' (ED-NOS) in DSM 4-TR but now has full eating disorder status. As with BN, the only change is a decrease in the threshold of binge-purge frequency from twice to once per week (Table 6.2). Due to its relatively recent inclusion as a full disorder (it remains under 'other' disorders in ICD 10), BED is relatively less studied, particularly in the paediatric population.

Epidemiology Previous inclusion under ED-NOS enables us to estimate that the lifetime prevalence of BED in community-based samples of 13–18-year-olds is 1.6%, making it the most common of the adolescent-eating disorders. It is also more common in females. The onset of BED is in later adolescence or early adulthood, with an average age of onset in the early to mid-twenties (Kessler et al. 2013).

Aetiology In the absence of studies of BED in adolescents, research in adults indicates that this disorder has a complex aetiology similar to the other eating disorders, where a combination of genetic factors, dieting, body dissatisfaction, low self-esteem, emotional eating and social factors all play a role. A key cognitive process involves binging leading to feelings of disgust, depression and shame, which further reinforces the adolescent's low self-esteem and cyclical pattern of binging.

Screening and Assessment

Screening and assessment for BED follows a similar framework to AN. Comorbid depression is common. Particularly in the case of binge eating disorder, adolescents may be significantly overweight or obese, and the medical history and examination may need a paediatric obesity-focused workup to include screening for: (1) developmental syndromes (e.g. Prader-Willi) with karyotyping if necessary; (2) metabolic syndrome and diabetes (lipids, blood glucose); (3) endocrine problems involving thyroid, growth or reproductive hormones; (4) gastrointestinal diseases; and (5) other anatomical abnormalities visible on imaging studies (e.g. polycystic ovaries, brain lesions or other pathology).

Treatment

Patients with BED are less likely to be physically compromised and so generally present to primary care services. Paediatric admission is rare. To date, there have been no RCTs that specifically address the treatment of BED in the adolescent population, and it is recommended that treatment planning is extrapolated from what works for an adult population, or for the adolescent-eating disorder, it most closely resembles. CBT-E or guided self-help may be useful approaches (Hay et al. 2014). However, given adolescents' developmental stage and relative vulnerability compared with adults, an adapted CBT-E approach with parent support is the most scaffolded and safest approach for the treatment of BED in adolescents. Group formats also hold promise, particularly for older adolescents, but this modality requires further research in this age group.

Conclusion

Feeding and eating difficulties frequently present in childhood and adolescence and need prompt identification and expert management to preserve physical and psychological development and avoid life-threatening situations.

References

Agras, S., Hammer, L., & McNicholas, F. (1999). A prospective study of the influence of eating-disordered mothers on their children. *The International Journal of Eating Disorders, 25*, 253–622.

Allen, K. L., Gibson, L. Y., NJ, M. L., Davis, E. A., & Byrne, S. M. (2014). Maternal and family factors and child eating pathology, risk and protective relationships. *Journal of Eating Disorder, 2*, 11.

American Psychiatric Association. (2014). *Diagnostic and statistical manual of mental disorders: DSM-5* (5th ed.). Washington, DC: American Psychiatric Association.

Anderluh, M. B., Tchanturia, K., Rabe-Hesketh, S., & Treasure, J. (2003). Childhood obsessive-compulsive personality traits in adult women with eating disorders: Defining a broader eating disorder phenotype. *The American Journal of Psychiatry, 160*(2), 242–247.

Arcelus, J., Mitchell, A. J., & Wales, J. (2011). Mortality rates in patients with anorexia nervosa and other eating disorders. *Archives of General Psychiatry, 68*(7), 724–731.

Arvedson, J. C. (2008, January 1). Assessment of pediatric dysphagia and feeding disorders: Clinical and instrumental approaches. *Developmental Disabilities Research Reviews, 14*(2), 118–127.

Bachle, C., Stahl- Pehe, A., & Rosenbauer, J. (2016). Disordered eating and insulin restriction in youths receiving intensified insulin treatment: Results from a nationwide population-based study. *International Journal of Eating Disorders, 49*(2), 191–196.

Bohn, K., Doll, H. A., Cooper, Z., O'Connor, M. E., Palmer, R. L., & Fairburn, C. G. (2008). The measurement of impairment due to eating disorder psychopathology. *Behaviour Research and Therapy, 46*, 1105–1110.

Bryant-Waugh, R. (2013, July 1). Avoidant restrictive food intake disorder: An illustrative case example. *The International Journal of Eating Disorders, 46*(5), 420–423.

Cardona Cano, S., Tiemeier, H., Van Hoeken, D., Tharner, A., Jaddoe, V. W., Hofman, A., Verhulst, F. C., & Hoek, H. W. (2015, September 1). Trajectories of picky eating during childhood: A general population study. *The International Journal of Eating Disorders, 48*(6), 570–579.

Carruth, B. R., Ziegler, P. J., Gordon, A., & Barr, S. I. (2004). Prevalence of picky eaters among infants and toddlers and their caregivers' decisions about offering a new food. *The Journal of the American Dietetic Association, 104*, 57–64. https://doi.org/10.1016/j.jada.2003.10.024.

Casey, P. H., Szeto, K., Lensing, S., Bogle, M., & Weber, J. (2001, April 1). Children in food-insufficient, low-income families: Prevalence, health, and nutrition status. *Archives of Pediatrics & Adolescent Medicine, 155*(4), 508–514.

CDC. (2013). *Eating disorders prevalence for children by sex and age*. National Youth Fitness Survey. Retrieved from https://www.nimh.nih.gov/health/statistics/prevalence/eating-disorders-among-children.shtm. Accessed 10 Jan 2017.

Chatoor, I. (2002, April 30). Feeding disorders in infants and toddlers: Diagnosis and treatment. *Child and Adolescent Psychiatric Clinics of North America, 11*(2), 163–183.

Chatoor, I., Hamburger, E., Fullard, R., & Fivera, Y. (1994). *A survey of picky eating and pica behaviors in toddlers*. Scientific proceedings of the annual meeting of American Academy of Child and Adolescent Psychiatry, 10', 50.

Chatoor, I., Loeffler, C., McGee, M., & Menvielle, E. (1998). *Observational scale for mother-infant interaction during feeding*. Washington, DC: Children's National Medical Center.

Chial, H. J., Camilleri, M., Williams, D. E., Litzinger, K., & Perrault, J. (2003, January 1). Rumination syndrome in children and adolescents: Diagnosis, treatment, and prognosis. *Pediatrics, 111*(1), 158–162.

Davies, W. H., Satter, E., Berlin, K. S., Sato, A. F., Silverman, A. H., Fischer, E. A., Arvedson, J. C., & Rudolph, C. D. (2006, September 1). Reconceptualizing feeding and feeding disorders in interpersonal context: The case for a relational disorder. *Journal of Family Psychology, 20*(3), 409–417.

Dovey, T. M., Staples, P. A., Gibson, E. L., & Halford, J. C. (2008, May 31). Food neophobia and 'picky/fussy'eating in children: A review. *Appetite, 50*(2), 181–193.

Dubois, L., Farmer, A. P., Girard, M., & Peterson, K. (2007, July 1). Preschool children's eating behaviours are related to dietary adequacy and body weight. *European Journal of Clinical Nutrition, 61*(7), 846–855.

Eisler, I., Simic, M., Hodsoil, J., Asen, E., et al. (2016). A pragmatic randomised multi- Centre trial of multifamily and single family therapy for adolescent anorexia nervosa. *BMC Psychiatry, 16*(1), 422.

Fairburn. (2008). *Cognitive behaviour therapy and eating disorders* (p. 316). Chichester: The Guilford Press.

Fairburn, C. G., & Beglin, S. J. (1994). Assessment of eating disorder psychopathology: Interview or self-report questionnaire? *International Journal of Eating Disorders, 16*, 363–370.

Fan, Y., Li, Y., Liu, A., Hu, X., Ma, G., & Xu, G. (2010). Associations between body mass index, weight control concerns and behaviors, and eating disorder symptoms among non-clinical Chinese adolescents. *BMC Public Health, 10*, 314. https://doi.org/10.1186/1471-2458-10-314.

Feldman, R., Keren, M., Gross-Rozval, O., & Tyano, S. (2004, September 30). Mother–child touch patterns in infant feeding disorders: Relation to maternal, child, and environmental factors. *Journal of the American Academy of Child and Adolescent Psychiatry, 43*(9), 1089–1097.

Ferguson, C. J., Munoz, M. E., Garza, A., & Galindo, M. (2012). Concurrent and prospective analysis of peer, television and social media influences on n body dissatisfaction, eating disorder symptoms and life satisfaction in adolescent girls. *Journal of Youth and Adolescence, 43*(1), 1–14. https://doi.org/10.1007/s106=964-012-9898-9.

Forman, S. F., McKenzie, N., Hehn, R., Monge, M. C., Kapphahn, C. J., Mammel, K. A., Callahan, S. T., Sigel, E. J., Bravender, T., Romano, M., & Rome, E. S. (2014, December 31). Predictors of outcome at 1 year in adolescents with DSM-5 restrictive eating disorders: Report of the national eating disorders quality improvement collaborative. *Journal of Adolescent Health, 55*(6), 750–756.

Goldstein, D. J., Wilson, M. G., Thompson, V. L., Potvin, J. H., & Rampey, A. H. (1995, May 1). Long-term fluoxetine treatment of bulimia nervosa. Fluoxetine bulimia nervosa research group. *The British Journal of Psychiatry, 166*(5), 660–666.

Goncalves, S., Silva, M., Rue Gomes, A., & Machado, P. (2012). Disordered eating among pre-adolescent boys and girls: The relationship with child and maternal variables. *Nutrients, 4*, 273–285.

Gowers, S. G., Clark, A. F., Roberts, C., Byford, S., Barrett, B., Griffiths, A., et al. (2010). A randomised controlled multicentre trial of treatments for adolescent anorexia nervosa including assessment of cost- effectiveness and patient acceptability- the TOuCAN trial. *Health Technology Assessment, 14*(15), 1–56.

Grylli, V., Hafferl-Gattermayer, A., Wagner, G., Schober, E., & Karwautz, A. (2005). Eating disorders and eating problems among adolescents with type 1 diabetes: Exploring relationships with temperament and character. *Journal of Pediatric Psychology, 20*(2), 197–206.

Gull, W. (1873). *'Anorexia Nervosa (Apepsia Hysterica, Anorexia Hysterica)'*: Paper to the Clinical Society of London.

Harrison, K. (2000). The body electric: Thin-ideal media and eating disorders in adolescents. *Journal of Communication, Summer, 50*, 119–143.

Hay, P., Chinn, D., Forbes, D., Madden, S., Newton, R., Sugenor, L., Touyz, S., & Ward, W. (2014, November). Royal Australian and New Zealand College of Psychiatrists clinical practice guidelines for the treatment of eating disorders. *Australian & New Zealand Journal of Psychiatry, 48*(11), 977–1008.

Herpertz- Dahnmann, B., Schwarte, R., Krei, M., Egberts, K., Warnke, A., Wewetzer, C., & Dempfle, A. (2014). Day-patient treatment after short inpatient care versus continued inpatient treatment in adolescents with anorexia nervosa (ANDI): A multicentre, randomised, open-label, non-inferiority trial. *The Lancet, 383*(9924), 1222–1229.

Herpertz-Dahlmann, B., van Elburg, A., Castro-Fornieles, J., & Schmidt, U. (2015). ESCAP expert paper: New developments in the diagnosis and treatment of adolescent anorexia nervosa —A European perspective. *European Child & Adolescent Psychiatry, 24*, 1153–1167.

Hudson, L. D., & Court, A. J. (2012). What paediatricians should know about eating disorders in children and young people. *Journal of Paediatrics and Child Health, 48*(10), 869–875.

Jacobi, C., Schmitz, G., & Agras, W. S. (2008). Is picky eating an eating disorder? *International Journal of Eating Disorders, 41*(7), 626–634.

Jacobs, M. J., Roesch, S. A., Wonderlich, R., Crosby, L., Thornton, D. E., Wilfley, W. H., Berrettini, H., Brandt, S., Crawford, M. M., Fichter, K. A., et al. (2009, March). Anorexia nervosa trios: Behaviour profiles of individuals with anorexia nervosa and their parents. *Psychological Medicine, 39*(3), 451–461.

Joy, E., Kussman, A., & Nativ, A. (2016). 2016 update on eating disorders in athletes: A comprehensive narrative review with a focus on clinical assessment and management. *British Journal of Sports Medicine, 50*, 154–162.

Kessler, R., Berglund, P. A., Chiu, W. T., Deitz, A. C., et al. (2013). The prevalence and correlates of binge eating disorder in the WHO World Mental Health Surveys *Biological Psychiatry, 73*(9), 904–913.

Kirkey, S. (2012). Picky eaters could join ranks of mentally ill. January 24, 2012. [Accessed March 2017]. Available from http://nationalpost.com/news/canada/picky-eaters-could-join-ranks-of-mentally-ill

Klump, K. (2013). Puberty as a critical risk period for eating disorders: A review of human and animal studies. *Hormones and Behavior, July, 64*(2), 399–410.

Kotler, L. A., Cohen, P., Davies, M., Pine, D. S., & Walsh, B. T. (2001, December 31). Longitudinal relationships between childhood, adolescent, and adult eating disorders. *Journal of the American Academy of Child and Adolescent Psychiatry, 40*(12), 1434–1440.

Le Grange, D., Lock, J., Agras, W. S., Bryson, S. W., & Jo, B. (2015, November). Randomized clinical trial of family-based treatment and cognitive-behavioral therapy for adolescent bulimia nervosa. *Journal of the American Academy of Child and Adolescent Psychiatry, 54*(11), 886–894.

Linscheid, T. R., Budd, K. S., & Rasnake, L. K. (2003). Pediatric feeding disorders. In M. C. Roberts (Ed.), *Handbook of pediatric psychology* (pp. 481–498). New York: The Guildford Press.

Lock, J., & Le Grange, D. (2012). *Treatment manual for Anorexia nervosa: A family based approach* (2nd ed.). New York: Guilford Press.

Lock, J., Le Grange, D., & Booil, J. (2010). Randomised clinical trial comparing family based treatment to adolescent focused individual therapy for adolescents with anorexia nervosa. *Archives of General Psychiatry, 67*(10), 1025–1032.

Lock, J., laVia, M. C., & AACAP, C. Q. I. (2015). Practice parameters for the assessment and treatment of children and adolescents with eating disorders. *JACAAP, 54*(5), 414–425.

Maloney, M. J., McGuire, J. B., & Daniels, S. R. (1988). Reliability testing of a children's version of the eating attitude test. *Journal of the American Academy of Child and Adolescent Psychiatry, 27*(5), 541–543.

Mascola, A. J., Bryson, S. W., & Agras, W. S. (2010). Picky eating during childhood: a longitudinal study to age 11 years. *Eating behaviors, 11*(4), 253–257.

McNicholas, F., Dooley, B., Keogh, L., & Lydon, A. (2010). Eating problems in Irish children and adolescence- EPICA. *Irish Journal of Psychological Medicine, 27*(4), 172–178.

Micali, N., Hagberg, K. W., Petersen, I., & Treasure, J. L. (2013). The incidence of eating disorders in the UK in 2000–2009: Findings from the general practice research database. *BMJ Open, 3*, e002646.

Micali, N., De Stavola, G., Ploubidis, E., Simonoff, E., Treasure, J., & Field, A. E. (2015). Adolescent eating disorder behaviours and cognitions: Gender specific effects of child, maternal and family risk factors. *The British Journal of Psychiatry, 204*(4), 320–327.

Morgan, J., Reid, F., & Lacey, H. (2000). The SCOFF questionnaire: A new screening tool for eating disorders. *The Western Journal of Medicine, Mar, 172*(3), 164–165.

Murphy, R., Straebler, S., Cooper, Z., & Fairburn, C. G. (2010). Cognitive behaviour therapy for eating disorders. *The Psychiatric Clinics of North America, 33*(3), 611–627.

Myers, T. C., Wonderlich, S. A., Crosby, R., Mitchell, J. E., Steffen, K. J., Smyth, J., & Miltenberger, R. (2006). Is multi-impulsive bulimia a distinct type of bulimia nervosa: Psychopathology and EMA findings. *The International Journal of Eating Disorders, 39*(8), 655–661.

Norris, M. L., Spettigue, W. J., & Katzman, D. K. (2016). Update on eating disorders: Current perspectives on avoidant/restrictive food intake disorder in children and youth. *Neuropsychiatric Disease and Treatment, 12*, 213.

Pearson, S. C., Wonderlich, S. A., & Smith, G. T. (2015). A risk and maintenance model for bulimia nervosa: From impulsive action to compulsive behaviour. *Psychological Review, 122*(3), 516–535.

Prochaska, J. O., Redding, C. A., & Evers, K. E. (2008). The transtheoretical model and stages of change. In K. Glanz, B. K. Rimer, & K. Viswanath (Eds.), *Health behavior and health education* (4th ed., p. 105). San Francisco: Jossey-Bass. ISBN 978-0-7879-9614-7.

RCPsych. (2012). *Junior MARSIPAN: Management of really sick patients under 18 with Anorexia nervosa (CR 168).*

Rhodes, P., Baillie, A., Brown, J., & Madden, S. (2005). Parental efficacy in the family-based treatment of anorexia: Preliminary development of the parents versus anorexia scale (PVA). *European Eating Disorders Review, 13*, 399–405.

Robin, A. L., Siegel, P. T., Koepke, T., Moye, A. W., & Tice, S. (1994, April). Family therapy versus individual therapy for adolescent females with anorexia nervosa. *Journal of Developmental and Behavioral Pediatrics, 15*(2), 111–115.

Rydell, A. M., Dahl, M., & Sundelin, C. (1995, June 1). Characteristics of school children who are choosy eaters. *The Journal of Genetic Psychology, 156*(2), 217–229.

Sanchez, K., Spittle, A. J., Allinson, L., & Morgan, A. (2015, September 1). Parent questionnaires measuring feeding disorders in preschool children: A systematic review. *Developmental Medicine and Child Neurology, 57*(9), 798–807.

Schreck, K. A., Williams, K., & Smith, A. F. (2004). A comparison of eating behaviors between children with and without Autism. *Journal of Autism and Developmental Disabilities, 34*, 433–438.

Society of Adolescent Health and Medicine- SAHM. (2015). Position paper of the society for adolescent Health and medicine: Medical management of restrictive eating disorders in adolescents and young adults. *Journal of Adolescent Health, 56*(1), 121–125.

Stein, A., Woolley, H., & Cooper, S. D. (1994, May 1). Fairburn CG. An observational study of mothers with eating disorders and their infants. *Journal of Child Psychology and Psychiatry, 35*(4), 733–748.

Stice, E., Agras, W. S., & Hammer, L. D. (1999). Risk factors for the emergence of childhood eating disturbances: A 5 year prospective study. *The International Journal of Eating Disorders, 25*(4), 375–387.

Strandjord, S. E., Sieke, E. H., Richmond, M., & Rome, E. S. (2015, December 31). Avoidant/restrictive food intake disorder: Illness and hospital course in patients hospitalized for nutritional insufficiency. *Journal of Adolescent Health, 57*(6), 673–678.

Strober, M., Freeman, R., & Morell, W. (1997). The long-term course of severe anorexia nervosa in adolescents: Survival analysis of recovery, relapse, and outcome predictors over 10–15 years in a prospective study. *The International Journal of Eating Disorders, 22*(4), 339–360.

Swanson, S. A., Scott, S. M., Crow, J., & Le Grange, D. (2011). Prevalence and correlates of eating disorders in adolescents: Results from the National Comorbidity Survey Replication Adolescent Supplement. *Archives of General Psychiatry, 68*(7), 701–713.

Timimi, S., Douglas, J., & Tsiftsopoulou, K. (1997, May 1). Selective eaters: A retrospective case note study. *Child: Care, Health and Development, 23*(3), 265–278.

Trace, S. E., Baker, J. H., Penas- Liedo, E., & Bulik, C. M. (2013). The genetics of eating disorders. *Annual Review of Clinical Psychology, 9*, 589–620.

Uher, R., & Rutter, M. (2012, June 1). Classification of feeding and eating disorders: Review of evidence and proposals for ICD-11. *World Psychiatry., 11*(2), 80–92.

Utzinger, L. M., Haukebo, J. E., Simonich, H., Wonderlich, S. A., Cao, L., Lavender, J. M., Mitchell, J. E., & Engel, S. G. (2016, July). Crosby RD a latent profile analysis of childhood trauma in women with bulimia nervosa: Associations with borderline personality disorder psychopathology. *The International Journal of Eating Disorders, 49*(7), 689–694. https://doi.org/10.1002/eat.22532. Epub 2016 Apr 1.

Van Tine, M. L., McNicholas, F., Safer, D. L., & Agras, W. S. (2017, August 31). Follow-up of selective eaters from childhood to adulthood. *Eating Behaviors, 26*, 61–65.

White, M., & Epston, D. (1990). *Narrative means to therapeutic ends*. New York: W. W. Norton. ISBN 978-0393700985.

Williams, K., Riegel, K., & Kerwin, M. (2009). Feeding disorders of infancy or early childhood. How often is it seen in feeding programs? *Journal of Child Health Care, 38*, 123–136.

Yilmaz, Z., Hardaway, J. A., & Bulik, C. M. (2015). The genetics and epigenetics of eating disorders. *Advances in Genomics and Genetics, 5*, 131–150.

Zerwas, S., & Bulik, C. (2011). Genetics and epigenetics of eating disorders. *Psychiatric Annals, 41*(11), 532–538.

Chapter 7
Adjustment to Medical Illness

Roshni L. Koli, Sherry Gaillard, Heather Tamaye, Joyce Wong, and Wendi Hirsch

Introduction

A medical condition, especially a chronic or life-threatening illness, can have a profound impact on children and their families. It is estimated that in the past 20 years chronic illness in children has more than doubled, so helping children to understand and process their feelings about their illness is imperative (Eccleston et al. 2012). Recent studies recognize parents' critical role in positively or negatively influencing their child's adjustment to a chronic illness (Eccleston et al. 2012; Campbell et al. 2017). Additional factors influencing this adjustment include the age or developmental stage of the child, parental or family stressors, and family dynamics. One way to help children and their families adapt to an illness is to promote active coping skills. The concept of coping can be described as the ability to manage or overcome life's challenges with limited, or without, distress. This is often difficult to do with children and adolescents, especially during a medical illness. Children can experience fear, worry, and pain and may not always know how best to manage these feelings. The published literature recognizes that helping children and their families with effective coping strategies is beneficial and can optimize recovery and improve treatment outcomes (Eccleston et al. 2012; Coakley and Wihak 2017; Mechtel and Stoeckle 2017; Schonfeld and Demaria 2015).

R. L. Koli (✉) · S. Gaillard · W. Hirsch
Kapiolani Behavioral Health Services, Kapiolani Medical Center for Women and Children, Honolulu, HI, USA
e-mail: Sherry.gaillard@kapiolani.org; Wendi.major@kapiolani.org

H. Tamaye · J. Wong
Child Life Department, Kapiolani Medical Center for Women and Children, Honolulu, HI, USA
e-mail: Heather.tamaye@kapiolani.org; JoyceWo@kapiolani.org

A. P. S. Guerrero et al. (eds.), *Pediatric Consultation-Liaison Psychiatry*,
https://doi.org/10.1007/978-3-319-89488-1_7

Developmental Aspects

Jean Piaget's (1896–1980) model of cognitive development can be used as a framework for introducing coping strategies to children. The second stage of this model is termed the *preoperational* period and generally occurs between the ages of 2–6 and 7. During this stage, children use their imagination and language to help understand the world from their own point of view (Berger 2005). Due to their inability to differentiate reality from fantasy, they can be easily confused and may be prone to anxiety (Mechtel and Stoeckle 2017). Providing age-appropriate education about a medical illness and its treatment through play, including explaining what to expect and answering children's questions, can help to ease their anxiety. Utilizing a certified child life specialist (CCLS), especially in the case of a new diagnosis or procedure, can be very helpful. Before a procedure, a CCLS can provide a tour of the operative suite and allow the child to touch and play with medical supplies to become familiar with what to expect and in turn reduce a child's apprehension over the situation (Mechtel and Stoeckle 2017).

By the time children reach the third stage, which is called the *concrete operational* period typically occurring between the ages of 6 or 7 and 11 or 12, they can think logically and have a sense of reason (Berger 2005). They can take into consideration another person's perspective beyond their own. They can only process facts and are incapable of thinking abstractly (Mechtel and Stoeckle 2017). Providing children with education through storytelling and then having them draw a picture about the story several days before a procedure allows them to have some time to process the information and can reduce or prevent anxiety (Mechtel and Stoeckle 2017). Among children and adolescents, females seem to be at somewhat higher risk (2:1 ratio) for anxiety than males, although both genders seem to be at equal risk for depression (American Psychiatric Association 2013). Therefore, it is important to assist all children and their families in managing potentially impairing emotions that arise from awareness of their illness.

Family Aspects

Parental mental health problems and marital conflict, financial strain, and child behavior problem issues can interfere with a child's ability to cope effectively with a significant illness (Schonfeld and Demaria 2015). Consulting on a child with a medical illness involves working with the entire family to help each person cope with the changes to the family system. There is strong evidence that including the parents in the treatment plan will improve outcomes for the child (Coakley and Wihak 2017). Campbell et al. (2017) found that parental use of "coping-promoting" behaviors (i.e., positive coping statements or humor) is predictive of optimal coping in children; parents engaging in "distress-promoting" behaviors (i.e., appearing anxious or worried and making negative or catastrophic comments) are a predictor for distress in children. Given the impact that parents can have on helping or hindering a child's ability to cope with a medical illness, it is essential to work with the entire family to optimize daily functioning.

Coping Styles and Mechanism

In western cultures, cognitive behavioral therapy (CBT) techniques are the cornerstone intervention for children coping with stress, anxiety, or depression (Coakley and Wihak 2017). This approach involves helping the child to become aware of their self-talk and to recognize how it can either be beneficial or not. Often, thoughts can be self-critical and self-defeating. By learning to reframe or restate their thoughts, children can alter their feelings about themselves or a situation and subsequently their behavior. Thinking that they will be in pain will likely increase their perception of pain and cause distress and avoidant behavior. Extensions of CBT, such as problem-solving therapy, which utilizes CBT skills to look at ways to help a child find solutions to a problem instead of perseverating on the problem, have been described. Eccleston et al. (2012) reported utilizing problem-solving therapy with both children and their parents as an effective approach to reducing distress among children with a chronic condition.

Other coping strategies or therapies commonly utilized by children with a chronic illness are diaphragmatic breathing, hypnosis, journaling, distraction, and art, music, or play therapy (Coakley and Wihak 2017).

Alternatively, in eastern cultures, a key coping intervention is mindfulness meditation. Kabat-Zinn (1994) explains it as a Buddhist practice, where one exists in the present and pays attention to their consciousness purposely without judgment. Many find this to be challenging, especially with numerous demands in each day. However, if one can center him/herself in the moment, it can be freeing and a cleansing of self. It involves breathing, "letting go," and self-acceptance. It is a learning to be with one's self (Chopra 1997). Some believe traditional western psychotherapy and meditation practices work well together (Epstein 1995).

Differential Diagnosis and Screening for Anxiety, Depression, and Distress in Chronic Medical Conditions

Case Vignette 7.1

In your role as the child and adolescent psychiatrist at your local Children's hospital, you attend pediatric oncology rounds. During rounds, an attending pediatric oncologist brings up his concerns regarding a 7-year-old male child with newly diagnosed acute lymphoblastic leukemia. Your colleague is concerned about his hospitalized patient's episodes of disruptive behavior that have been occurring more frequently, in particular, prior to procedures and during physical exams. He also wonders how the family is coping.

After explaining to the family the rationale for behavioral health involvement, the oncologist asks you to provide a formal consult.

Adults with chronic medical conditions, such as inflammatory bowel disease (IBD; i.e., Crohn's disease and ulcerative colitis), experience greater rates, compared with healthy individuals, of depression and anxiety. These higher rates of anxiety and depression are seen after disease onset. Individuals with active IBD may be nearly twice as likely to have symptoms of anxiety and depression when compared to individuals with inactive disease (Loftus et al. 2011). These findings are like those seen in pediatric populations. Children with Crohn's disease are at significantly increased risk of developing persistent anxiety or depression (defined as a duration of greater than 1 year) and are more likely to receive psychotropic intervention (Mikocka-Walus et al. 2016).

These studies emphasize the importance of screening for anxiety, depression, and quality of life at the onset of a chronic illness and throughout treatment, with attention to times when there is an exacerbation of illness.

Case Vignette 7.2

Prior to evaluating the patient and family, you start with gathering information from the patient's bedside nurse. She states that beginning the night before a planned procedure, the patient becomes irritable, tearful, and often has difficulty sleeping. On the morning of a procedure, the patient often remains irritable and will sometimes yell, "I don't want to be in the hospital anymore!"

Given your knowledge about the high rates of anxiety, depression, and emotional distress for pediatric oncology patients and their families, you wonder if a screening tool has been administered at any point during the illness.

Screening for psychosocial distress in children with cancer and their families has become a national standard put forth by the Commission on Cancer and the American College of Surgeons (https://www.facs.org/quality-programs/cancer/coc/standards). Additionally, in 2007 the Institute of Medicine published a report entitled *Cancer Care for the Whole Patient: Meeting Psychosocial Needs* which emphasizes the importance of screening patients for distress and psychosocial health needs as a critical first step to providing high-quality cancer care. For children with cancer, parental distress, which is generally considered normal reaction, is usually increased at the time of diagnosis. However, parental distress can be persistent and may be impairing in vulnerable caregivers. Parental distress can, in turn, affect coping and adjustment in a child (Kearney and Salley 2015). Children often experience and respond to distress differently than adults. Factors that may influence a child's emotional distress include type of cancer, frequency of hospitalizations, and rate of complications (Kurtz and Abrams 2010). Early identification of distress and referral to appropriate services is key in optimizing child and family well-being.

There are several tools that can be used to screen for distress in children with chronic medical conditions and their families. The distress thermometer is frequently used in the adult population and has been adapted for use with parents

(Haverman et al. 2013). The Psychosocial Assessment Tool (PAT) is a parent-completed psychosocial risk screener that triages patients into three different categories based on level of distress and risk factors. The three categories are universal, targeted, and clinical/treatment. Examples of universal interventions include social work, patient navigator, and CCLS consults. Targeted interventions may include supportive counseling, additional patient/family resources, and medical play for behavioral difficulties in children. Finally, clinical interventions represent the highest level of the screening process, typically indicating the potential need for formal consult by the pediatric consult-liaison team, crisis intervention, potential psychotropic medication use, and potential of risk management and/or patient relations involvement. Interventions are based upon the PAT risk level, with formal behavioral health intervention reserved for those individuals triaged to the clinical/treatment group. This screening and triage system is based on trauma-informed care for children and families in a medical setting (www.healthcaretoolbox.org) and is available in multiple languages. It is used most often in the oncology setting; however, there are also versions available for the neonatal and pediatric intensive care units.

A brief, multidimensional, and developmentally tailored tool for measuring health-related quality of life is the Pediatric Quality of Life Inventory (PedsQL™4.0), available at http://www.pedsql.org/index.html.

Case Vignette 7.3

You speak with the patient navigator, who shares that she recently administered a PAT to the patient's parents. With this screen, she learned that the patient's mother had recently lost her own sister to breast cancer. The patient's father endorsed his own history of depression. Both parents endorsed a high level of distress over the patient and for themselves. The patient navigator is very grateful for your assistance in this case.

You initially meet with the patient and his parents together and explain your role as a child and adolescent psychiatrist. The patient's parents express appreciation for your visit and describe their concerns that their son has not seemed like himself since his admission to the hospital 2 weeks ago. After gathering information regarding the patient's history of present illness, developmental, social, and family history, you suggest that some individual time with the patient may be helpful. The patient's parents agree and step out of the room.

Based on your knowledge of developmental coping, you suggest playing a game to help the patient feel more comfortable. While playing a card game, the patient tells you about some of his worries. He asks you some questions about cancer. He informs you that, when he must be "put to sleep" for a procedure, he fears that he won't wake up. He also describes worrying about being in pain and losing his hair.

While these concerns seem reasonable given the patient's medical illness and developmental age, you decide to screen more thoroughly to ensure that he is not presenting with an anxiety or depressive disorder.

He tells you about his favorite activities, including swimming, soccer, and video games. He describes some difficulty falling asleep at night and not feeling as hungry as usual. You believe that these symptoms are related to various disruptions in the hospital and medication side effects, respectively, rather than to depression. He smiles and laughs at times throughout your session. There is no worthlessness, hopelessness, or guilt. He denies any safety concerns. He denies any history of anxiety prior to the current illness or in any other context besides the medical procedures.

Since he is at high risk for delirium due to his medical illness and its treatment, you also do a more thorough cognitive assessment, even though you believe that an Adjustment Disorder is a more likely diagnosis.

You test the patient's orientation, registration, short term recall, and attention. He does well on these measures, and you decide against administering a more thorough cognitive screen, such as the Montreal Cognitive Assessment (MoCA).

You meet separately with the patient's parents to discuss how they are coping with the patient's hospitalization. The patient's mother expresses appropriate sadness and grief over her sister's death 3 months ago and worries about how the patient will do in treatment. The patient's father expresses that he has been feeling more sad and worried about how the patient is doing. He also describes some difficulty with his own sleep, decreased appetite, weight loss, low energy, and poor motivation. He has noticed that he has also had more difficulty concentrating at work. He denies any safety concerns. He requests a referral for his own counseling to better cope with his son's illness, and you refer him to the adult psychiatry clinic associated with your hospital.

Later, you meet with the patient and his parents together again to recommend supportive psychotherapy, and you discuss the multidisciplinary team approach to providing the patient and family with additional support. You also briefly discuss the role of the CLS and how this person may be able to further bolster the patient's coping. You offer to return later in the week to follow up with the patient and family. Both patient and family appear much more relaxed after your visit.

You consult the hospital's nurse specializing in integrative services and CLS to discuss a multidisciplinary approach to helping this patient and family. The integrative services nurse plans to offer "healing touch" the night prior to a procedure and aromatherapy for help with relaxation. The CLS plans to offer diagnosis teaching and assistance in coping with procedural anxiety utilizing distraction. You plan to continue providing individual and family therapy on a regular basis.

Hospital-Based Services to Facilitate Adjustment

Child Life Services

The hospital can be an unfamiliar and stressful environment for children and their families. work. As members of an interdisciplinary medical team, certified child life specialists (CCLS) and child life service staff practice family-centered care with a particular focus on the social, emotional, and developmental needs of children in the hospital to optimize their coping with illness, injury, and/or hospitalization. All

Table 7.1 Common child life program interventions

Preadmission visits/tours
Surgical preparation
Procedural support
Education about diagnoses
Medical play
Family support
Academic support services

CCLSs are trained to assess patients and identify any potential stressors that a child may face during hospitalization or even in reaction to a diagnosis. A CCLS will create a plan of care that is built upon a child and family's preexisting coping skills and introduce additional methods to cope with various stressors. The aim of this care plan is focused on building resilience in young individuals.

In the USA, child life services are not billable; yet, most pediatric hospitals employ these professionals. Although the structure, scope, and scale of a child life department may vary among hospitals, some of the ubiquitous services offered by child life programs are summarized in Table 7.1.

Preadmission visits or tours are frequently offered to familiarize children with the hospital setting and prepare them and their families for their stay. *Procedural and surgical preparation* (covered further in Chap. 11) incorporates developmentally appropriate language and visual aids with an aim to decrease overall anxiety and prevent trauma. It also helps to build trust between patients, families, and providers. *Procedural support* can come in the form of a calming presence, distraction techniques, or preemptively informing patients of common sensory experiences. *Education about diagnoses* communicates developmentally appropriate and accurate medical information using an approach geared toward the patient's understanding. A CCLS ensures that hospitalized children understand the reason for their admission and what to expect during their stay. *Medical play* allows children to prepare for, or reenact, medical interventions to gain a sense of mastery over their situation.

Developmentally appropriate play is one of the primary modalities used to promote positive coping. A CCLS ensures access to play opportunities in the hospital and engages pediatric patients in purposeful play to facilitate emotional expression, learning about hospital procedures, progression toward developmental milestones, sensory stimulation, socialization, comfort, distraction, a sense of normalcy, and sheer fun.

CCLS frequently operate a playroom that is designed to accommodate children of all ages and capabilities. These rooms are often staffed by assistants and supported by hospital volunteers, and they represent safe spaces where no medical procedures or interventions are allowed. Because children often feel a sense of loss of control during hospitalization, playrooms are designed to provide play options that are fully directed by the patient. This setting also offers opportunities to socialize with peers and alleviate boredom. These spaces may host to special events such as celebrity guest visits and seasonal parties. In these spaces, families often access several programs and services, which may include music, art, dance, and pet therapies. Some hospitals also incorporate a teen lounge and family resource room.

A child's hospitalization and recovery can impact various family members in different ways. A CCLS works closely with family members to understand their unique needs as well. Particularly when a child's behavior impedes medical care, a CCLS can provide parenting support and tools that work within the family structure. Depending on the severity of behavioral health concerns that are present in the hospital setting, a CCLS may work in coordination with members of a psychiatry consult-liaison team. Additionally, the CCLS acts to provide as much comfort and support to each family member regardless of their age. Close attention is paid to siblings, especially during critical moments, such as during end of life planning of a pediatric patient.

A CCLS is trained to speak with dying children about death and will often help the child express their wishes. When a child's death is imminent or has occurred, the CCLS facilitates family bereavement and legacy activities as an opportunity for memory making. The CCLS may also visit the child's school to speak with classmates to quell fears and misconceptions about the death of the patient.

Educational Support

Child life professionals understand that maintaining the connection between a child and their school is of utmost importance. Children need support in accessing their school work during their hospitalization and may also need additional services when transitioning back to the classroom. Therefore, child life staff often work in conjunction with teachers from the local school district to provide educational services to patients.

These services may be coordinated by an educational liaison, who is often a member of child life team. These services may include informing the school of any new accommodations, such as tutoring, needed to accommodate the medical condition.

Some medical centers maintain hospital-based classrooms, which allow patients to resume their role as a student while continuing their inpatient treatment, which may combine school subjects and cognitive rehabilitation principles, and which offer opportunities for socialization and a sense of normalcy.

When hospitalized children return to school, reintegration support is often provided to those patients who have experienced extended absences due to their medical condition. A CCLS may be able to visit patients' classes to educate their peers on relevant diagnoses, clarify any misconceptions, and coach school personnel on the new medical needs of the child.

CCLS are invaluable in identifying and helping to manage the emotional and behavioral aspects of a child's care during a hospitalization. They may be able to recognize when a child is not coping well before other members of the multidisciplinary team and can offer a variety of first-line supports. They also may alert the treatment team to patients that would benefit from formal behavioral health evaluation.

Hospital-Based Integrative Care

As healthcare evolves, increasing numbers of families are seeking more comprehensive medical treatment. Integrative care is the practice of all appropriate therapeutic, evidence-based approaches to optimize health and healing. It refers to the provision of complementary and alternative therapies, in addition to conventional treatment, with the goal of providing holistic care.

Chapter 21 covers this topic in further detail. While Chap. 21 focuses on the consultant's role in assessing complementary and alternative therapies requested by patients in an international context, this current chapter highlights the role of complementary and alternative therapies that are often provided by hospitals to facilitate adjustment to medical illness.

Holistic Nursing

Holistic nursing is an approach that creates a caring space within oneself to promote unconditional *presence for* healing, removes barriers to the healing process, facilitates the patient's personal growth, assists with recovery from illness or transition to a peaceful death, strives for wholeness and well-being for the patient and family, and involves collaboration with the patient and family in a way that facilitates their leading the way to wellness.

Specific Therapies

While families want to have state-of-the-art medical care that offers the best chance of cure, they also often want gentle, natural opportunities for healing that are creative and fun and that are likely to engage children. Some complementary and alternative therapies commonly offered in pediatric hospitals are listed in Table 7.2.

Healing Touch

Healing Touch (HT), and the later addition of Reiki, aims to promote relaxation, sleep, and pain relief. Receiving Healing Touch, compared to reading a book or engaging in developmentally appropriate play, may improve pain, anxiety, and fatigue in pediatric oncology patients (Wong et al. 2012).

Table 7.2 Integrative services modalities in hospitals

Healing touch/reiki
Aromatherapys
Yoga/meditation
Preterm infant massage

Aromatherapy

Aromatherapy is the use of essential oils (pure aromatic compounds extracted from plants, flowers, trees, and seeds) to promote wellness, relaxation, and relief of fatigue and nausea/vomiting. Smelling stimulates the olfactory nerve and connections to the limbic system, where personal memories are stored. To optimize safety in pediatric patients, an allergy assessment is recommended, and only the inhalation method is utilized.

Yoga

Yoga is an ancient art and science developed in India and later in Tibet. It means "integration" or "joining together" of body and mind with each other and the universe (Snyder and Lindquist 2014).

In pediatrics, simple yoga poses are offered in a playful manner, sometimes using animals and objects as references. Meditation can be offered in the form of storytelling, rhymes, and games. Mantras can be sung to a rhythm to accompany a child's yoga practice, which may be done individually at the bedside or in a group in the playroom.

Gentle movement, stretches, restorative poses, breathing awareness techniques, and meditation promote holistic healing, fun, and coping with the hospitalization.

Preterm Infant Massage

Preterm infant massage can help with weight gain, muscular development, circulation, sleep patterns, and relaxation. Positive effects on immunity, brain development, flexibility, coordination, and bone density have also been described (Field et al. 2010). Preterm infant massage can be offered in the NICU as part of normal developmental care and can be done by a variety of specially trained providers, including registered nurses and occupational therapists.

The Role of a Hospital Facility Dog

Numerous studies have demonstrated the positive impact of animal-assisted therapy on pain, anxiety, heart rate, and treatment adherence (Barker and Wolen 2008; Sobo et al. 2006; Morrison 2007) Unlike a therapy dog, a facility dog is professionally trained to the level of a service dog or guide dog and works full-time on site in a clinical role with a handler. This consistency allows facility dogs to be more fully integrated into care plans, and patients are better able to develop positive associations with hospital stays based on enjoyable interactions with these team members.

While the authors' home hospital, Kapi'olani Medical Center for Women and Children (KMCWC), had visiting therapy dogs for many years in 2006, it became one of the first children's hospitals in the USA to employ a full-time hospital facility dog. A highly trained 2-year-old golden retriever, "Tucker," was hand-selected and trained to work in the pediatric intensive care unit, general pediatrics wards, outpatient clinics, and emergency department. With improvement seen in patients' levels of anxiety and depression, treatment adherence, pain perception, and quality of life, Tucker served as an example of the benefits of animal-assisted therapy in comprehensive medical care.

Conclusion

In conclusion, while an acute or chronic medical condition can be devastating for children and their families, pediatric psychosomatic medicine plays an important role in treating and healing the "invisible wounds" that can sometimes cause the greatest distress. In addition to assessing for psychiatric comorbidities, the pediatric psychosomatic medicine consultant, in close collaboration with the disciplines described in this chapter, can provide a comprehensive formulation and recommend various modalities to promote healthy adjustment for the patient and family.

References

American Psychiatric Association. (2013). *Diagnostic and statistical manual of mental disorders* (5th ed.). Arlington: American Psychiatric Publishing.

Barker, S. B., & Wolen, A. K. (2008). The benefits of human-companion animal interaction: A review. *Journal of Veterinary Medicine Education, 35*, 487–495.

Berger, K. S. (2005). *The developing person: Through the life span* (6th ed.). New York: Worth Publishers.

Campbell, L., DiLorenzo, M., Atkinson, N., & Riddell, R.P. (2017). Systematic review: A systematic review of the interrelationships among children's coping responses, children's coping outcomes, and parent cognitive-affective, behavioral, and contextual variables in the needle-related procedures context. *Journal of Pediatric Psychology,42*, 611–621.

Chopra, D. (1997). *The path to love: Spiritual strategies for healing*. New York: Three Rivers Press.

Coakley, R., & Wihak, T. (2017). Evidence-based psychological interventions for the management of pediatric chronic pain: New directions in research and clinical practice. *Children, 4*(9), 1–18.
Eccleston, C., Palermo, T.M., Fisher, E., & Law, E. (2012). Psychological interventions for parents of children and adolescents with chronic illness. *Cochrane Database of Systematic Reviews, 8,* CD009660.
Epstein, M. (1995). *Thoughts without a thinker*. New York: Basic Books.
Field, T., Diego, M., et al. (2010). Preterm infant massage: A review. *Infant Behavior & Development, 33*(2), 115–124.
Haverman, L., Von Oers, H. A., et al. (2013). Development and validation of the distress thermometer for parents of a chronically ill child. *The Journal of Pediatrics, 163*(4), 1140–1146.
Kabat-Zinn, J. (1994). *Wherever you go there you are: Mindfulness meditation in everyday life*. New York: Hyperion.
Kearney, J. A., & Salley, C. G. a. (2015). Standards of psychosocial care for parents of children with cancer. *Pediatric Blood & Cancer, 62*(5), S632–S683.
Kurtz, B., & Abrams, A. N. (2010). Psychiatric aspects of pediatric cancer. *Child and Adolescent Psychiatric Clinics of North America, 19*(2), 401–421.
Loftus, E. V., Jr., Guérin, A., Yu, A. P., et al. (2011). Increased risks of developing anxiety and depression in young patients with crohn's disease. *The American Journal of Gastroenterology, 106*, 1670–1677.
Mechtel, M., & Stoeckle, A. (2017). Psychosocial care of the pediatric oncology patient undergoing surgical treatment. *Seminars in Oncology Nursing, 33*(1), 87–97.
Mikocka-Walus, A., Knowles, S. R., et al. (2016). Controversies revisited: A systematic review of the comorbidity of depression and anxiety with inflammatory bowel diseases. *Inflammatory Bowel Diseases, 22*(3), 752–762.
Morrison, M. L. (2007). Health benefit of animal-assisted interventions. *Complementary Health Practice Review, 12*, 51–62.
Schonfeld, D., & Demaria, T. (2015). Providing psychosocial support to children and families in the aftermath of disasters and crises. *Pediatrics, 136*(4), e1120–e1130.
Snyder, M., & Lindquist, R. (2014). In M. Tracy (Ed.), *Complementary and Alternative Therapies in Nursing*. New York: Springer.
Sobo, E. J., Eng, B., et al. (2006). Canine visitation (pet) therapy: Pilot study data on decrease in child pain perception. *Journal of Holistic Nursing, 24*, 51–57.
Wong, J., Ghiasuddin, A., Kimata, C., et al. (2012, June) The impact of healing touch on pediatric oncology. *Patients Integrative Cancer Therapies.* http://ict.sagepub.com/content/early/2012/06/11/1534735412446864

Chapter 8
Acute Mental Status Change

Steven R. Williams

A common reason for psychiatric consultation on a pediatric inpatient service is "acute mental status change". C&L psychiatrists are often called for "acute mental status change" because neither the pediatrician nor the family has an adequate explanation for such an anxiety-provoking situation, and both may have many unanswered questions. Acute mental status changes are often the consequence of the medical illness that necessitated the hospitalization. Furthermore, one in five children in the United States will have a seriously debilitating mental disorder (NIMH), and many of these children are admitted to a pediatric service for medical care. Considering the inherent stress of inpatient treatment, it is not surprising that many of these children have psychiatric illness exacerbations that manifest as "acute mental status change."

This request often connotes urgency and a need for prioritization when working on a busy C&L service. Acute mental status changes can be equated to acute vital sign changes, which often represent the proverbial "red flag" requiring an urgent evaluation and treatment. Acute manifestations of one of the more common DSM-5 diagnoses are more likely to be the best explanation for a given patient, but having a more detailed biopsychosocial understanding will lead to more effective treatment. Child and adolescent psychiatrists can assist pediatricians with the rarer medical etiologies that may be contributing to the acute mental status changes. The child psychiatrist will likely be more familiar with the basic DSM-5 diagnostic domains that will be utilized during the assessment. After all likely medical etiologies have been considered, one considers the utility, probability, and cost of evaluating the patient for rare medical etiologies that may be related to clinical findings. It is important to remember that a mental status examination is a cross-section evaluation and that more severe findings may distract the clinician from putting together a more thorough and longitudinal history and negatively impact the diagnostic

S. R. Williams (✉)
University of Hawaii, Honolulu, HI, USA
e-mail: williamss@dop.hawaii.edu

A. P. S. Guerrero et al. (eds.), *Pediatric Consultation-Liaison Psychiatry*,
https://doi.org/10.1007/978-3-319-89488-1_8

process. Besides the many medical etiologies that are associated with acute mental status changes and delirium, other psychiatric conditions to consider include stress-related disorders, substance use disorders, mood disorders, schizophrenia spectrum illness, and cognitive limitations. The vignettes in this chapter will illustrate the challenges associated with differentiating between and managing the various causes of "acute mental status change."

Case Vignette 8.1

An 8-year-old boy is evaluated in the pediatric ICU by a child psychiatrist because the parents are concerned about their son becoming "more confused." He had been admitted to the PICU 4 days earlier because of cellulitis of the leg leading to possible sepsis. The nursing staff have been scoring the Cornell Assessment of Pediatric Delirium (CAPD) (Traube et al. 2014) *twice a day for the past 3 days, with the most recent score being 10. You look at the algorithm from the PICU/PCU Delirium Clinical Pathway* (PICU/PCU Delirium Clinical Pathway-ICU Children's Hospital of Philadelphia) *and note that a score of equal or greater than 9 is a positive screen for delirium.*

The differential diagnosis for "confusion" is wide and has different meanings and likely etiologies in a preschooler versus an adolescent (Pediatric delirium – iacapap 2015). When considering confusion, is there a timeline context within which it developed? The more immediate medical history is likely the most important initial consideration in a hospital setting. Physicians sometimes forget to consider a patient's psychological response to a medical condition or its treatment. This may present as anxiety and an alteration in a child's perceptions associated with the drastic change in settings from the home to the inpatient environment. Initial, broad diagnostic considerations associated with confusion are delirium, anxiety, and psychosis. Do not underestimate how past and current psychosocial stressors can exacerbate the symptoms in these diagnostic domains.

The patient has a history of developmental delays, and he has been in a special education class since the first grade. His psychoeducational testing records reveal a full-scale intelligence quotient of 68 and a diagnosis of a reading disorder. Further details are obtained from the pediatric attending and the parents. The boy has spoken of an imaginary pet dog for the past 6 months, but what is more concerning is that he states he has been seeing and hearing the pet dog in the PICU for the past 2 days. The seeing and hearing of an imaginary pet dog is a new occurrence according to the parents. Having this information, you look at the eight questions on the CAPD and realize the answers may be skewed because of the child's baseline cognitive limitations.

This scenario now brings up the question of how children's cognitive development and abilities can affect their interpretation of occurrences in high stimuli environments. If this child is in a preoperational stage of development, he will have difficulty assimilating most of the new stimuli in a PICU setting. Therefore, it is possible that this patient's symptoms may simply be related to his intellectual developmental disorder. However, in the setting of the PICU, delirium becomes the most important diagnosis to consider.

Although the prevalence of delirium in a PICU is at least 20%, delirium is often under recognized in an ICU setting and is associated with significant morbidity and mortality (Traube et al. 2017). Therefore, caution is needed not to miss the diagnosis of delirium (Kelly and Frosch 2012). Most cases of pediatric delirium in the ICU occur within the first few days of being admitted to the ICU. This boy was admitted to the ICU 4 days ago. Additionally, children with developmental delays are at higher risk for delirium (Traube et al. 2017). Another risk factor for this child is that he has an infectious/inflammatory illness.

His vital signs are stable, and he has been sleeping through the night. The pediatric intensivist believes that the sepsis is improving with treatment.

On examination, the boy has a clear sensorium. He is consistently alert and oriented, but sometimes has difficulty communicating his needs. On occasion he makes minimal eye contact and there pauses with his interactions. His vocabulary is limited for his age. He relates well despite having an anxious affect. The boy describes feeling anxious related to being in a very unfamiliar setting and being away from his home and parents. You review the algorithm again and look at the acronym "BRAIN MAPS" (Bring oxygen, Remove/Reduce drugs, Atmosphere, Infection/mobilization/inflammation, New organ dysfunction, Metabolic disturbance Awake, Pain, and Sedation from http://www.chop.edu/clinical-pathway/picu-pcu-delirium-clinical-pathway accessed 1/10/2018) and realize the "Atmosphere" section applies to your patient. He usually wears glasses, and his parents have been spending a limited amount of time with him. He describes seeing and hearing the pet dog as more of a wish or desire rather than well-defined hallucinations. He expresses some uncertainty as to whether the dog is in the room. You are unable to identify any medication he is taking or other medical etiology that may explain any change in his mental status. He was not prescribed any steroids, benzodiazepines, or anticholinergics prior to, or during, this hospitalization. The attending pediatrician inquiries about the possible use of an antipsychotic medication. Your first thoughts are that the side effect profiles for antipsychotic medications can be quite significant, and therefore you would like to be more certain as to whether they are indicated.

Further consideration is given to the child's cognitive development and the significant stressor of being a patient in a PICU. You assess the patient to still be in the preoperational stage of cognitive development, and you believe that his anxiety has impacted his interpretations of stimuli. You also consider the benefits and risks associated with anxiolytic medications. You ultimately decide not to recommend any psychiatric medication but instead to encourage the patient's parents to spend more time with their son in the PICU and provide him his glasses. It was noted that as the parents reassured their son more, his anxiety lessened, and he was less preoccupied with his imaginary dog.

Psychosocial interventions that engage – to the degree possible in a general hospital or intensive care setting – the family and other supports can be particularly effective in addressing anxiety experienced by younger children confronted by separation from significant attachment figures.

You reevaluate the patient prior to discharge from the PICU and note that he is exhibiting only a minimal amount of anxiety. He continues to talk about his imaginary pet dog, but after using his eyeglasses and feeling supported by his parents, he denied seeing or hearing the dog. His parents and the PICU team are relieved to know that this characteristic is not unusual for a child with cognitive limitations in the preoperational stage of cognitive development. Your discharge diagnoses are adjustment disorder with anxiety and intellectual developmental disorder.

Looking up Piaget's four stages of development, you appreciate how a child goes from magical thinking to more logical thinking (preoperational to concrete operational stage). This developmental progression needs to be considered when assessing a child for psychosis.

Scrutiny for delirium was needed in this case. There is the possibility that this boy may have had a delirium related to his infection that resolved with the treatment of his cellulitis and sepsis. Medication-related factors and autoimmune-related factors did not play a role here. His normal sleep cycle and ability to be consoled made delirium less suspect. Unlike in adults, the severity of short- and long-term memory problems and delusions may not present as frequently with pediatric delirium, which often manifests as irritability, mood lability, and agitation (Grover et al. 2012), (Turkel et al. 2006). There is a role for recently developed and validated pediatric delirium rating scales such as the CAPD (Traube et al. 2014), which may be helpful for routine screening in high-risk settings such as the PICU. The CAPD has a sensitivity of 94% and a specificity of 79%. The management of delirium (Thom 2017) was considered in this case and included symptom-targeted treatment, such as increased contact with important attachment figures to reassure the patient and decrease his anxiety. Anxiety, especially in a young child, may not only contribute to the misinterpretation of stimuli and information given to the child but may magnify the misinterpretations, such that the child appears delirious or psychotic.

It is believed that there are multiple neural mechanisms that lead to delirium such as electrolyte imbalances, activation of inflammatory cytokines, cortisol excess, and changes with GABA and serotonin activity. When evaluating a patient for possible delirium, more priority is given to assessing conditions that might disrupt the balance of acetylcholine and dopamine (Gaudreau 2012).

However, in pediatric psychosomatic medicine, it is essential to also consider a child's cognitive abilities and their effect on the interpretation of stimuli. Whenever possible, reviewing any available psychological testing results may prove to be invaluable. Furthermore, sensory misperceptions can be misconstrued as psychotic symptoms; differentiating the two can be extremely challenging in patients with intellectual disabilities.

Case Vignette 8.2

The emergency room attending physician requests a psychiatric consultation for a 16-year-old girl who was brought to the emergency room by her parents because she was acting strange and out of character after coming home late from a party with her friends. The parents stated she appeared fearful, was staring into space, and was mumbling incoherently. They were very worried about her because she had never appeared like this before. You try to interview the girl, but she appears to be too frightened to answer your questions, and the only answer she provides is her name.

As is often the case in child and adolescent psychiatry, collateral information from those familiar with the patient can provide essential information. When indicated, additional diagnostic evaluations, including laboratory studies, may yield pertinent data. Standard studies to consider when a child or adolescent presents with "acute" mental status changes are serum chemistries, hepatic function enzymes, thyroid-stimulating hormone (TSH), antinuclear antibodies (ANA), urine drug screen, structural brain imaging, electroencephalogram (EEG), and infectious disease labs if there is a high level of suspicion for specific infections, i.e., human immunodeficiency virus (HIV). All studies must be tailored to the patient's presentation and must factor in the likely yield and cost of the study especially for relatively rare conditions (e.g., heavy metal poisoning and rare metabolic illnesses). One must keep in mind that, for young patients who do not have an obvious or likely etiology related to their acute mental status changes, the likelihood of finding another medical etiology is low. It is at this point when a wide psychiatric differential must be considered.

Her vital signs are significant for a heart rate of 106.

As basic as vital signs are, they can often be a tip off if they are abnormal. Changes in these parameters can give you clues to possible etiologies for the mental status changes such as central nervous system infections or substance use. Awareness of typical substance intoxication and withdrawal presentations can help to guide your management. Tachycardia and/or hypertension may be related to intoxication with amphetamines, cocaine, hallucinogens, cannabis, or other illicit drugs with associated delirium, psychosis, and mood symptoms (Ghuran et al. 2001). Tachycardia and/or hypertension can be observed in withdrawal from alcohol, benzodiazepines, barbiturates, and opiates. Intoxication with opiates is more associated with bradycardia than with tachycardia. Caffeine is the most common psychoactive drug in the world. Caffeine intoxication and withdrawal are now identified as a diagnosis in the DSM-5. Caffeine intoxication, while less likely to cause delirium, can present with anxiety and a change in vital signs. Caffeine may exacerbate anxiety, mood, and psychotic disorders. There have been case reports of caffeine-induced psychosis and mania. Energy drinks with high content caffeine have become popular, and if a younger adolescent or child were to drink an excessive amount, this could lead to acute mental status changes.

You question the parents further and find that she has not experienced any recent impairing psychiatric symptoms and has been doing well in high school. After inquiring further with the parents, you are unable to identify any recent stressors, mood symptoms, or schizophrenia spectrum illness symptoms. The parents are not aware of any recent head trauma. As best as can be ascertained, she is not taking any anticholinergic drugs. The parents have never suspected their daughter to be using any illicit substances. She is afebrile, and her blood pressure is normal. On physical examination, the patient's pupils are noted to be somewhat dilated. An electrocardiogram (ECG) reveals a sinus rhythm and a rate of 108 beats per minute. Laboratory studies, which include serum chemistry, TSH, CBC, liver enzymes, urine drug screen, and HCG, are within normal limits.

You wonder whether or not the patient has a medical condition that has not yet been identified and is presenting as a delirium or if she is experiencing new-onset psychotic symptoms. Despite the negative history, you continue to consider substance use as a possible contributor to the patient's presentation. You know that most standard urine drug screens do not check for some illicit substances such as hallucinogens (d-lysergic acid diethylamide (LSD) and psilocybin), bath salts, synthetic cannabinoids, ketamine, and 3,4-methylenedioxy-methamphetamine (MDMA). You understand that some of these can be tested for but realize that some of these labs may be expensive and may take a considerable amount of time to be completed. You consider whether you should obtain these additional labs and wait to base your recommendations on the result or suggest therapeutic interventions guided by the patient's symptoms.

Considering that she can only provide her name, you are extremely concerned that her acute presentation, altered sensorium, mydriasis, and tachycardia likely represent a delirium.

Considering that no other medical etiology has been identified and she has the neurologic finding of mydriasis, you order a head computerized tomography (CT) scan, which is found to be unremarkable.

She is admitted to the adolescent psychiatric unit because of her acute mental status changes. Her diagnosis remains uncertain. Later in the evening on the day of admission, the inpatient staff notices that she is speaking more and voicing paranoid beliefs. When you interview her the following day, she is coherent, with a clear sensorium and without any delusional thought content, and she denies any psychotic symptoms. Her vital signs are normal, and she no longer exhibits mydriasis. She is euthymic, and her insight and judgment are good. She then proceeds to tell you that she used LSD with her friends yesterday. A discussion takes place regarding the effects of LSD, substance abuse treatment, and how she feels about discussing recent events with her parents. You ponder whether you would have requested brain imaging if you were told beforehand that this patient was using LSD.

When adolescents without any significant psychiatric history present with acute onset mental status changes and the standard urine drug screen panel is negative, one needs to consider many other drugs, such as synthetic cannabinoids (K2 and Spice), bath salts, LSD, psilocybin, and many other hallucinogens, all of which can produce acute symptoms of psychosis. A patient may have tachycardia and mydriasis with the use of LSD. Structural brain imaging is warranted when young patients present with unexplained acute mental status changes and neurologic findings.

There has been an increase in the use of LSD in the United States and Europe recently. In 2015, an estimated 1.2 million people aged 12 or older were current users of hallucinogens in the United States (SAMHSA 2015 National Survey). According to the National Institute on Drug Abuse (2016), the lifetime prevalence rate for 12th grade students using LSD in 2016 was 4.9%. About 7 percent of emergency room visits in the United States related to illicit drug use are because of hallucinogens (National Estimates of Drug-Related Emergency Department Visits n.d.). LSD psychosis has been well described and has been used as a pharmacological model of psychosis in preclinical research (De Gregorio et al. 2016). LSD's mechanism of action is pleiotropic, involving serotonergic, dopaminergic, and glutamatergic receptors. It is known to stimulate D2, 5-HT2A, and 5-HT1A receptors. In addition to delusions and hallucinations, LSD can produce euphoria, synesthesia, and alterations in the state of consciousness. It stimulates the sympathetic system, causing tachycardia, elevated blood pressure, and mydriasis. Other signs and symptoms which are more severe and life-threatening may occur, depending on the dosage taken. A crucial part of the management is for the patient not to be exposed to excessive stimuli and to be in a supportive environment. Agitation may be treated with benzodiazepines. In the rare instance of hyperthermia and/or significant cardiovascular or respiratory compromise, appropriate supportive medical care will be needed.

Case Vignette 8.3
A 15-year-old boy is admitted to the pediatric inpatient service because of respiratory compromise related to his asthma. His pediatrician has asked for a psychiatric consultation because recently he has been failing in school, spending less time with his friends, engaging less with family members, and sometimes talking to himself. These behaviors were noted to begin approximately 4–6 months ago. His pediatrician thinks that the boy's more recent behavior may have contributed to his asthma medication nonadherence, which led to this admission. Of note, he had not recently been on oral steroid medications in the past several years prior to admission.

Approximately 10% of children have been diagnosed with asthma, and about one third of youth experience a mental disorder across their lifetime (Ries Merikangas and Nakamura 2009). This combination of chronic medical illness and mental disorder can lead to suboptimal treatment adherence and higher morbidity and mortality rates (Gardiner and Dvorkin 2006). As further discussed in a separate chapter, this pattern is often seen in other chronic childhood illnesses such as diabetes mellitus.

An adolescent's mental status can have a profound effect on the management of any illness. If the underlying causes of mental status changes are not adequately treated, it can be difficult to motivate an adolescent to adhere to a treatment regimen.

While meeting with the patient's parents, they tell you that he has been spending more time alone in his bedroom and looking at unusual websites on the Internet.

There is no significant family history of psychiatric illness and no suspicion of substance abuse. When interviewing the patient you note his flat affect and poverty of thought content. No hallucinations or delusions are endorsed. No acute mood symptoms are endorsed or observed. His thought process is linear. He reports finding minimal enjoyment with any activity, and he has difficulty describing his likes and dislikes. He admits that he does not take his asthma medication regularly, but he is unable to explain why. He appears to have limited insight regarding the recent changes in his behavior and the implications of not taking his asthma medications.

You rely on his mental status findings to make the decision of whether he is having active-phase symptoms of a schizophrenia spectrum disorder. He has denied hopelessness, excessive guilt, suicidal ideation, or worthlessness.

Feeling that his history is more consistent with the prodromal phase of schizophrenia rather than a major depressive episode, you wonder whether antipsychotic medication should be started now without the patient fulfilling DSM-5 criteria for schizophrenia, because he has predominantly negative symptoms rather than active-phase symptoms. His poor insight and judgment are impacting his asthma treatment, and therefore you discuss the benefits and risks of starting an antipsychotic medication. The patient and his parents prefer not to have any psychiatric medication prescribed. The following day, while the patient is still on the pediatric inpatient service, his mother calls you, insisting that her son be seen as soon as possible because he has "lost touch with reality." You see him that day on the pediatrics floor. While his asthma is clinically improved, the boy is now elaborating on how the Central Intelligence Agency (CIA) was using special radio waves to communicate with him when he was in his bedroom. He describes his beliefs with complete conviction and insists that you not tell other people about what he has just told you because of possible consequences with the CIA. He describes an urgent need to return home so that he can continue to communicate with the CIA in his bedroom. Your first consideration is to ensure the safety of the patient and others. As you inquire further about his intentions, he states the CIA is asking him to assassinate one of his family members. More details are gathered regarding the onset and timeline of his symptoms, and you feel more confident about your impression of a schizophrenia spectrum illness. You assess that the patient's recent onset of delusional thoughts is influencing his judgment and may lead to dangerous behaviors.

It is extremely important to understand the themes in a patient's delusional thoughts in order to consider how the themes may influence a patient's behaviors, decision-making and judgment, particularly in the context of another medical illness. The patient and parents need psychoeducation emphasizing how mental illness may have a significant impact on adherence with the treatment of medical comorbidities and the need for more vigilance regarding taking his medication regularly.

You meet with the patient's parents and the primary pediatrics team to discuss possible diagnoses including schizophrenia and mood disorders with psychotic features. You realize that it is crucial that the patient's psychiatric disorder be adequately treated, in part to reduce the potential morbidity and mortality of the other medical illnesses. Knowing that steroids may exacerbate psychiatric symptoms, the pediatric team uses judicious doses of steroids to treat his asthma. His asthma symptoms were stabilized quickly on these low doses, and you further concluded that hospitalization could be easily prevented with medication adherence. You recommend that the primary pediatrics team transfer the patient to the inpatient psychiatric unit for further evaluation of first episode psychosis and to be started on a low dose of risperidone (Coentre et al. 2009) (National Institute for Health and Care Excellence UK 2016).

This case highlights the importance of closely monitoring children and adolescents in the prodromal phase of schizophrenia for the emergence of active symptoms. Individuals with co-occurring psychotic and other medical conditions may not only suffer from the baseline symptoms of each disorder but also from an overall worsening in status related to any suboptimal treatment adherence. Additionally, safety issues must always be considered, even if the patient has never entered the active phase of schizophrenia or exhibited the positive symptoms of schizophrenia such as hallucinations, delusions, or a thought disorder. Paramount to the monitoring is the use of a mental status examination. Most clinicians would begin an antipsychotic medication if the patient is in the prodromal phase of schizophrenia or carries a diagnosis of schizophreniform disorder, especially if the degree of impairment is significant. A key part of the treatment is starting antipsychotic medication and providing adequate psychoeducation. When choosing a medication, consideration needs to be given to the medication's side effect profile, such as metabolic syndrome, potential for EPS, and sedation. Part of the management includes completing a baseline abnormal involuntary movement scale (AIMS) and obtaining fasting lipids and a hemoglobin A1c.

You have a discussion with the patient and the parents, and you direct them to the local first episode psychosis clinic for further evaluation and treatment. You also give the parents information from the RAISE website from the National Institute of Mental Health (NIMH >> Fact Sheet: First Episode Psychosis) and educate them further about schizophrenia spectrum illness versus *mood disorder spectrum illness* (Gochman et al. 2011; Cannon et al. 1999; https://www.nimh.nih.gov/health/topics/…/fact-sheet-first-episode-psychosis.shtm).

Case Vignette 8.4

You are asked to consult on a 17-year-old girl in the ICU who had overdosed on acetaminophen 3 days earlier. There is a history of the patient being depressed and psychotic just prior to her overdose. The reason for the consultation is to help distinguish her psychotic symptoms from possible symptoms of delirium. Her liver enzymes and serum ammonia are elevated, and she appears confused and restless. She had been started on N-acetylcysteine 6 hours after ingesting the acetaminophen. Over the past day, she has voiced her belief that she is the worst person in the world and expresses feelings of guilt and wanting to die. There is no previous history of contact with a mental health-care provider or substance use. According to her parents, she had recently become severely depressed over the breakup with her boyfriend. She was experiencing guilt of psychotic proportions, such as stating she had treated her boyfriend in ways that were far from true. Since her admission to the ICU, she takes frequent naps during the day and is awake most of the night.

*When you meet with the patient, she tells you that she is responsible for horrific events that are occurring around the world, and she does not deserve to live. On examination, while she is unable to describe her mood, she appears sad with a blunted affect and easily tears. She denies experiencing any hallucinations. She has difficulty recalling recent events, and her attention and concentration, as assessed with serial 3 s and stating the months of the year backwards, are significantly impaired. The patient can provide her name, but she is unsure of her location and the current year. You realize that this patient is exhibiting some of the cardinal findings – notably a disturbance in attention and awareness and additional cognitive disturbances (*e.g., *disorientation) – of delirium; considering the timeline for the onset of her symptoms and a readily identifiable cause, you strongly suspect the diagnosis of delirium due to hepatic encephalopathy. The Confusion Assessment Method (CAM)* (Gusmao-Flores 2012) *is completed by an ICU nurse and found to be positive for delirium. In addition, an EEG demonstrates diffuse slowing of the background rhythm.*

A proposed mechanism for delirium due to hepatic encephalopathy involves elevated plasma ammonia leading to increased plasma glutamine. This excess glutamine creates an osmotic stress on astrocytes in the brain and resultant astrocyte swelling. Based on this conceptualization, a reduction in plasma ammonia would lead to a decrease in plasma glutamine and thereby lead to an improvement in sensorium (iacapap.org/wp-content/uploads/1.5-DELIRIUM-2015.pdf; Brusilow and Cooper 2011).

You are having difficulty evaluating her thought content. Her guilt does appear to be of psychotic proportions and with a theme that is consistent with her history and affect. However, you realize that it is very difficult to assess a patient's thought content when the patient does not have a clear sensorium. Considering the history leading up to her hospitalization and the limited MSE findings, you include major depression with psychotic features as a possible diagnosis, in addition to delirium.

Notwithstanding this additional diagnostic possibility, you explicitly recommend against any antidepressant medication, particularly given her hepatic status. You work with the medical team to insure treatment of underlying causes of delirium.

The patient is started on lactulose to treat the hyperammonemia. Subsequently, the sensorium improves as the plasma ammonia decreases.

The most important interventions for pediatric delirium include treatment of its etiology (or etiologies, as may often be the case) and frequent and supportive reorientation. The consulting psychiatrist can help the family and healthcare team to appreciate that agitation and distress can often result from disorientation, particularly in an unfamiliar setting and around unfamiliar people. Indeed, it is difficult to "go overboard" in efforts to provide frequent reorientation, and it is helpful for others to appreciate that delirium is not unlike being in a half-awake/half-asleep state or in a state of recovery from anesthesia, where what is learned even just a little while ago may not easily be remembered.

The mnemonic "IWATCHDEATH" also applies to possible etiologies for pediatric delirium: *i*nfection, *w*ithdrawal, *a*cute metabolic, *t*rauma, *C*NS Pathology, *h*ypoxia, *d*eficiencies (B12, thiamine, folic acid), *e*ndocrinopathies, *a*cute vascular, *t*oxic or drugs, and *h*eavy metals.

The risks and benefits of using an antipsychotic medication, such as haloperidol, for agitation is considered. If the patient exhibits significant psychomotor agitation, a low dose of IV haloperidol could be given with the expectation of observing only a minimal amount of EPS. An ECG should be performed beforehand with monitoring of the QTc.

Antipsychotic medications are more often used for the hyperactive subtype of pediatric delirium than for the hypoactive subtype. The hyperactive subtype is characterized by psychomotor agitation, affective lability, hallucinations, delusions, restlessness, and unstable vital signs. The hypoactive subtype of pediatric delirium is characterized by withdrawn behavior, apathy, inattention, limited responsiveness, and psychomotor retardation. Historically, haloperidol has been used for pediatric delirium, but there is now literature supporting the use of second-generation antipsychotic (SGA) medication such as quetiapine, olanzapine, risperidone, and ziprasidone (Joyce et al. 2015). The conclusion is that second-generation antipsychotic medications are effective and safe to control the symptoms of delirium in children and adolescents (Turkel et al. 2012). The choice of the SGA medication will depend on how the adverse side effects of a particular SGA will impact on the medical complications related to the delirium. Risperidone would not be used in this patient because of her compromised hepatic metabolism. Another example would be that quetiapine and olanzapine have more anticholinergic and sedating effects. An observational study of two cases of adolescent delirium suggested that hyperactive delirium was more responsive to haloperidol and that mixed/hypoactive delirium was more responsive to risperidone (Karnik et al. 2007).

By day 5 of her hospitalization, the patient's liver and ammonia lab values have significantly improved and the delirium has resolved. She is now able to give you a coherent narrative about the breakup with her boyfriend and how it affected her mood. The Beck Depression Inventory (NIMH, https://www.nimh.nih.gov/health/statistics/…/major-depression-among-adolescents.shtml) (Dolle et al. 2012) *yields a score of 32. On the MSE, she does not endorse any delusional thought content, and she does not appear to have any psychotic symptoms. Her sensorium is clear, and she is not having any cognitive difficulties. She is given a diagnosis of major depression. She appears to be moderately to severely depressed, but presently not acutely suicidal and with future orientation. After meeting with the parents and the patient, they agree with your recommendation of implementing interpersonal psychotherapy and beginning fluoxetine* (Birmaher and Brent 2007). *You explain that interpersonal psychotherapy for depressed adolescents is an evidence-based treatment and has demonstrated effectiveness for the treatment of depression in this age group* (Mufson and Sills 2006).

Case Vignette 8.5

A 16-year-old boy is admitted to the surgical service with multiple fractures related to being in a motor vehicle accident while driving at an excessive speed. He suffered only minimal head trauma. His parents inform the surgical team that for the two-week period just prior to the admission he was noticeably irritable, sleeping much less than normal, distractible, and announcing plans to pursue several demanding careers. Two days after admission, the surgical attending, thinking that the patient may be manic, requested a psychiatry consult.

Before seeing the patient, you examine his diagnostic studies. You find that his head CT and other labs are within normal limits but notice that no thyroid studies or drug screens have been performed. Before even seeing the patient, you realize that part of the differential diagnosis may be hyperthyroidism or a substance use disorder. A history is obtained from the patient and the parents. The more significant findings on the mental status exam are pressured speech, distractibility, an expansive affect, grandiosity in wanting to obtain several graduate degrees, and poor insight and judgment. He has little understanding of the relationship between his driving and the reason for the car accident and how he may pose a danger to others on the road. He views himself as not making mistakes. His sensorium is clear. On physical exam, there are no focal neurologic deficits, and his thyroid is of normal size. A urine drug screen and TSH are ordered. The drug screen is negative, with the caveat, as you recall, that if he were using some drugs 2–3 days prior to the urine test, the test may easily come back negative. His TSH level is normal.

Hyperthyroidism affects approximately 2.5% of the US population and may present with psychosis or delirium. Hyperthyroidism can present with manic type symptoms such as emotional lability, insomnia, delusions, hallucinations, and paranoia. Also of note is that hyperthyroidism in adults is more likely to manifest as an "affective" psychosis than a nonaffective psychosis (Lee and Hutto 2008).

You gather a history from the parents, and they report that their son was depressed for approximately 1 month when he was 14 years old. The patient's parents deny any suspicion of substance use. They have recently noticed some unexplained weight loss, increased sweating, and jitteriness. There is an uncle who has been described as having severe mood symptoms, but never formally diagnosed with a mood disorder. You have the parents complete a Mood Disorder Questionnaire–Adolescent Version for their son, and the result is a score of 11, which is significant for a bipolar spectrum disorder.

Most patients who are finally given a diagnosis of bipolar disorder initially had a depressive episode before a manic episode (Youngstrom et al. 2009).

The surgeon had ordered low doses of prn haloperidol and lorazepam, which were given. You meet with the patient and parents and provide psychoeducation on the patient's diagnosis of bipolar I disorder and its treatment (Dolle et al. 2012). *You review that a pharmacologic algorithm for the treatment of manic and mixed episodes in adolescent bipolar disorder patients (age 12 and older) includes the following:*

- *Evaluation with the Young Mania Rating Scale – Clinician or Parent version.*
- *With psychosis – risperidone with lithium or divalproex. If poor response or side effects to severe, consider replacing risperidone with olanzapine, quetiapine, aripiprazole, or asenapine.*
- *Without psychosis – risperidone and lithium. May consider lithium only. Quetiapine may be superior to divalproex. Consider olanzapine, aripiprazole, or asenapine.*
- *If the patient is obese or has diabetes, recommend not giving olanzapine.*
- *Consider comorbid diagnoses that would benefit from pharmacologic treatment.*
- *If the patient is refractory with the above medications, consider the use of clozapine or electroconvulsive therapy.*
- *Maintenance treatment with either lithium, divalproex, or aripiprazole.*

The DSM-5 criteria for a manic episode are further discussed in Chap. 3, and presentations of mania in children and adolescents are reviewed in the literature (IACAPAP 2012). The risk of having a depressive episode soon after a manic episode is significant. It is for this reason that patients and family members are educated about the early signs and symptoms of depression and the need for the psychiatrist to more closely monitor the symptoms over the ensuing next few months. The pathophysiology and molecular mechanisms involved with bipolar disorder continues with research related to mitochondrial dysfunction, oxidative stress, glutamatergic neurotransmission, and the regulation of CRMP2 (Kim et al. 2017; Proceedings of the National Academy of Sciences 2017). The more common maintenance medications used for adolescent bipolar disorder are lithium, divalproex, and aripiprazole. The selection of a medication is based on the sex of the patient, side effect profile that the patient and parents agree with, presence of a blood relative with a similar diagnosis that has responded well to a particular medication, and any comorbid psychiatric diagnoses that are likely to improve with a particular medication. Major concerns are the long-term thyroid and renal complications when using lithium, metabolic syndrome (obesity, hyperlipidemia, diabetes), and tardive dyskinesia with the second-generation antipsychotic medications, polycystic ovary disease with valproate, and other complications with other anticonvulsants. When taken as maintenance medications for extended periods, the antipsychotic medications have more significant sequelae than the other medications (NIMH, http://www.nimh.nih.gov/health/publications/bipolar-disorder…children). The need to keep the patient's circadian rhythm and sleep pattern stable cannot be overemphasized. Psychosocial treatments include multifamily psychoeducation groups, family focused therapy, Interpersonal and Social Rhythm Therapy for Adolescents, cognitive behavioral therapy, and interpersonal psychotherapy.

The parents and the patient were educated about the risks and benefits of lithium, divalproex, and aripiprazole as maintenance medications. He was placed on a low dose of risperidone and lithium (Findling 2016) *with the intention of tapering and discontinuing the risperidone after the resolution of the manic symptoms and continuing with lithium at therapeutic blood levels as a maintenance medication.*

Acute Mental Status Changes

The emphasis on "acute" is extremely important in guiding the prioritization of one's differential diagnosis. There is a correlation between how acute the mental status changes are and the likelihood of identifying an etiology, whether it be a significant biological or psychosocial stressor. A crucial part of the evaluation is to differentiate an acute psychotic disorder or psychosis associated with a mood disorder from a delirium. This differentiation is critical because of the greater likelihood of finding a medical etiology related to delirium and being able to treat it. In an inpatient setting, where the psychiatric symptoms are usually more acute and disruptive, rating scales for the mental status are useful in following the patient's clinical course and in guiding treatment decisions. Treatment interventions for acute mental status changes can be both biological and psychosocial.

References

Birmaher, B., & Brent, D. (2007). Practice parameter for the assessment and treatment of children and adolescents with depressive disorders. *Journal of the American Academy of Child & Adolescent Psychiatry, 46*(11), 1503–1526.

Brusilow, S. W., & Cooper, A. J. (2011). Encephalopathy in acute liver failure resulting from acetaminophen intoxication: New observations with potential therapy. *Critical Care Medicine, 39*(11), 2550–2553.

Cannon, M., Jones, P., Huttunen, M. O., et al. (1999). School performance in Finnish children and later development of schizophrenia: A population-based longitudinal study. *Archives of General Psychiatry, 56*(5), 457–463.

Coentre, R., Silva-dos-Santos, A., Lopes, J., et al. (2009). Initial medical work-up in first-episode psychosis – RCAAP. *Early Intervention in Psychiatry, 3*(1), 10–18.

De Gregorio, D., Comai, S., Posa, L., et al. (2016). d-Lysergic Acid Diethylamide (LSD) as a model of psychosis: Mechanism of action and pharmacology. *International Journal of Molecular Sciences, 17*(11)Pii, E1953. https://doi.org/10.3390/ijms17111953.

Dolle, K., Schulte-Korne, G., O'Leary, A. M., et al. (2012). The Beck depression inventory-II in adolescent mental health patients: Cut-off scores for detecting depression and rating severity. *Psychiatry Research, 200*(2–3), 843–848.

Findling, R. L. (2016). Evidence-based pharmacologic treatment of pediatric bipolar disorder. *The Journal of Clinical Psychiatry, 77*(Suppl), e2.

Gardiner, P., & Dvorkin, L. (2006). Promoting medication adherence in children. *American Family Physician, 74*(5), 793–798.

Gaudreau, J. (2012). Insights into the neural mechanisms underlying delirium. *American Journal of Psychiatry, 169*(5), 450–451.

Ghuran, A., van der Wieken, L., & Nolan, J. (2001). Cardiovascular complications of recreational drugs. *British Medical Journal, 323*(7311), 464–466.

Gochman, P., Miller, R., & Rapoport, J. (2011). Childhood-onset schizophrenia: The challenge of diagnosis. *Current Psychiatry Reports, 13*(5), 321–322.

Grover, S., Kate, N., Malhotra, S., et al. (2012). Symptom profile of delirium in children and adolescents – Does it differ from adults and elderly? *General Hospital Psychiatry, 34*(6), 626–632.

Gusmao-Flores, et al. (2012). The confusion assessment method for the intensive care unit (CAM-ICU) and intensive care delirium screening checklist (ICDSC) for the diagnosis of delirium: A systematic review and meta-analysis of clinical studies. *Critical Care, 16*, R115.

https://www.nimh.nih.gov/health/topics/…/fact-sheet-first-episode-psychosis.html

IACAPAP. (2012). Mood disorders chapter E.2. Bipolar disorder in children and adolescents.

Joyce, C., et al. (2015). *Journal of Child and Adolescent Psychopharmacology, 25*(9), 666–670.

Karnik, N. S., Joshi, S. V., Paterno, C., et al. (2007). Subtypes of pediatric delirium: A treatment algorithm. *Psychosomatics, 48*(3), 253–257.

Kelly, P., & Frosch, E. (2012). Recognition of delirium on pediatric hospital services. *Psychosomatics, 53*, 446–451.

Kim, Y., Santos, R., Gage, F., et al. (2017). Molecular mechanisms of bipolar disorder: Progress made and future challenges. *Frontiers in Cellular Neuroscience, 11*, 30.

Lee, C., & Hutto, B. (2008). Recognizing thyrotoxicosis in a patient with bipolar mania: A case report. *Annals of General Psychiatry, 7*, 3.

Mufson, L., & Sills, R. (2006). Interpersonal psychotherapy for depressed adolescents (IPT-A): An overview. *Nordic Journal of Psychiatry, 60*(6), 431–437.

National Estimates of Drug-Related Emergency Department Visits. (n.d.). HHS Publication No. (SMA) 13-4760, DAWN Series D-39. Rockville, MD.

National Institute for Health and Care Excellence, UK. (2016). *Psychosis and schizophrenia in children and young people: recognition and management.*

NIMH >> Bipolar Disorder in Children and Teens: http://www.nimh.nih.gov/health/publications/bipolar-disorder…children

NIMH >> Major Depression Among Adolescents: https://www.nimh.nih.gov/health/statistics/…/major-depression-among-adolescents.shtml

Pediatric delirium – iacapap 2015 Chapter I.5 IACAPAP textbook of child and adolescent mental health.

Pediatric delirium – iacapap. iacapap.org/wp-content/uploads/1.5-DELIRIUM-2015.pdf.

PICU/PCU Delirium Clinical Pathway-ICU Children's Hospital of Philadelphia. www.chop.edu/clinical-pathway/picu-pcu-delirium-clinical-pathway

Probing the lithium-response pathway in hiPSCs implicates the phosphoregulatory set-point for a cytoskeletal modulator in bipolar pathogenesis. *Proceedings of the National Academy of Sciences*, 2017, 201700111.

Ries Merikangas, K., Nakamura, E., & Kessler, R. (2009). Epidemiology of mental disorders in children and adolescents. *Dialogues in Clinical Neuroscience, 11*(1), 7–20.

Thom, R. (2017). Pediatric Delirium. *American Journal of Psychiatry, Residents' Journal, 12*(2), 6–8.

Traube, C., Silver, G., Kearney, J., et al. (2014). Cornell assessment of pediatric delirium: A valid, rapid, observational tool for screening delirium in the PICU. *Critical Care Medicine, 42*(3), 656–663.

Traube, C., Silver, G., Gerber, L. M., et al. (2017). Delirium and mortality in critically ill children: Epidemiology and outcomes of pediatric delirium. *Critical Care Medicine, 45*(5), 891–898.

Turkel, S. B., Trzepacz, P. T., & Tavare, C. J. (2006). Comparing symptoms of delirium in adults and children. *Psychosomatics, 47*(4), 320–324.

Turkel, S. B., et al. (2012). *Journal of Child and Adolescent Psychopharmacology, 22*(2), 126–130.

Youngstrom, E., Freeman, A., & Jenkins, M. (2009). The assessment of bipolar disorder in children and adolescents. *Child and Adolescent Psychiatric Clinics of North America, 18*(2), 353–359.

Chapter 9
"Other Medical" Presentations and Considerations in Pediatric Consultation-Liaison Psychiatry

Taryn Park, Ian Kodish, and Anthony P. S. Guerrero

This chapter covers some of the more common consultation-liaison psychiatry scenarios, including the patient with "somatic" symptoms of uncertain etiology requiring a thorough evaluation for "other medical" etiologies and the patient with behavioral symptoms more clearly attributable to "other medical" or "biological" (in the biopsychosocial formulation) etiologies. The consultant can play a key role in adequately investigating differential possibilities, in addressing all relevant aspects of the biopsychosocial formulation, in establishing an expected course of recovery, and in insuring that the child and family feel supported. The case vignettes will review the traditional somatic symptom and related disorders as well as other situations where the psychiatrist can help guide the team in considering other medical etiologies for behavioral symptoms.

Somatic Symptom and Related Disorders

Case Vignette

Jane is a 14-year-old female, who was brought in to the local emergency department (ED) by her parents due to new-onset seizure-like episodes which started about 2 days ago. Jane has suffered from recurrent headaches and nonspecific abdominal

T. Park (✉) · A. P. S. Guerrero
Department of Psychiatry, University of Hawai'i John A. Burns School of Medicine, Honolulu, HI, USA
e-mail: ParkT@dop.hawaii.edu; GuerreroA@dop.hawaii.edu

I. Kodish
Department of Psychiatry and Behavioral Sciences, University of Washington School of Medicine, Seattle, WA, USA
e-mail: ian.kodish@seattlechildrens.org

A. P. S. Guerrero et al. (eds.), *Pediatric Consultation-Liaison Psychiatry*,
https://doi.org/10.1007/978-3-319-89488-1_9

pain since middle childhood. Her parents describe the recent episodes as whole-body tonic-clonic-like movements lasting several minutes occurring on several occasions over the past couple of days. They deny any associated confusion, syncope, or loss of bladder control preceding, during or following the episodes. Both parents describe the patient as shy and withdrawn, and as a child she experienced some difficulty with separation. Jane describes that the episodes involve a rhythmic jerking of her entire body, an accompanying sensation that it is "happening to her," and a feeling that she is a victim in her own body. With a high suspicion that Jane's symptoms are not due to a seizure, the admitting physician orders both a video electroencephalogram (EEG) and psychiatry consultation. Video EEG monitoring reveals no seizure activity. The psychiatric consultant provides a diagnosis of conversion disorder (functional neurological symptom disorder (FNSD)), with attacks. This diagnosis is explained to both parents and Jane, and the importance of establishing mental health care is emphasized. Prior to discharge, both primary care and psychiatric follow-up appointments are scheduled.

Conversion disorder, or FNSD, in the broader category of somatic symptom and related disorders (which also includes somatic symptom disorder, illness anxiety disorder, psychological factors affecting other medical conditions, and factitious disorder), can present in youth and are diagnosed with the same criteria used for adults. The most common somatic complaints in the pediatric population are pain, fatigue, and gastrointestinal problems, but symptoms can present as complex neurological problems and other severe medical disorders (Kodish 2016; Janssens et al. 2009). During the evaluation process, it is important to perform a comprehensive medical assessment while avoiding unnecessary tests and procedures (Ibeziako and Bujoreanu 2011). The primary diagnostic feature for FNSD is the presence of neuromuscular or sensory impairments that are incompatible with basic anatomy and pathophysiology (Kodish 2016; Ibeziako and Bujoreanu 2011). Symptoms may persist for longer (persistent) or shorter (acute episode) than 6 months and a precipitating psychological stressor may or may not identifiable. The impairment can present suddenly with significant changes in symptom severity and a variable and episodic course (Kodish 2016).

When the diagnosis of FSND is made, it should be communicated explicitly to patients and their families. Providers should clearly discuss the variance between the presenting symptoms and physical exam and laboratory findings and should validate the patient's experience as real and treatable. Validating patients' distress caused by symptoms is important because they may feel unwanted or even blamed for "faking" an illness. Providers should encourage parents to also validate the patient's experience and distress. At the same time, it is equally important to communicate basic expectations for maintaining or progressing toward normative functioning such as walking, communicating, performing activities of daily living, as well as attending school and social activities. Patients and families should be reassured that the prognosis in children is good, that symptoms can resolve fully and quickly, and that impairments can resolve within 3 months of diagnosis (Kodish

2016; Ibeziako and Bujoreanu 2011). There may be reluctance in accepting this diagnosis or the idea that the symptoms have a prominent psychological component; parents may insist on further diagnostic evaluation, multiple primary care visits, or referrals to specialists before they are willing to accept the diagnosis of FSND (Kodish 2016).

It is recommended that providers have some patient interviews separate from parents, and vice versa. These encourage both patient and parents to frankly communicate their feelings and perspective about the impairments without concern of judgment. This open dialogue can help both diagnostically as well as therapeutically, as verbal expression of emotions is a more adaptive form of communication than somatization. This also gives the provider an opportunity to fully assess safety and to address any misconceptions the child or families may have, including that others believe the patient is fabricating the signs and symptoms of an illness (Kodish 2016).

A multidisciplinary approach to treatment is key. Primary care providers (PCPs) play an important role in symptom management. Patients often present to their PCP with symptoms or following an ED evaluation. A behavioral health provider or neurologist can help patients and families understand the underlying cause of symptoms as well as provide reassurance regarding the safety and importance of a neuropsychiatric approach to treatment. Continued involvement of mental health providers should be arranged to facilitate behavioral interventions and provide ongoing psychoeducation to patients and families (Kodish 2016; Ibeziako and Bujoreanu 2011).

Behavioral strategies should address two areas: increasing the adaptive functioning of the child and decreasing symptom reinforcers in the environment. Ideally, treatment takes place in the child's home environment, as hospitalization can reinforce impairments. Treatment should progress in a step-wise fashion, with clear and measurable goals toward self-efficacy. Parents and providers should encourage and praise the patient's demonstration of improvement in function, while seeking to identify any unintentional environmental reinforcers. Providers should be aware that parents may struggle to discontinue actions that reinforce symptoms in their child. Parents may need guidance on how to balance emotional support and validation while setting consistent expectations (Kodish 2016).

Paroxysmal nonepileptic events (PNEs) are described as sudden, involuntary changes in behavior, sensation, or consciousness resembling epileptic seizures but are not accompanied by abnormal ictal discharges in the brain (Park et al. 2015). "PNEs" overlap somewhat with another term – psychogenic nonepileptic seizures – that has a similar acronym (PNES). For the purposes of this discussion, we will focus on PNEs with likely psychiatric etiologies and attempt to avoid terminology that might suggest that either the patient's distress is not "real" or is purely and noncontroversially attributable to a "psychological" cause.

PNEs can occur in all age groups and are common in children. Early and accurate diagnosis of PNEs in children is imperative: to avoid unnecessary and potentially harmful treatments, to allow engagement in appropriate treatment, to mitigate functional impairment, and to prevent the patient from internalizing and overidentifying with the wrong diagnosis, potentially affecting his/her self-image (Park et al. 2015). A careful history and physical examination can be helpful in sorting through the differential possibilities (Kotagal et al. 2002). It is recommended that, when interviewing and communicating with a child, the provider helps to create an environment where the child feels comfortable expressing him- or herself (Cornaggia et al. 2016).

It is important to fully characterize the episodes in terms of frequency, duration, appearance, associated symptoms, and the context in which they occur to aid in differentiating the potential causes (Takasaki et al. 2016). Unresponsiveness without motor manifestations is a common feature of PNEs (Kotagal et al. 2002). Episodes that occur in the same context, exclusively in the presence of others, frequently and for long duration, and with memory of the event are highly probable for PNEs. Additionally, lack of event-related injury is another diagnostic feature. Certain physical features of the episode can also be revealing. PNEs are often asynchronous such as a bicycling motion. Eye closure with or without opposition to opening and vocalizations that are often comprehensible, coherent, and inclusive of emotional content are more descriptive of PNEs. Patients may also respond to verbal and distracting stimuli during and immediately after the episodes (Takasaki et al. 2016).

Presentation and symptoms often vary based on the child's age. Children 6 years and younger often exhibit normal infant behavior such as repetitive grimacing, mouth twisting, crossing legs with cold sweats, and tonic-clonic movement. Episodes may occur more than once a day and on average may last about 1 min. Also common in this age group are myoclonic jerking and periodic limb movement. For these children, subjective symptoms such as dizziness, headache, and chest discomfort were reported. These occurred alone and in combination with tonic-clonic movement of the extremities. Adolescent patients with PNEs describe dizziness, blackouts (that need to be differentiated from vasogenic syncope), and cold sweats, which proceed to generalized tonic-clonic movements or loss of consciousness (Park et al. 2015).

Several risk factors and associated features have been identified for PNEs. Psychiatric risk factors for their development include somatization, anxiety sensitivity, and posttraumatic stress disorder (Plioplys et al. 2016). Internalizing disorders such as depression and anxiety are often present (Sawchuk and Buchhalter 2015). Additional risk factors for both PNEs and internalizing disorders include female sex, older age youth, adversities, and somatization (Plioplys et al. 2016). In the pediatric population, numerous psychiatric diagnoses have been identified as risk factors. These include depression and other mood disorders, anxiety, school phobia, separation anxiety, panic disorder, attention-deficit/hyperactivity disorder (ADHD), history of abuse, posttraumatic stress disorder, cognitive impairment, and learning disorders (Takasaki et al. 2016). Commonly identified stressors include peer issues, family conflict, learning difficulties, and bullying (Sawchuk and Buchhalter 2015).

General assessment for PNEs includes routine blood chemistry/basic metabolic profile, serum antiepileptic drug levels to assess adherence if one is prescribed, toxicology screen, EEG, and imaging in select cases (Plioplys et al. 2007). Video EEG is often cited as the "gold-standard" diagnostic tool (Sawchuk and Buchhalter 2015). It is beneficial to initiate mental health evaluation in parallel with a neurological assessment to avoid a delay in diagnosis (Plioplys et al. 2007; Cole et al. 2014). Delays in accurate diagnosis can lead to inappropriate treatment with antiepileptic medications, which can result in problems with learning and behavior due to their adverse effects (Park et al. 2015; Cornaggia et al. 2016).

Patients and families are more accepting of a diagnosis of PNEs when educated properly (Sawchuk and Buchhalter 2015). When educating patients and families about the nature of PNEs, it important for patients and families to understand that this is a medical condition that benefits from psychiatric consultation and liaison. Providers should emphasize to patients and their families that the patients neither are "faking" their symptoms nor are they to blame. Psychoeducation and psychotherapy can reduce symptom intensity and frequency and can result in partial to full remission of symptoms (Kodish 2016).

As with FSND, a multidisciplinary approach to the assessment and treatment of PNEs is recommended and includes the primary care provider, the mental health consultant, the pediatric neurologist, and school staff. Short-term goals are to decrease the frequency and duration of events and return the patient to typical daily activities. These goals are achieved by critically assessing the current antiepileptic drug treatment and initiating psychopharmacologic agents if appropriate. A behavioral approach, focused on reducing reinforcement of the events, is recommended. Psychotherapy assists the patient in identifying, verbalizing, and communicating feelings that may be perpetuating these episodes. Parent guidance and/or family therapy sessions may promote parental facilitation of adaptive communication of feelings by the patient and other family members. It is also important to work collaboratively with schools, so they too have an accurate understanding of the child's condition and can support the intervention, possibly through a behavioral plan (Plioplys et al. 2007).

Other Medical Causes of Common Psychiatric Symptoms: Example of Traumatic Brain Injury (TBI)

Case Vignette

Johnny is a 1 1/2-year-old male who is admitted to the children's hospital 2 days ago for a new-onset focal seizure not associated with a fever. Neuroimaging studies revealed a subdural hematoma, and subsequent investigations, including an ophthalmological exam and skeletal survey, confirmed the suspicion of child abuse. The pediatric team requests a child and adolescent psychiatry consultation. They note that the child is very irritable, and the young teenage mother has difficulty in consoling him. The team wonders whether you may be able to help in "assessing and helping the family".

You state that you are happy to help, but you are careful to ensure that other appropriate referrals have been made to appropriately address the other concerns. Child protective services has been contacted, and the worker is scheduled to meet with the family later in the day. A security plan has been implemented to keep the child and family safe from the alleged perpetrator (the mother's ex-boyfriend). The hospital's child abuse team, led by a pediatrician with expertise in this area, has also become involved.

You meet with the child and the mother, who agreed to the consultation. You clarify your role as a physician consultant for the child, rather than a forensic evaluator or direct care provider for any adult family member. Your history reveals that the child had previously been developmentally normal, with a generally peaceful temperament. You recognize the various factors that may be contributing to the child's current irritability, including the unfamiliar setting and the likely emotional trauma of the abuse. In addition, and especially after your discussion with the pediatric neurologist, you believe that the head injury may be an important contributing factor to the behavioral change. Part of your recommendations includes a plan to provide long-term follow-up and monitoring of the child's behavior over time.

Severe traumatic brain injury (TBI) is defined as amnesia lasting for 7 days or a Glasgow Coma Scale (GCS) score of 3–8, while mild injury is classified as amnesia lasting less than 7 days or a GCS score of 13–15 (Max et al. 1997). The patient' age at the time of injury is an important prognostic factor. Younger children may present similarly to older youth in the acute setting. However, younger children who suffer severe injury seem to experience greater and longer-term cognitive and behavioral consequences. For children who experience injury at an early age, the extent of executive functioning deficits and behavioral disturbances may not reveal themselves until the environmental expectations exceed the child's abilities. This difference may not become apparent until the child is older (Max et al. 1997). Similarly, the severity of behavioral problems tends to be worse in those who have sustained severe injury in childhood as compared to in adulthood. Early-onset injuries are more likely to result in maladaptive behaviors. Despite normal-appearing cognitive function, injury during early childhood can lead to disrupted social development and behavioral self-regulation (Kodish 2016; Ibeziako and Bujoreanu 2011).

It is notable that pre-injury psychiatric disorders are common in children who sustain traumatic brain injuries. One hypothesis to explain this finding is that children with externalizing disorders are more likely to engage in risk-taking behaviors and, as a result, to sustain traumatic brain injuries. Epidemiological data support this hypothesis, as pre-injury psychiatric diagnoses often include attention-deficit/hyperactivity disorder, oppositional defiant disorder, or conduct disorder. Internalizing disorders are much less likely (Max et al. 1997).

It is crucial to note the severity of injury, as this aspect can also impact prognosis and recovery. Indirect measures of severity indicate that patients with more severe injury experience more neurocognitive and behavioral problems, but even mild injury can adversely impact a child's concentration, personality, and academics

(Hooper et al. 2004). Neurocognitive symptoms can include staring spells, memory difficulties, and temper outbursts. While some neurological symptoms, such as headache, tend to improve over subsequent months, other neurocognitive symptoms may persist or increase. It is possible for problems with both memory and attention to worsen in the months following an injury (Hooper et al. 2004). Deficits in working memory seen in those with severe traumatic brain injury generally improve in the year post-injury, but there may be a persistence or even late decline. Deficits in executive function are well documented in the literature. Difficulties in attentional-inhibitory control can result in distractibility and inability to remain on task for lengthy periods of time. There is also a direct relationship between the severity of injury and deficits in planning and problem solving. These deficits are more apparent in problems with moderate to high complexity. It has also been observed that, even one year after the injury, children who have suffered a severe injury have difficulty summarizing or formulating an interpretation of a story (Levin and Hanten 2005).

While the most salient neuropsychiatric features following TBI are neurocognitive in nature, emotional and behavioral symptoms can be present as well (Luis and Mittenberg 2002). Patients may experience sleep difficulties and lowered frustration tolerance. It does not appear that mild injuries are associated with a significant increase in psychiatric disorders. However, compared to mild injury, severe traumatic brain injury is associated with higher rates of more serious psychiatric sequela such as mood and anxiety disorders and personality change (Hooper et al. 2004). Furthermore, in comparison with other types of trauma such as orthopedic injuries, there is a connection between severe traumatic brain injury and externalizing symptoms as far out as 18 months post-injury (Chapman et al. 2010). Another factor that predicts development of a subsequent mood or anxiety disorder is post-injury stress level (Luis and Mittenberg 2002).

Problems with social skills and social-behavioral regulation have been observed, which present as difficulty identifying emotions and perceiving intentionality and a lack of awareness of the effect of one's behavior on others (Levin and Hanten 2005). Problems with inhibition have also been observed 2 years post-injury in the context of a secondary ADHD. The term "secondary ADHD" has been applied when the diagnosis of ADHD has been made in patients who previously sustained a traumatic brain injury. Secondary ADHD is more commonly diagnosed in patients who have sustained severe TBI and occurs in as many as one third of cases and less so after mild or moderate injury. Secondary ADHD may or may not persist after the injury. Identifying these children can help to inform prognosis. It has been found that, among children who have suffered a severe TBI, those with secondary ADHD experience more difficulties in adaptive and intellectual functioning than those without this diagnosis. Family functioning may also be adversely affected in those with this condition (Max et al. 2004).

Compared to those with milder injury, children with more severe TBI tend to take longer to return to school and experience increased rates of educational problems such as learning and behavioral difficulties. This discrepancy highlights the importance of planning transition back to school for children who have suffered severe traumatic brain injuries. Inpatient physicians play a key role in preparing families for potential problems secondary to the injury and in coordinating care with the primary care provider upon discharge. A successful handoff between the inpatient and outpatient team should communicate enough data about the child's neurological symptoms, neurocognitive functioning, and behavioral problems so these can be tracked in the outpatient setting throughout recovery (Hooper et al. 2004).

Other factors including family psychiatric history, socioeconomic status (SES), and pre- and post-injury family functioning can also influence recovery (Max et al. 1997). More specifically, SES, family functioning, and permissive parenting styles can contribute to deficits in executive functioning (Chapman et al. 2010).

The above case illustrates an opportunity for the CL psychiatrist to be helpful not only in the acute inpatient but also in the outpatient/long-term follow-up setting. While the vignette presents an example of an obvious head injury, we suggest that the astute CL clinician should screen for a history of head injury in comprehensively assessing all patients with behavioral symptoms.

Iatrogenic/Substance Issues

Case Vignette

Jake is an 8-year-old boy who was brought in to the local ED by his parents for a fever and confusion. Jake could not provide much history given his altered mental state. His parents tell you that he was in his usual state of good health until earlier that day, at which time they noticed that he appeared confused. They took his temperature and found that he had a fever. Jake does not have a significant past medical or psychiatric history, and he does not take any medications. His mother has a diagnosis of generalized anxiety disorder, for which she is prescribed sertraline. She reports that, when she went to take her daily dose, she noticed that a significant quantity of her sertraline tablets was missing. In the ED, Jake has a fever and is tachycardic. His pupils are dilated, and he is also diaphoretic, with flushed skin. His musculoskeletal exam reveals clonus, rigidity, and increased deep tendon reflexes. He is disoriented and mildly agitated. Suspecting serotonin syndrome, given his mother's report and physical examination findings, the attending physician consults psychiatry "to assist with managing delirium and the effects of a psychotropic medication," treats the patient with intravenous fluids and a benzodiazepine, and provides supportive care over the next several days, after which the symptoms resolve.

Psychiatrists need to be aware of psychotropic medications' risk in producing serious and potentially life-threatening side effects. Medication side effects are commonly encountered in CL settings, where patients may either be ill enough to warrant treatment in a medical unit or where patients are vulnerable to experiencing side effects because of their other medical illnesses.

Selective serotonin reuptake inhibitors (SSRIs) and serotonin-norepinephrine reuptake inhibitors (SNRIs) are commonly used agents for the treatment of anxiety and depression in the pediatric patient population. Their adverse effects and toxicity are relatively low, but acute, intentional, and unintentional exposure in the pediatric population is high. Most acute overdoses of SSRIs and SNRIs do not result in serotonin syndrome. There are several other medications, across different classes and with different indications, that also affect intrasynaptic serotonin levels (Kant and Liebelt 2012). These include monoamine oxidase inhibitors, tricyclic antidepressants, opioids, over-the-counter cough and cold medicines, and illicit drugs (Phan et al. 2008). Serotonin syndrome can result when these agents are taken in isolation and in combination with SSRIs and SNRIs (Kant and Liebelt 2012).

Serotonin syndrome is classified as a clinical triad of altered mental status, autonomic hyperactivity, and neuromuscular excitation. Diagnosis is made via history of known or suspected ingestion of a serotonergic agent and characteristic symptoms and physical examination findings. Mild cases present with tachycardia, shivering, diaphoresis, and mydriasis. In moderate cases, hypertension and hyperthermia may be present, along with other autonomic signs such as hyperactive bowel sounds. Neurologic symptoms such as hyperreflexia and clonus, which are often greater in the lower extremities, as well as agitation, may also be observed. In severe cases, patients may present with severe hypertension and tachycardia, seizures, delirium, or unconsciousness. They may also demonstrate muscle rigidity and hypertonicity, also greater in the lower extremities (Kant and Liebelt 2012).

The differential diagnosis overlaps with that of neuroleptic malignant syndrome and includes anticholinergic syndrome and malignant hyperthermia. Treatment includes discontinuation of the offending serotonergic agent and supportive care to address autonomic instability and agitation. Symptomatic measures, such as intravenous fluids and benzodiazepines, may be indicated. After discontinuation of serotonergic agent and initiation of treatment, most cases resolve in about 24 h (Kant and Liebelt 2012).

Conversely, serotonin discontinuation syndrome can occur in those who have been taking an SSRI or SNRI over a period of time and abruptly discontinue usage. While it is a withdrawal type of reaction, SSRIs and SNRIs neither cause dependence or addiction; therefore, the term "discontinuation syndrome" is preferred to "withdrawal" when describing this phenomenon. Discontinuation syndrome may also occur during rapid taper of an SSRI or SNRI. All SSRIs or SNRIs have been known to cause discontinuation syndrome, although symptom severity is variable, and the likelihood of an occurrence is greater in agents with shorter half-lives. Commonly reported symptoms in children include dizziness, lightheadedness, drowsiness, poor concentration, nausea, headache, and fatigue, with dizziness being the most frequent. More distressing symptoms include headache, ataxia, and insomnia. Most symptoms are mild, and severity is often inversely related to the SSRI's half-life. For example, discontinuation symptoms with fluoxetine, a commonly prescribed antidepressant for children, may not be severe. Discontinuation syndrome is often short-lived. Symptoms may occur 1–3 days after discontinuation of the SSRI or SNRI, and no active treatment is required for mild symptoms. If symptoms are moderate in severity, symptomatic treatment may be warranted. In the case of severe discontinuation syndrome, resumption of the medication with a more gradual taper can resolve the symptoms. When prescribing SSRIs and SNRIs, patients and families should be educated about both the potential adverse effects and the possibility of discontinuation symptoms (Hosenbocus and Chahal 2011).

Neuroleptic malignant syndrome (NMS), another serious psychotropic medication side effect that generally warrants medical hospitalization, presents as elevated temperature, "lead pipe" rigidity, altered mental status, autonomic dysfunction, and elevated creatine kinase in the context of antipsychotic use (Ty and Rothner 2001; Rasimas and Liebelt 2012). Additional features include leukocytosis, tachypnea, delirium, and diaphoresis (Croarkin et al. 2008). The true incidence of NMS is unclear, as less severe episodes may not be diagnosed or reported. Of note, most cases of NMS occur with dosing in the typical therapeutic range, rather than in overdose. NMS often occurs during the first 2–4 weeks of treatment and after a recent dose increase but it can also occur after long-term use of a neuroleptic medication (Rasimas and Liebelt 2012). Risk factors for the development of this syndrome include prior episodes of NMS, agitation, dehydration, high doses of neuroleptic medication, rapid increase in dose, intramuscular administration, and polypharmacy (Ty and Rothner 2001; Croarkin et al. 2008).

NMS appears mediated by dopamine, specifically D_2 receptor blockade (Croarkin et al. 2008). This diagnosis should be considered in the evaluation of fever of unknown origin (Joshi et al. 1991). When concerned about NMS, pediatric providers should consider the differential diagnoses of malignant hyperthermia, heat stroke, neuroleptic-induced parkinsonism, serotonin syndrome, atropinism, and central nervous system infection (Ty and Rothner 2001). While providers should probe for a specific history of neuroleptic use, it is important to keep in mind that other dopaminergic agents such as antiemetics like prochlorperazine and metoclopramide – not infrequently encountered in the medical setting – can also produce NMS (Edwards 1991).

Identification of risk factors in the patient history and early recognition are important. The offending agent should be discontinued and symptomatic interventions initiated (Ty and Rothner 2001; Abu-Kishk et al. 2004). Rehydration can prevent renal failure, and dialysis should be considered. Levodopa/carbidopa and bromocriptine can be considered to reverse the hypodopaminergic state, extrapyramidal symptoms of rigidity, and consequent hyperthermia and rhabdomyolysis. Dantrolene can also be considered to treat the skeletal muscle rigidity, hyperthermia, and rhabdomyolysis (Ty and Rothner 2001; Joshi et al. 1991). Benzodiazepines can be utilized for agitation (Ty and Rothner 2001). In refractory cases, electroconvulsive therapy can also be considered (Abu-Kishk et al. 2004).

Other times, the CL psychiatrist may be called to address behavioral symptoms that are side effects of medications prescribed for other medical conditions.

Case Vignette

A 6-year-old girl admitted to the hospital for chemotherapy for acute lymphoblastic leukemia reports hearing voices of demons telling her to kill herself. Although she seemed initially to adjust well to her diagnosis and treatment, her behavior suddenly changed, and she is sometimes sobbing inexplicably. As the requested psychiatric consultant, you review her list of medications and note that she has recently been started on a steroid regimen.

While most of the literature describes the adverse psychiatric effects of corticosteroid treatment in the adult population, this class of agents is integral to the management of many pediatric illnesses. Case series have revealed that as many as 50% of children receiving steroid treatment have experienced behavioral and affective adverse effects. In general, the most commonly observed symptoms include anxiety, fear, tearfulness, indifference, lethargy, insomnia, irritability, agitation, labile mood, pressured speech, and restlessness. Hypomania/mania, depression, or mixed states are the most common psychiatric disturbances (Warrington and Bostwick 2006). Suicidality should be assessed for in children being treated with steroids. Psychotic symptoms, such as persecutory delusions and auditory hallucinations, may also be present (Stuart et al. 2005). Cognitive deficits, including problems with declarative or verbal memory altered consciousness and disorientation, have also been documented (Warrington and Bostwick 2006; Stuart et al. 2005).

Generally, dosage appears to be the most important risk factor to consider. Higher doses are associated with increased rates of psychiatric adverse effects. However, there is not a direct dose-response effect. Case reports in pediatric populations reveal daily oral corticosteroid doses ≥40 mg of prednisone equivalents were associated with severe psychiatric adverse effects. There are no clear differences between particular corticosteroids, but there is some data to suggest dexamethasone may be associated with more psychiatric adverse reactions than prednisolone in pediatric populations (Stuart et al. 2005). Timeline in treatment is not a reliable predictor, as adverse effects can occur at initiation and cessation of treatment (Warrington and Bostwick 2006). However, data on children and adolescents has revealed that psychiatric adverse effects typically emerge within days of treatment initiation (Stuart et al. 2005).

If a patient experiences adverse psychiatric effects with steroid treatment, discontinuation or reduction in dose is the primary recommendation (Warrington and Bostwick 2006). Treatment with an alternative corticosteroid agent can also be considered (Stuart et al. 2005). For those patients who have received high doses or long courses of steroid treatment, cautious taper is recommended to prevent withdrawal. Withdrawal symptoms after prolonged corticosteroid use are mediated by the hypothalamic-pituitary-adrenal axis. The most common psychiatric symptoms are depression, anxiety, and fatigue, but mania and delirium have also been described (Warrington and Bostwick 2006). Suicidal ideation during corticosteroid treatment has been reported in children and adolescents, but there is insufficient data to draw conclusions about suicidality during discontinuation of treatment (Stuart et al. 2005). Pharmacologic options for the treatment of affective and psychotic symptoms when corticosteroid treatment must be continued include mood stabilizers such as lithium, carbamazepine, and antipsychotic agents. The adult literature recommends treatment with lithium, but this may be impractical for the pediatric population (Ularntinon et al. 2010). Case reports have detailed the utility of risperidone in the treatment of steroid-related mood and psychotic symptoms in the pediatric nephrology and oncology settings (Ularntinon et al. 2010; Bag et al. 2012).

Because of the prevalence and utility of treatment with corticosteroids across a wide range of conditions, pediatric providers should be familiar with potential psychiatric adverse effects. Patients and parents should be counseled about these potential adverse effects. Providers should proactively probe for psychiatric symptoms at follow-up, as patients and parents may not spontaneously report these problems (Ularntinon et al. 2010).

Sleep Disturbances: An Often-Under-appreciated Contributor to Behavioral Symptoms

We close this chapter by considering sleep disturbances as an example of an often-under-appreciated yet important "biological" factor in formulations explaining the origin of behavioral symptoms.

Case Vignette
Carson is a 12-year-old boy with type 1 diabetes mellitus who was admitted after a recent episode of diabetic ketoacidosis. His parents describe Carson as being chronically inattentive and often distracted during independent assignments, but he has become increasingly irritable over the past week and even intermittently refuses to comply with his diabetic care. They also report that his teachers have commented on Carson's irritable mood. Carson reports feeling fatigued during the day, and he and his parents report that he does not have a consistent bedtime. After dinner, Carson has the freedom to engage in any leisure activity, including watching television, playing video games, or jumping on the trampoline in the backyard. The family removed the television from his bedroom about 3 weeks ago and only recently implemented a household rule of Carson relinquishing his cellular telephone at 8:00 PM every night. Carson and his parents are educated on ideal sleep hygiene practices. Additional behavior changes are recommended, including a set bedtime of 9:00 PM and wake time of 7:00 AM, restriction of all electronics, and physical exercise in the hour before bedtime. Also, a bedtime routine was established, which would start 30 min before bedtime and include showering, changing into his pajamas, and brushing his teeth.

Insomnia describes difficulty with sleep initiation, sleep maintenance or early morning awakenings, or inability to resume sleep. Sleep problems – insomnia being the most common – can affect 25–30% of children (Nunes and Bruni 2015; Badin et al. 2016). Some predisposing factors include being the first born and/or only child, maternal psychopathology or depression, ineffective caregiver management of nocturnal awakenings, nighttime feeding, and co-sleeping. Providers should pay attention to conditions such as depression, ADHD, autism spectrum disorder, epilepsy, and Tourette syndrome (Nunes and Bruni 2015).

A thorough history, including details on sleep routine and characteristics of sleep and wake states, is important for diagnosis. The BEARS tool (Owens and Dalzell 2005) can be used to screen for sleep difficulties in the pediatric population. Asking about **B**edtime Issues, **E**xcessive daytime sleepiness, **A**wakenings during the night, **R**egularity and duration of sleep, and **Snoring** can aid in detecting disordered sleep patterns. Utilizing a sleep journal for 2 weeks is another helpful option. This allows some assessment of circadian rhythm patterns and amount of sleep. There are other validated questionnaires that can be utilized to assess sleep quality and that also take into account a child's age. Options include the Brief Infant Sleep Questionnaire (Sadeh 2004) and the Sleep Disturbance Scale for Children (Bruni et al. 1996). Sleep patterns can also be monitored externally. Actigraphy utilizes a wristwatch-appearing device that monitors body movements to evaluate sleep-wake rhythms. Polysomnography, considered the gold standard for examining sleep, utilizes an electroencephalogram and other physiologic parameters to analyze sleep architecture, respiratory events, and body movements (Nunes and Bruni 2015).

The specific type of sleep difficulty can vary with age. Behavioral issues are common etiologies for sleep problems in infants, including behavioral insomnia and night time feedings. Behavioral problems are also common in toddlers. Another consideration would be age-appropriate nocturnal fears. In adolescence, the most common sleep difficulty is insomnia due to delayed sleep phase (Pelayo and Dubik 2008).

Treatment can include both behavioral and pharmacologic approaches. Healthy sleep hygiene practices are an important first step in the management of disordered sleep. Parents may require education on what constitutes healthy sleep hygiene. Key aspects include a regular and consistent bedtime appropriate for the child's age, avoiding high-caffeine food and drinks, a comfortable nighttime environment, a bedtime routine, and a consistent wake up time (Nunes and Bruni 2015).

Dietary considerations should be discussed. Food and drinks that contain caffeine and alcohol should be avoided during daytime hours and especially at night. Nicotine and marijuana are other substances to ask patients and families about which affect sleep quality. Timing of activities is another important consideration. Moderate exercise during the day can have a positive impact on sleep. In the 3 h before initiation of an established bedtime routine, the child should engage in relaxing, rather than physically strenuous, activities to avoid overstimulation in the period before bed.

Families should be encouraged to eliminate electronic use at least 1 h before bedtime (Nunes and Bruni 2015). Television watching, especially in children's bedrooms, has become increasingly prevalent. Television watching has been repeatedly associated with inadequate or disrupted sleep. In general, greater television watching and the presence of a television in the bedroom are associated with a decreased amount of sleep (Cespedes et al. 2014).

Other aspects of the bedroom environment should also be assessed and adjusted to encourage good sleep hygiene. The room should be at a comfortable temperature, have adequate ventilation, and be quiet and dark at night. Providers should recommend against using the bedroom for punishment, such as time out, as children will develop a negative association with the room. A bedtime routine of consistent activities that prepare the child for sleep should be repeated every night. Aspects can include hygiene activities, reading a story, or spending time with parents and turning off lights. It is also recommended that the routine be started at a reasonable time to allow for completion of activities in a calm manner (Nunes and Bruni 2015).

Behavioral therapy is another approach to treating insomnia. The main goal is to eliminate the negative associations that have developed and led to insomnia. Behavioral therapy can be utilized in children as young as 6 months old. There are multiple approaches to behavioral therapy, and a discussion between provider and parents should identify which option is the best fit for the child. Therapy approaches include extinction, gradual extinction, positive routines, planned bedtime, programmed awakening, cognitive restructuring, relaxation techniques, sleep restriction, and stimulus control. When implemented properly, behavioral therapies can improve daily functioning, mood, sleep, and parental marital satisfaction (Nunes and Bruni 2015). Cognitive-behavioral therapy for insomnia (CBT-I) utilizes cognitive-behavior strategies to treat insomnia. It is the first-line treatment in adults with some efficacy in children as well. The goal of this form of treatment is to correct the features that perpetuate insomnia; these features include physiological, behavioral, environmental, and psychological aspects. Key components of CBT-I include stimulus control, sleep restriction, sleep hygiene, cognitive therapy, behavioral relaxation, and relapse prevention (Badin et al. 2016).

In addition to sleep hygiene and behavioral interventions for the management of insomnia, there are pharmacologic options as well. However, there are no medications approved by the US Food and Drug Administration for the treatment of insomnia in children. Pharmacologic treatment can be considered when behavioral interventions do not yield adequate results or when parents cannot properly implement behavioral strategies. It is recommended that pharmacologic treatments be implemented in conjunction with behavioral therapy and that they be time limited (Nunes and Bruni 2015). Among primary care providers, the most common reason to initiate pharmacologic treatment is for sleep onset delay (Honaker and Meltzer 2016).

The following considerations can help guide the initiation of pharmacologic sleep interventions. The medication should target a specific symptom or a primary sleep disorder and should consider age and neurodevelopmental level. Commonly used pharmacologic agents include antihistamines such as hydroxyzine and diphenhydramine, alpha agonists such as clonidine, melatonin, L5-hydroxytryptophan, benzodiazepines, and tricyclic antidepressants (Nunes and Bruni 2015). Antihistamines are the over-the-counter pharmacologic agents most commonly recommended by pediatric primary care providers, while alpha 2 agonists are the most commonly prescribed medications (Honaker and Meltzer 2016). Except for clonazepam, benzodiazepines are not commonly used in the treatment of sleep disorders in children (Pelayo and Dubik 2008).

It can be helpful to consider psychiatric comorbidities when initiating pharmacologic treatment for insomnia. Alpha agonists such as clonidine are the most common sleep aid in children with comorbid ADHD. Trazodone is often prescribed for sleep problems in children with mood or anxiety diagnoses. While they are not sleep aids, antidepressants such as mirtazapine are also prescribed for children with comorbid mood and sleep disorders (Badin et al. 2016).

Parents should be educated about the possible adverse reactions and potential for paradoxical reactions when using hypnotic medications and about the importance of dosing and timing of administration (Pelayo and Dubik 2008).

Aside from insomnia, there are a wide range of sleep problems and disorders that can occur in children. Unusual sleep behaviors can be attributed to nightmares and other parasomnias. Conditions like restless legs syndrome, periodic limb movement disorder, and obstructive sleep apnea can disrupt sleep. Excessive daytime sleepiness can be caused by narcolepsy and Kleine-Levin syndrome. A more in-depth review of these disorders and their treatment are available to the reader (Gringras 2008).

Conclusions

In summary, we believe that the consultation-liaison psychiatrist has a potentially important role in helping the medical team to conscientiously approach the challenge presented by pediatric patients who present with "somatic" symptoms with a likely psychiatric diagnosis or who present with "behavioral" symptoms likely caused by other medical conditions, psychiatric medications, or medications prescribed for other medical conditions. The unifying theme is that in these situations, it is essential to have a thoughtful and systematic approach to considering other medical conditions. We suggest that the consultation-liaison psychiatrist (adapted from Guerrero and Matsu 2007):

A. Adequately consider differential diagnoses.

   1. Correctly identify the chief complaint (without being inappropriately biased toward psychiatric etiologies at the exclusion of other medical etiologies).
   2. Identify mechanisms behind the chief complaint to establish an initial list of differential diagnoses (again, to avoid being narrowly focused on only psychiatric etiologies).
   3. Carefully elicit and examine other coexisting signs and symptoms to test the hypotheses.
   4. Ask "Why now?" to evaluate further which hypotheses best explain why the patient is currently having the symptoms.

B. Specifically consider life-threatening conditions.

   5. Observe abnormalities in mental status and vital signs while specifically considering the most life-threatening explanations (e.g., unexplained hypertension and bradycardia, possibly associated with a space-occupying brain lesion; unexplained tachycardia, possibly associated with substance or medication toxicity; etc.).

C. Consider child development and specific pediatric conditions.

   6. Apply knowledge of child development to the interpretation of presenting symptoms (e.g., preverbal children may manifest pain as unusual behavioral symptoms such as head-banging).
   7. Consider specific pediatric illnesses in the differential diagnosis (e.g., genetic syndromes associated with certain behavioral phenotypes; infections that are statistically probable in children and adolescents such as Epstein-Barr virus infections for depression, streptococcal infections for obsessive-compulsive spectrum disorders; etc.).

D. Advocate for optimal general medical care.

8. Consider the rarity of certain psychiatric conditions relative to the other medical conditions being ruled out (e.g., many of the somatic symptom and related disorders are, from a statistical standpoint, relatively rare compared to other medical conditions).
9. Consider other medical conditions that may be comorbid or underrecognized in the context of a psychiatric condition or challenging psychosocial circumstance.
10. Use liaison skills in managing bias and countertransference and working with the general medical team.

E. Effectively communicate and listen.

11. Consider asking families what they fear may happen to their child to guide supportive explanation.
12. Listen to other people's suggestions about diagnostic possibilities.

Given the complex nature of many of these cases, we recommend that the consulting psychiatrist follow these patients closely and work closely with the medical team. Finally, in determining whether a patient can be safely discharged from an inpatient or emergency setting, we recommend performing a final checklist:

1. Have other medical conditions been adequately ruled out?
2. Have patient/family concerns about what they "are most worried is causing these symptoms" been addressed (otherwise, the patient may soon present again to the hospital)?
3. Have threats to the patient's safety, including abuse/neglect, been adequately ruled out through individual and family interview?
4. Have the patient and family been "prescribed" a face-saving expected course of recovery?
5. Is there a follow-up plan?

Especially in the context of complex presentations with multifactorial or uncertain etiologies, the consultation-liaison psychiatrist plays an essential role in ensuring safe and appropriate care.

References

Abu-Kishk, I., Toledano, M., Reis, A., Daniel, D., & Berkovitch, M. (2004). Neuroleptic malignant syndrome in a child treated with an atypical antipsychotic. *Journal of Toxicology. Clinical Toxicology, 42*, 921–925.

Badin, E., Haddad, C., & Shatkin, J. P. (2016). Insomnia: The sleeping Giant of pediatric public health. *Current Psychiatry Reports, 18*, 47.

Bag, O., Erdogan, I., Onder, Z. S., Altinoz, S., & Ozturk, A. (2012). Steroid-induced psychosis in a child: Treatment with risperidone. *General Hospital Psychiatry, 34*, 103.e5–103.e6.

Bruni, O., Ottaviano, S., Guidetti, V., Romoli, M., Innocenzi, M., Cortesi, F., & Giannotti, F. (1996). The sleep disturbance scale for children (SDSC) construction and validation of an instrument to evaluate sleep disturbances in childhood and adolescence. *Journal of Sleep Research, 5*(4), 251–261.

Cespedes, E. M., Gillman, M. W., Kleinman, K., Rifas-Shiman, S. L., Redline, S., & Taveras, E. M. (2014). Television viewing, bedroom television, and sleep duration from infancy to mid-childhood. *Pediatrics, 133*, e1163–e1171.

Chapman, L. A., Wade, S. L., Walz, N. C., Taylor, H. G., Stancin, T., & Yeates, K. O. (2010). Clinically significant behavior problems during the initial 18 months following early childhood traumatic brain injury. *Rehabilitation Psychology, 55*, 48–57.

Cole, C. M., Falcone, T., Caplan, R., Timmons-Mitchell, J., Jares, K., & Ford, P. J. (2014). Ethical dilemmas in pediatric and adolescent psychogenic nonepileptic seizures. *Epilepsy & Behavior, 37*, 145–150.

Cornaggia, C. M., di Rosa, G., Polita, M., Magaudda, A., Perin, C., & Beghi, M. (2016). Conversation analysis in the differentiation of psychogenic nonepileptic and epileptic seizures in pediatric and adolescent settings. *Epilepsy & Behavior, 62*, 231–238.

Croarkin, P. E., Emslie, G. J., & Mayes, T. L. (2008). Neuroleptic malignant syndrome associated with atypical antipsychotics in pediatric patients: A review of published cases. *The Journal of Clinical Psychiatry, 69*, 1157–1165.

Edwards, M. S. (1991). Neuroleptic malignant syndrome. *Pediatrics, 88*, 1074.

Gringras, P. (2008). When to use drugs to help sleep. *Archives of Disease in Childhood, 93*, 976–981.

Guerrero, A. P. S., & Matsu, C. R. (2007). Chapter 24: Children and Adolescents. In H. Leigh & J. Streltzer (Eds.), *Handbook of Consultation-Liaison Psychiatry* (pp. 316–340). New York: Springer.

Honaker, S. M., & Meltzer, L. J. (2016). Sleep in pediatric primary care: A review of the literature. *Sleep Medicine Reviews, 25*, 31–39.

Hooper, S. R., Alexander, J., Moore, D., Sasser, H. C., Laurent, S., King, J., Bartel, S., & Callahan, B. (2004). Caregiver reports of common symptoms in children following a traumatic brain injury. *NeuroRehabilitation, 19*, 175–189.

Hosenbocus, S., & Chahal, R. (2011). SSRIs and SNRIs: A review of the discontinuation syndrome in children and adolescents. *Journal of the Canadian Academy of Child and Adolescent Psychiatry, 20*, 60–67.

Ibeziako, P., & Bujoreanu, S. (2011). Approach to psychosomatic illness in adolescents. *Current Opinion in Pediatrics, 23*, 384–389.

Janssens, K. A., Oldehinkel, A. J., & Rosmalen, J. G. (2009). Parental overprotection predicts the development of functional somatic symptoms in young adolescents. *The Journal of Pediatrics, 154*, 918–923.e1.

Joshi, P. T., Capozzoli, J. A., & Coyle, J. T. (1991). Neuroleptic malignant syndrome: Life-threatening complication of neuroleptic treatment in adolescents with affective disorder. *Pediatrics, 87*, 235–239.

Kant, S., & Liebelt, E. (2012). Recognizing serotonin toxicity in the pediatric emergency department. *Pediatric Emergency Care, 28*, 817–821. quiz 822-4.

Kodish, I. (2016). Functional neurological symptom disorder in youth. *Pediatric Annals, 45*, e356–e361.

Kotagal, P., Costa, M., Wyllie, E., & Wolgamuth, B. (2002). Paroxysmal nonepileptic events in children and adolescents. *Pediatrics, 110*, e46.

Levin, H. S., & Hanten, G. (2005). Executive functions after traumatic brain injury in children. *Pediatric Neurology, 33*, 79–93.

Luis, C. A., & Mittenberg, W. (2002). Mood and anxiety disorders following pediatric traumatic brain injury: A prospective study. *Journal of Clinical and Experimental Neuropsychology, 24*, 270–279.

Max, J. E., Lindgren, S. D., Knutson, C., Pearson, C. S., Ihrig, D., & Welborn, A. (1997). Child and adolescent traumatic brain injury: Psychiatric findings from a paediatric outpatient specialty clinic. *Brain Injury, 11*, 699–711.

Max, J. E., Lansing, A. E., Koele, S. L., Castillo, C. S., Bokura, H., Schachar, R., Collings, N., & Williams, K. E. (2004). Attention deficit hyperactivity disorder in children and adolescents following traumatic brain injury. *Developmental Neuropsychology, 25*, 159–177.

Nunes, M. L., & Bruni, O. (2015). Insomnia in childhood and adolescence: Clinical aspects, diagnosis, and therapeutic approach. *Jornal de Pediatria, 91*, S26–S35.

Owens, J. A., & Dalzell, V. (2005). Use of the 'BEARS'sleep screening tool in a pediatric residents' continuity clinic: A pilot study. *Sleep Medicine, 6*(1), 63–69.

Park, E. G., Lee, J., Lee, B. L., Lee, M., & Lee, J. (2015). Paroxysmal nonepileptic events in pediatric patients. *Epilepsy & Behavior, 48*, 83–87.

Pelayo, R., & Dubik, M. (2008). Pediatric sleep pharmacology. *Seminars in Pediatric Neurology, 15*, 79–90.

Phan, H., Casavant, M. J., Crockett, S., Lee, A., Hall, M. W., & Nahata, M. C. (2008). Serotonin syndrome following a single 50 mg dose of sertraline in a child. *Clinical Toxicology (Philadelphia, Pa.), 46*, 845–849.

Plioplys, S., Asato, M. R., Bursch, B., Salpekar, J. A., Shaw, R., & Caplan, R. (2007). Multidisciplinary management of pediatric nonepileptic seizures. *Journal of the American Academy of Child and Adolescent Psychiatry, 46*, 1491–1495.

Plioplys, S., Doss, J., Siddarth, P., Bursch, B., Falcone, T., Forgey, M., Hinman, K., Lafrance, W. C., Jr., Laptook, R., Shaw, R. J., Weisbrot, D. M., Willis, M. D., & Caplan, R. (2016). Risk factors for comorbid psychopathology in youth with psychogenic nonepileptic seizures. *Seizure, 38*, 32–37.

Rasimas, J. J., & Liebelt, E. L. (2012). Adverse effects and toxicity of the atypical antipsychotics: What is important for the pediatric emergency medicine practitioner. *Clinical Pediatric Emergency Medicine, 13*, 300–310.

Sadeh, A. (2004). A brief screening questionnaire for infant sleep problems: Validation and findings for an internet sample. *Pediatrics, 113*(6), e570–e577.

Sawchuk, T., & Buchhalter, J. (2015). Psychogenic nonepileptic seizures in children – psychological presentation, treatment, and short-term outcomes. *Epilepsy & Behavior, 52*, 49–56.

Stuart, F. A., Segal, T. Y., & Keady, S. (2005). Adverse psychological effects of corticosteroids in children and adolescents. *Archives of Disease in Childhood, 90*, 500–506.

Takasaki, K., Diaz Stransky, A., & Miller, G. (2016). Psychogenic nonepileptic seizures: Diagnosis, management, and bioethics. *Pediatric Neurology, 62*, 3–8.

Ty, E. B., & Rothner, A. D. (2001). Neuroleptic malignant syndrome in children and adolescents. *Journal of Child Neurology, 16*, 157–163.

Ularntinon, S., Tzuang, D., Dahl, G., & Shaw, R. J. (2010). Concurrent treatment of steroid-related mood and psychotic symptoms with risperidone. *Pediatrics, 125*, e1241–e1245.

Warrington, T. P., & Bostwick, J. M. (2006). Psychiatric adverse effects of corticosteroids. *Mayo Clinic Proceedings, 81*, 1361–1367.

Part III
Contemporary Value-Building Roles Spanning Multiple Specialties and Healthcare Settings

Chapter 10
Principles of Biopsychosocial Formulation and Interventions in the Pediatric Medical Setting

Kevin K. Tsang, Serena A. Fernandes, and Patricia Ibeziako

Consultation-liaison (CL) providers commonly fulfill multiple roles beyond simply direct care (Carter et al. 2014). Effective consultation and liaison work includes (a) direct assessment and provision of evidence-based interventions for medically-psychologically involved patients and their families, (b) continued advancement of systems-based quality improvement and clinical pathway development, and (c) multidisciplinary collaboration and education, ranging from in-hospital providers to schools. Without a clear conceptualization of the factors contributing to the presenting concern, it is exceedingly difficult to develop a structured and focused management plan, and the clinician's efforts can easily become overly diffuse.

The role of the biopsychosocial formulation is to concisely communicate a comprehensive synthesis of the multiple elements that led to a patient presenting at clinic or hospital with a problem. Understanding these past and recent contributors should logically inform the recommendations for care of that patient. In other words, the formulation offers a working hypothesis about the etiology and sustaining factors of a presenting concern while also theorizing an individualized treatment plan (Winters et al. 2007).

An accurate biopsychosocial formulation provides a basis for psychoeducation (i.e., explanation of psychological presentations and treatments) with patients and their families as well as multidisciplinary providers within and outside the hospital setting. Such formulation provides validation for symptoms of concern while allowing increased empathy and understanding of contributing factors, without overreliance or undue emphasis on any one contributor (e.g., psychological factors in the absence of biological or social concerns) or potential stigma of an oversimplified understanding of a psychiatric diagnosis. The challenge of biopsychosocial

K. K. Tsang (✉) · S. A. Fernandes · P. Ibeziako
Department of Psychiatry, Boston Children's Hospital/Harvard Medical School, Boston, MA, USA
e-mail: kevin.tsang@childrens.harvard.edu; serena.fernandes@childrens.harvard.edu; patricia.ibeziako@childrens.harvard.edu

A. P. S. Guerrero et al. (eds.), *Pediatric Consultation-Liaison Psychiatry*,
https://doi.org/10.1007/978-3-319-89488-1_10

formulation is to provide a narrative that describes "the important people or events that shaped the person into a unique individual" (Ross 2000) and that allows others to better understand and engage that individual. If a formulation simply summarizes a case or lacks cohesion, it is no longer an effective tool for communicating an understanding of the patient and subsequent care plan. Furthermore, biopsychosocial formulation differs from differential diagnosis (Winters et al. 2007).

An effective biopsychosocial formulation decreases stigma while simultaneously providing understandable psychoeducation regarding the etiology of the presenting concern. From this developed synthesis and understanding of contributing biopsychosocial factors, guidance on how to address the presenting concern from multiple trajectories can be presented.

The Fundamentals of Biopsychosocial Formulation

Biological Contributors include congenital conditions, Family genetic vulnerabilities such as psychiatric illness, temperament, neurodevelopmental delays or disorders, medication, and/or other substance use effects and side effects, and the biological consequences of acute and chronic medical conditions (such as a concussion or inflammatory conditions).

Psychological Factors may include the patient's psychiatric conditions, educational level, understanding of illness and care plan, personality characteristics and defense mechanisms, approach to coping with stressors, degree of distress tolerance, and capacity for effective self-regulation and problem-solving.

Social Contributors to consider include dependent relationships, available social supports such as family members or friends, how these family members or friends experience the patient's illness or problem, financial stressors, community/school/workplace contributors and response to the problem, and the cultural context that informs one's understanding of the psychiatric/medical illness. Cultural factors may also include spiritual/religious attributions about symptoms and acute and chronic experiences of oppression or devaluation associated with illness, gender, race, sexuality, etc.

Developmental Biological, psychological, and social domains must also be considered in the context of development. Norms for biology, psychology, and social/cultural considerations all evolve at different developmental stages. For example, the ways in which an individual accesses social support (and what social supports are primary and available, such as the shift from parents to peers to spouse) inherently change across the lifespan; physiology changes with puberty and self-concept; and problem-solving changes with adolescent development. Additionally, several contributors may cross multiple domains, such as early attachment, temperament, and executive functioning history.

The 4Ps (Predisposing, Precipitating, Perpetuating, and Protective)

Biopsychosocial formulation can also be generated with consideration of predisposing, precipitating, perpetuating, and protective factors, commonly referred to as the 4Ps. *Predisposing* factors take into consideration the historic vulnerabilities and behavioral patterns that inform the current problem. *Precipitating* factors include current or recent stressors that appear to have contributed to the problem. *Perpetuating* factors are those that maintain the presenting concerns. Lastly, *protective* factors are strengths that suggest possible support or resilience that may positively affect the outcome of the current problem.

Vignette 10.1

Presenting Problem and Reason for Consultation

Tracy is a 16-year-old female presenting with weight loss over the past 3 months. Medical workup identifies no concern for inflammation, obstruction, or infectious concerns. Her family is deeply concerned about her continued pain and debilitated functioning and is desperate to help her get better. Consult question to CL psychiatry from gastroenterology admitting service: Evaluation of suspected functional abdominal pain and management recommendations.

In obtaining a comprehensive intake, CL practitioners interview several informants, including the patient, the patient's caregiver(s), nurses, social workers, and medical providers working to provide patient care. The following history is provided:

History of Presenting Illness

Tracy was in her usual state of good health until approximately 3 months ago when she became ill with an episode of gastroenteritis lasting 3 days. Since that time, she has had persistent periumbilical pain and nausea for which she has attempted to compensate by cutting out "heavy foods," but over time her caloric restriction has increased. She presents to the emergency department yesterday with dizziness, evidence of dehydration, and approximately 10% weight loss over the past 3 months. Medical workup thus far has identified no physiologic cause for her pain and nausea.

Developmental History

Tracy was born following a full-term pregnancy and Cesarean delivery. Early temperament is described as slow-to-warm. Developmental milestones were on time, except she received services for speech concerns, which reportedly improved by age four and did not require continued services in school.

Past Medical History
Largely unremarkable. At 8 years of age, tonsils and adenoids were removed with no complications or concerns. At 12 years of age, she sprained her ankle but recovered with no concerns.

Past Psychiatric History
No formal diagnoses or treatment history. She is described by her mother as high-achieving and always sensitive to others' pain. Tracy describes feeling anxious about what the abdominal pain may signify and endorses increased irritability with pain experience but denies other worries or mood changes.

Family Medical History
Maternal grandmother has Alzheimer's disease. Paternal aunt was diagnosed with irritable bowel syndrome.

Family Psychiatric History
There is a maternal family history of anxiety and a paternal extended family history of alcohol use disorder. Parents deny any personal psychiatric history. Tracy's brother is described as typically developing with no emotional or behavioral problems.

Social History
Tracy is the younger of two children born to her parents. Her brother is 18 years old. She reportedly seeks and is sought for friendships. Although reticent to discuss, Tracy discloses during the interview that she had one past romantic relationship with one of her brother's male friends. This relationship lasted 3 months and ended sometime last month. She denies sexual activity and denies that her parents or brother were aware of this relationship. She denies any concerns for relational aggression. She reports some jealousy from peers while she was dating this older male, and she reports peer victimization in the form of name-calling and rumors from female peers at school about the nature of the romantic relationship being sexual. She reports worrying that her parents and brother will find out about this relationship and these rumors, some of which were on social media.

School History
Tracy attends 11th grade at a public high school. She receives straight As with honors. There is no history of being retained or advancement in academic grade. There is no history of learning concerns.

Mental Status Exam
On examination, Tracy appears underweight, is casually dressed in a blouse and skirt, and appears adequately kept. She is slow-to-warm, complaining of fatigue, but engages with greater reciprocity as the examination continues. Speech is clear and coherent. Language is appropriate to age. She describes her mood as "anxious" about ongoing medical workup, and she is worried about what the doctors will find. Affect is constricted and overall congruent to mood. Thoughts are logical and goal-directed. Judgment regarding personal safety is good by history. Insight regarding current anxieties is fair.

Biopsychosocial Formulation

Tracy is a 16-year-old female presenting with concern for weight loss, dizziness, and dehydration in the context of 3 months of abdominal pain. Tracy's experience of persistent abdominal pain appears to have occurred after a significant gastroenteritis, which resolved. No other acute medical processes of concern are identified. Her experience of anxiety around continued periumbilical pain, in the context of her cautious slow-to-warm temperament, and family history of anxiety and alcohol uses suggest some vulnerability toward anxious ideation. Restriction of caloric intake, decreased functioning over time, and increased attention to abdominal pain concerns likely exacerbate any experience of gastrointestinal discomfort. Furthermore, additional recent social stressors, including recent end of surreptitious romantic relationship, peer victimization around this relationship, and concerns about family discovery of this romantic relationship for this interpersonally sensitive adolescent may contribute to additional psychosocial burden. In the absence of new medical findings, Tracy's persistence of pain was likely triggered by initial gastroenteritis but sustained by anxiety, social stressors, decreased functioning and oral intake, and Tracy's limited understanding of factors contributing to her pain and limited ability so far to manage this physical discomfort.

Feedback as Intervention

As in the above-noted vignette, the goal of a biopsychosocial formulation is not simply to summarize the history. The formulation answers the question, "Why this concern, and why now?" and concisely provides relevant information related to the condition at hand and a logical rationale for treatment recommendation moving forward. Equipped with this information, the CL provider is better able to provide psychoeducation while reducing stigma related to the psychosocial factors contributing to her physical symptoms and increasing clarity around factors contributing to and maintaining the presenting concern. Effective formulation helps to bridge patient, family, and provider understanding and builds a common language within which to consider a problem.

With formulation in hand, the consultant must determine how to best communicate back to the medical team and family. Goldman et al. (2010) describe a *family conference* as an opportunity for the medical and psychosocial provider teams to meet with the patient/family to review multidisciplinary findings, impressions, and recommendations, working "toward a consensus with the family about the treatment plan" (p. 43). Ideally, the above-noted formulation would pair directly with the primary medical team's formulation thus far and would thereby increase the consistency of and faith in the team's findings. By providing a thoughtful explanation and treatment recommendations for the symptoms of concern, the formulation would also reduce the teams' anxieties or affect associated with the psychological aspects of this case. It goes without saying that providing a clear and concise explanation for multiple contributors to the presenting illness along with a reasonable and understandable treatment approach helps to reduce provider and patient/family anxiety.

Vignette 10.1 Outcomes

The gastroenterology and psychiatry teams met with Tracy and her parents to review their findings. The gastroenterology team noted the negative medical workup and rationale for no further medical concerns. They described the concern of initial physiologic insult from the gastroenteritis without evidence of an ongoing acute medical process. Both the gastroenterology and psychiatry teams were aware that reviewing negative medical findings does not often provide reassurance to families. Instead, they spent most of the conversation identifying positive contributors and sustaining factors based on the developed biopsychosocial formulation. Information was presented to Tracy and her parents in a developmentally and culturally informed manner to support their understanding of the multifactorial contributions to Tracy's current pain. Furthermore, the formulation described allowed Tracy and her parents to better understand and come to agreement with recommendations for psychotherapy, a structured and stepwise approach to increasing caloric intake, and gradual rehabilitation of daily functioning.

Through a non-stigmatizing but logical and well-developed biopsychosocial formulation, the gastroenterology and psychiatry teams were able to collaborate in helping Tracy and her family understand the relationship between the initial medical insult and now persistent pain. More importantly, helping Tracy and her family understand this formulation supported her taking recovery-focused steps that were inherently different from what they expected upon coming to the hospital and that reduced the cost and risk burdens of unnecessary medical procedures and inappropriate treatment.

From Formulation to Intervention

In conducting a psychiatric assessment, the clinician first understands the illness presentation and then examines surrounding domains of functioning. Bronfenbrenner's (1979) model of bioecological systems theory (BST) is a common model for understanding multiple and overlapping domains in which a person and presenting concern exist (Figure 10.1). Within the BST, the *individual* is understood to exist within various systems that surround them. The *microsystem* includes those that directly impact the individual and their development. Examples include immediately involved family members, school staff, medical providers, and religious institutions or places of worship. The *mesosystem* describes interactions between these various microsystems, including providers, caregivers, and institutions. The *exosystem* describes those settings within which the individual does not directly interact but which may influence the mesosystem or microsystem. Examples

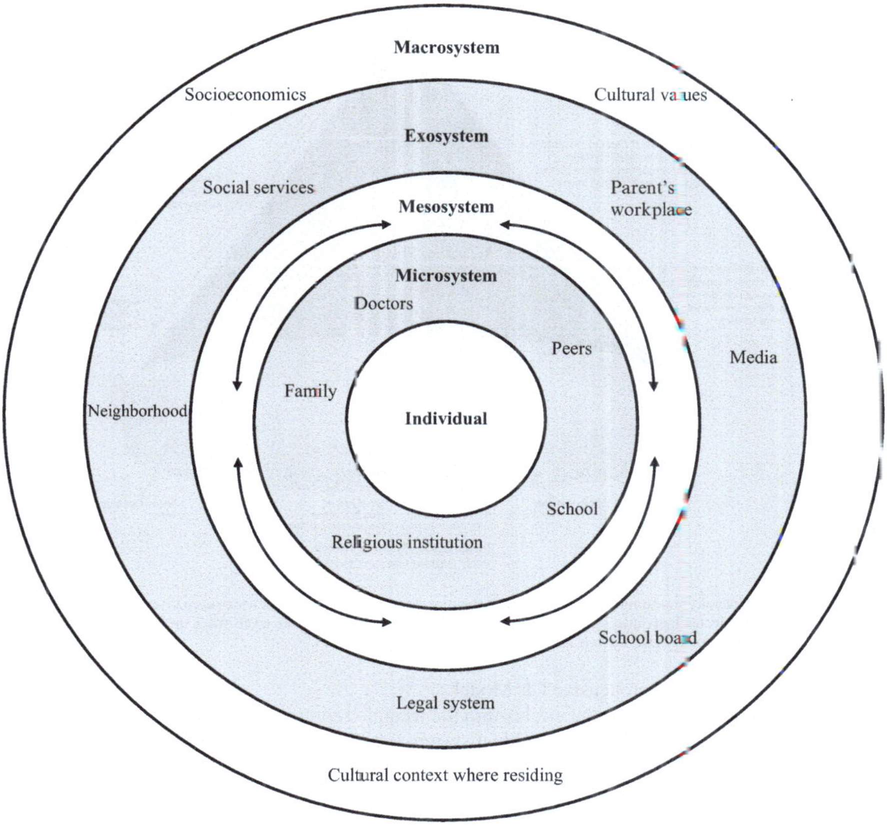

Fig. 10.1 Illustration of Bronfenbrenner's Bioecological Systems Theory (BST)

include parental work setting, social services available in a community, and the influence of media or neighbors. The *macrosystem* describes the broader cultural factors – including cultural norms of the individual's country and cultural heritage or values – that inform the included systems.

Utilizing biopsychosocial formulation to develop effective intervention beyond psychoeducation, however, requires more than just identifying and describing interactions between bioecological systems. Different models have been proposed to formulate the appropriate level of response based on the clinical formulation. For example, Kazak (2006) proposed a stratified model for assessing and determining intervention for health-related stressors in medically ill children and their families. The pediatric psychosocial preventative health model (PPPHM) proposes a differential response from universal (psychoeducation and advocacy for all children and their families presenting with acute or chronic illness) to targeted (providing more specific psychoeducation, monitoring, and microsystem-related support for at-risk families) to clinical/treatment (provision of traditional mental health services

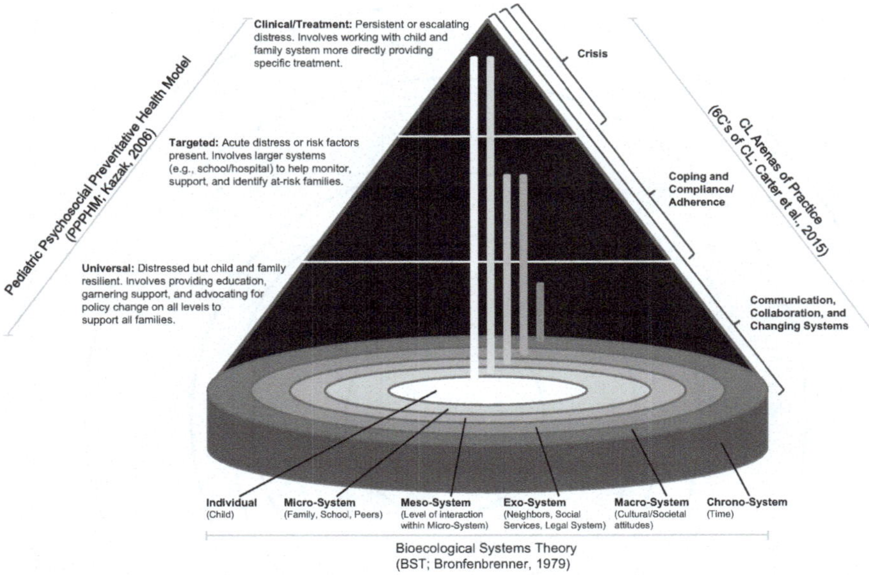

Note: Columns projecting from the circles into the triangle represent the levels at which each system is addressed. For example, the Individual system (child) is targeted at all three treatment/care levels while the Macrosystem is involved primarily at the Universal level.

Fig. 10.2 Integrated Comprehensive CL Model
Note: Columns projecting from the circles into the triangle represent the levels at which each system is addressed. For example, the Individual system (child) is targeted at all three treatment/care levels while the Macrosystem is involved primarily at the Universal level

including more comprehensive assessment and intervention). Additionally, a recent model proposed by Carter et al. (2017) suggests a combined model for presenting BST with PPPHM, including the "Six C's of CL" (Figure 10.2). This additional model includes various levels of CL intervention, from crisis (targeting the individual and microsystem), coping, compliance/adherence, communication, collaboration, and changing systems.

Effective use of biopsychosocial formulation can help to shape the focus of specific interventions. At times the role of a CL clinician is to manage the direct safety concern or crisis. At other times, the focus is on broader systems concerns. Consider the following example:

Vignette 10.2

Presenting Problem

Thomas is a 9-year-old male admitted with diabetic ketoacidosis (DKA). He was in his usual state of health until the day of admission, when he woke up with recurrent vomiting. His parents report having difficulties managing his diabetes mellitus. Thomas is very anxious about the finger pricks to check his blood glucose. As a result, they chase him around the house for hours to obtain his blood glucose and administer his insulin injections. Over the last couple of weeks, they have resorted to only giving him injections while he is asleep.

Past Medical History

Thomas was diagnosed with type 1 diabetes mellitus at age 5 years. He had frequent ear infections at age 3 years; these infections were treated with oral antibiotics only. He has no prior history of DKA and has had no previous hospitalizations.

Developmental History

Thomas was born following a full-term pregnancy and Cesarean delivery. There were no perinatal complications. He achieved all developmental milestones on time. His parents describe him as temperamentally anxious especially about social interactions at school and potential embarrassment. He is also described as "sensitive" to other people's distress.

Past Psychiatric History

There is no history of formal psychiatric diagnosis or treatment.

Family Medical and Psychiatric History

Thomas's maternal aunt has type 1 diabetes mellitus. His paternal grandfather, who is deceased, had a history of prostate cancer. A paternal uncle has an unspecified anxiety disorder. There is no known family history of any type of psychiatric treatment or of suicide attempts.

Social History

Thomas lives with his biological parents and two younger sisters, who are 3 and 5 years old. Parents describe good family relationships, although there has been increasing conflict around how to manage Thomas's diabetes. He has two best friends but is described as inhibited and anxious around social interactions and, as such, does not make friends easily.

Education History

He is currently in the third grade and receives good grades. In the last 2 weeks, he missed 15 days of school due to his illness and is anxious and fearful about returning to school and worried about catching up on schoolwork. The school nurse describes staff worry and discomfort about his diabetes care and reports that the current plan is to send him from school to the emergency department whenever his blood sugars are elevated.

Mental Status Exam

Thomas is neatly dressed in shorts and a t-shirt and appears small for age. His speech and language are within normal limits. He describes his mood as "scared," and his affect is constricted. Thought content is notable for worries about receiving needle shots for diabetes management and for fears of sleeping. Thought process is goal oriented. There are no symptoms of psychosis or suicidality.

Formulation with 4Ps

Thomas is a 9-year-old boy with a history of type 1 diabetes mellitus and no formal psychiatric history who presents with DKA and concerns for nonadherence to diabetes care. Thomas's nonadherence appears to result from a combination of the following factors. Predisposing factors include genetic vulnerabilities to diabetes and anxiety; Thomas's own baseline anxiety, including needle phobia; and parental worries about his diabetes care and management. Precipitating factors include Thomas's increasing diabetes management needs, increased anxieties related to his needle phobia and peer judgment, parental anxieties as his participation in diabetes care has decreased, and increased school personnel reactivity to his diabetes care. Perpetuating factors include the ongoing impact of significant variation in his blood glucose levels due to persistent challenges in management, worsening of trauma associated with insulin due to nighttime insulin sticks, and increased feelings of parental distress given need to chase Thomas for his diabetes care. Protective factors include invested and caring parents, supportive school receptive to medical education, and Thomas's own interest and engagement in treatment during this admission. Treatment recommendations should therefore include treatment of anxiety and needle phobia and support for Thomas's parents via behavioral training, to decrease trauma response, to empower Thomas and parents to participate together in diabetes care, and to promote appropriate limit setting. Coordination between Thomas's medical providers and school would also be beneficial to develop a plan to support his continued participation in school and reduced emergency department visits if possible.

Biopsychosocial Formulation Blending in 4Ps (See Fig. 10.3)
Thomas is a 9-year-old male with a history of type 1 diabetes mellitus and no formal psychiatric history who presents with DKA and concerns for nonadherence to diabetes care. He presents with genetic predisposition to anxiety, an anxious temperament, and history of mild to moderate school and social anxiety. Additionally, despite development of diabetes at an early age, at some point a needle phobia developed, which has only worsened over time and which now significantly contributes to diabetes nonadherence. His parents, recognizing the need for continued diabetes management, have now resorted to chasing Thomas and administering his insulin when he is asleep. These developments have, in a vicious cycle, only increased his anxieties, needle fears, and mistrust of parents in supporting his sense of safety. His school's increased reactivity and limited familiarity and comfort with diabetes management further exacerbates the feelings of distrust and heightened reactivity to his routine insulin care. Treatment recommendations therefore include desensitization for needle phobia, anxiety disorder treatment, support for Thomas's parents with behavioral parent training around insulin administration, and care coordination between medical providers and school-based caregivers.

Vignette 10.2 Outcomes

This formulation helped the psychiatric provider to recognize challenges requiring multiple levels of intervention for Thomas. Immediate concerns included supporting Thomas in receiving his necessary insulin despite a highly reinforced phobic

	Biological	**Psychological**	**Social**
Predisposing	*Family history of anxiety* *Family history of diabetes* *Thomas anxious temperament*	*Needle phobia*	*Parental anxieties about Thomas health*
Precipitating	*Diabetes Mellitus requiring Insulin*	*Trauma exposures with nighttime insulin injections* *Thomas's catastrophic thinking around needle shots*	*School/peer pressures* *Parents uncertain about administering insulin*
Perpetuating	*Impact of blood glucose variance with hypoglycemic and hyperglycemic episodes*	*Thomas's anxious avoidance of his diabetes management*	*Parents chasing Thomas around for insulin and nighttime insulin administration*
Protective	*Thomas's average to above average cognitive functioning*	*Parents interest in psychoeducation and engagement in improving diabetes care*	*Invested and educated parents* *Supportive School*

Fig. 10.3 Integrating Biopsychosocial and 4Ps Factors

response to needles. Psychoeducation to his parents about needle phobia and anticipatory anxiety was also an early focus of treatment. Parent behavioral training, behavioral interventions, and exposure-based desensitization reduced Thomas's anxiety around diabetes care over time. Beyond the crisis management, coping, compliance/adherence, communication, and collaboration were also identified as key pieces in supporting future outcomes for Thomas. The psychiatry and endocrinology providers reached out to the school to identify challenges in managing Thomas's behaviors in the school and provided appropriate education about diabetes management in the school setting. The psychiatry and endocrinology team also reached out to the primary care physician, who could serve as an additional resource for the parents and school in collaborating on a developmentally appropriate plan for Thomas's ongoing diabetes care.

These interventions, driven by a comprehensive but concise and coherent biopsychosocial formulation, helped to significantly reduce the likelihood of future diabetic crisis for Thomas and helped his parents to feel more comfortable and supported in managing his diabetes care. Furthermore, because of school and primary care physician involvement, not only do Thomas and his family have a better chance of developing a consistent approach to medical adherence across settings, but his anxiety was also likely to be more consistently and more effectively addressed. Reduced emotional reactivity at school also means he will be less likely to miss school unnecessarily. Well-developed formulation supports not only understanding the current problem but also additional areas of positive impact on the patient's future functioning.

Conclusion

This chapter provides an overview of the utility of biopsychosocial formulation, approaches to developing a formulation, and examples of application of formulation to guide intervention in CL settings. Establishing a clear and concise narrative of the theorized convergence of multiple contributors allows for improved communication and provision of education to families and providers alike in understanding how the problem came to be and the rationale for proposed treatment. Furthermore, applying biopsychosocial formulation to understanding the multiple potential roles for a CL provider allows for efficient utilization of intervention efforts, from the crisis and direct care level to more systemic and advocacy-based approaches.

References

Bronfenbrenner, U. (1979). *The ecology of human development: Experiments by nature and design*. Cambridge, MA: Harvard University Press.

Carter, B. D., Thompson, S. M., & Townsend, A. N. (2014). Pediatric consultation-liaison in the children's hospital: The psychological hospitalist. In M. C. Roberts, B. S. Aylward, & Y. P. Wu (Eds.), *Clinical practice of pediatric psychology: Cases and service delivery* (pp. 63–77). New York: Guilford Press.

Carter, B. D., Kronenberger, W. G., Scott, E. L., Kullgren, K. A., Piazza-Waggoner, C., & Brady, C. E. (2017). Inpatient pediatric consultation-liaison. In M. Roberts & R. Steele (Eds.), *Handbook of pediatric psychology* (5th ed., pp. 105–118). New York: Guilford.

Goldman, S. J., Shaw, R. J., & DeMaso, D. R. (2010). The pediatric psychosomatic medicine assessment. In R. J. Shaw & D. R. DeMaso (Eds.), *Textbook of pediatric psychosomatic medicine* (pp. 33–45). Washington, DC: American Psychiatric Publishing, Inc.

Kazak, A. (2006). Pediatric psychosocial preventative health model (PPPHM): Research, practice, and collaboration in pediatric family systems medicine. *Families, Systems and Health, 24*, 381–395.

Ross, D. E. (2000). A method for developing a biopsychosocial formulation. *Journal of Child and Family Studies, 9*(1), 1–6.

Winters, N. C., Hanson, G., & Stoyanova, V. (2007). The case formulation in child and adolescent psychiatry. *Child and Adolescent Psychiatric Clinics of North America, 16*, 111–132.

Chapter 11
Pre-procedure Evaluation and Psychological Screening of Children and Adolescents in Pediatric Clinics

Trude Reinfjell and Trond H. Diseth

Background

Severe and/or chronic medical disease, congenital malformations, or functional impairments in children significantly increase the risk of psychological, psychosocial, and familial difficulties (Diseth 2006). Affected children experience significant uncertainty, daily worry, and anxiety. Family members have to adapt to changes in everyday life, the medical situation, and associated emotional rigors.

Moreover, 90% of medically ill children have experienced at least one traumatic event—3.14 events on average (Stuber et al. 2003)—and are at increased risk for developing posttraumatic stress and dissociative symptoms (Diseth 2006). Many children have had a serious or life-threatening illness from early childhood and have undergone multiple, often protracted hospitalizations, which may have involved separations, scary experiences, and repeated stressful medical procedures. Also, children with less serious chronic conditions, but who must still undergo invasive and painful medical treatment, may develop posttraumatic stress symptoms (Diseth 2006). Several studies show that both parents and siblings report higher incidence of posttraumatic stress symptoms than sick children themselves (Alderfer et al.

T. Reinfjell (✉)
Department of Psychology, Norwegian University of Science and Technology, Trondheim, Norway

Department of Child and Adolescent Psychiatry, St. Olavs University Hospital, Trondheim, Norway
e-mail: Trude.Reinfjell@ntnu.no

T. H. Diseth
Section for Psychosomatics and CL-Child Psychiatry, Department of Clinical Neurosciences for Children, Division of Paediatric and Adolescent Medicine, Oslo University Hospital, Oslo, Norway

Institute of Clinical Medicine, Faculty of Medicine, University of Oslo, Oslo, Norway

A. P. S. Guerrero et al. (eds.), *Pediatric Consultation-Liaison Psychiatry*,
https://doi.org/10.1007/978-3-319-89488-1_11

2003; Diseth and Emblem 2017), indicating that childhood illness has a tremendous impact on children's families.

In pediatric settings, pain is often a significant ongoing concern for both children and their parents. Medical procedures are often painful, unexpected, and accompanied by heightened situational stress and anxiety; Zeltzer and Zeltzer (2016) emphasize that if pain is not well managed initially, children can experience posttraumatic stress symptoms due to memory recall of invasive procedures during treatment. Pain is especially problematic in younger children, and it is necessary to consider a child's age, developmental level, cognitive and communication skills, previous pain experiences, and associated beliefs when planning treatment (Morton 1997; Srouji et al. 2010; Cohen et al. 2008). Despite its frequency, pain is still often underestimated and undertreated in infants, children, and adolescents (McGrath and Frager 1996; Vatne et al. 2010). Managing procedural pain, nausea, and other symptoms requires interventions based on the child's development (Srouji et al. 2010). Vatne et al. (2010) point out that it is difficult for young children to talk about difficult topics in a "traditional" conversation. Therefore, children would be at risk of having their symptoms and problems remaining underdiagnosed and undertreated.

Clinical experience suggests that improving routines for painful or intimidating procedures and focusing on abilities and needs would create more predictability for children (Gjems and Diseth 2011). Children will also experience more control if they are well prepared for what is going to happen before, during, and after the procedure. Several studies have shown that preparation using hypnosis or cognitive behavioral interventions, for example, reduces anxiety, helplessness, and stress during medical procedures (Srouji et al. 2010; Stuber 1996; Lindheim and Helgeland 2017) and increases coping and feelings of control. It is often useful to give children an active role and to use different play materials, dolls, and drawings to prepare them for painful procedures or operations. Older children and adolescents may perceive increased control over the situation if they can listen to their favorite music or available relaxation tapes (LeRoy et al. 2003).

Factors Affecting Pre-procedure Evaluation

The Impact of Developmental Level on Children's Ability to Understand Their Illness and Treatment Procedures

Children's and adolescents' understanding of their illness depends on developmental factors, such as their ability to gain knowledge and to understand and reflect upon their situation. Emotional and cognitive development therefore has implications on how to inform children about their illness (Eiser 1985; Reinfjell et al. 2007), and the content and process of what is communicated must depend on the child's developmental level, maturity, and life experience (Vatne et al. 2010). Children's reactions to their disease situation and their ability to understand it will be affected by how they perceive the situation. It is therefore essential that professionals be aware of children's views to know how to inform them about their disease and necessary medical interventions (LeRoy et al. 2003; Vikan 1988).

Preschoolers

With some variations, preschoolers (3–4 years) are often considered to have a concrete mindset. Children of this age can therefore find it difficult to think "under" direct observable events. Children's specific experiences with illness and death play a role in how they perceive events.

Case 11.1
A 3-year-old boy was recently diagnosed with cancer. His grandfather had died of cancer 6 months before. Standing in the hospital corridor, he suddenly asks the nurse "Do I get the same medicines as my grandfather got?" The nurse comfortingly told the boy that she understood that he perhaps thought a lot about his grandfather. She said, "You have cancer and you're wondering if you will get the same medicine that your grandfather got? I think it is very good that you ask me about things that you are wondering about. Have you thought a lot about this?" The nurse informed the boy further: "Your grandpa had a different cancer than you have, and unfortunately the medicine he had did not work for that kind of cancer. But for the cancer you have, we have a medicine that can help you, and that is important to remember."

Here the nurse creates a situation where the boy can ask questions, express his fears, and receive emotional support. In this example, the child shows a greater level of maturity because of his concrete experience of illness and death, and this experience will naturally affect his perception of his own illness. A previous study found that children as young as 4 and 5 years old are capable of talking about illness and their explanations and understanding become more complex with more maturity (Myant and Williams 2005).

Five- and six-year-olds can think about the cause of disease, although their explanations are limited. They tend to understand illness as the result of the body coming in physical contact with something that is then internalized. While children accept that the disease is localized inside their body, they believe the cause is external. Thus, they do not quite understand that disease is a result of an error in body function. One study found that some children between the ages of 4 and 6 attributed the cause of illness to magic or witchcraft, while other children thought of illness as a form of punishment (Bibace and Walsh 1980).

Preschool children may also believe that they themselves are the cause of both their own and others' diseases. This belief is because of their still limited understanding of relationships between things and events. Many seriously ill children undergo intensive and painful treatment procedures. Because they often do not understand the relationship between disease and treatment, they tend to perceive treatment as being independent of the disease. Some children even experience treatment as a punishment, which results in their losing control and influence over their own life (Vikan 1988; Bibace and Walsh 1980). However, children can understand reality if they are informed of the facts in an age-appropriate way.

Children's understanding of illness becomes more sophisticated as they age (Myant and Williams 2005; Bibace and Walsh 1980). In later preschool age, children have a larger vocabulary, which makes it easier to communicate emotions and to understand and regulate emotions. Language has a major impact on the way children cope with and express their emotions.

It can be useful to provide preschool-age children with appropriate information about treatment procedures and to give them the opportunity to ask questions. Healthcare providers should treat children's cues as important therapeutic opportunities (Vatne et al. 2012). The following active distraction methods can be useful for children in this age group (Srouji et al. 2010): blowing bubbles, playing with toys, and talking about their families and about other things in their life. Deep breathing methods are also helpful for older children. Parents and healthcare professionals can also use more passive distraction techniques such as reading age-appropriate books or singing songs.

Early School Age (6–10 Years)

In early school age (6–10 years), children develop a greater understanding of the causes of disease and a better grasp of reality. They can understand, for example, that illness can be "caught" from another individual (Eiser 1985). They can, therefore, have a more proactive and preventive approach to disease. They also begin to distinguish themselves from their disease and can therefore understand that treatment is intended to help them (Brewster 1982). Moreover, children over 10 years are more likely to accept the potential long-term benefits of treatment. Schoolchildren increasingly use cognitive strategies such as telling themselves that they can manage or thinking of something else. While 5-year-olds need help to use cognitive strategies, 10-year-olds can use them spontaneously (Brenner et al. 1997). Children of early school age mostly cite their parents as a source of emotional support, while older children most often cite their friends.

Older School-Age Children (10–18 Years)

Older schoolchildren (ages 10 years and up) can understand abstract concepts and the relationships between them. At this age they can now localize disease etiology within the body: for example, a poorly functioning organ (Myant and Williams 2005). Understanding of the relationship between disease, treatment, and prevention increases throughout adolescence. From age 14 years, children begin to understand the interdependence of mental and other physical and how disease can be influenced by psychological factors such as stress. They often turn to friends for support to deal with emotionally difficult situations. This is also an age characterized by emotional fluctuations. A serious chronic disease can be particularly traumatic when it presents itself during adolescence. Most adolescents have some knowledge of their disease and realize that they are seriously ill. Meanwhile, they are often less able, in comparison to young adults, to share this knowledge. In addition, many adolescents may experience little social support if they are gaining independence from their families but have not yet established close relationships outside of the family. They may perceive their disease as a crisis that they have to deal with alone (Eiser 1985).

Several Vignettes

A teenage girl who had just started radiotherapy after relapse asks the nurse: "What will happen if the radiation treatment does not work?"

In the latter vignette, it could be that this girl received specific information about what will happen, but her direct question shows that she experiences unpredictability (Reinfjell et al. 2007). It is important to find out what might lie behind these children's questions. Perhaps it is the fear of dying. It is very important that adults not dismiss such questions from children because of their own fear and uncertainty. It is important to ensure a private setting for procedures, since adolescents sometimes deny pain in front of family and friends. Moreover, it is important to allow them to choose the type of distraction and also whether they would like friends and family to be present (Srouji et al. 2010).

General Approaches

Overall, verbal information given to children should be developmentally appropriate, simple, realistic, and honest (LeRoy et al. 2003). Children take in complex information gradually, and concrete experiences help them to integrate more advanced information. Therefore, informing children about illness must be regarded as a process, even in the short term. The first phase of treatment is often characterized by crisis, chaos, and confusion, which can leave children with overwhelming impressions. Information will need to be repeated. Information must be very simple and concrete at first but can eventually be developed and expanded (Reinfjell et al. 2007).

Vignette 11.1
An 11-year-old girl is receiving treatment for cancer. Notwithstanding the stressfulness of the hospitalization, the parents, in describing their experience, state: "What has been particularly good in the meeting with the hospital was when they explained our daughter's illness to her. The nurse read to our daughter from a selected children's book about chemotherapy and used language that our daughter could understand."

This vignette illustrates the importance of accurate yet personalized information, which plays a key role in the treatment of seriously ill children. Lack of information can cause uncertainty, anger, and anxiety. The feeling of losing control may also be curbed through good information. It is important that children get the necessary information and facts about their disease to encourage a concrete understanding; often this is accomplished using relevant books, graphic images, and puppets. Eiser (1998) stresses the importance of updating information when there are changes in treatment, such as relapse, and points out that this is often overlooked. The same principle applies to issues in relation to side effects of treatment. Children with serious medical diseases undergoing intensive treatment procedures and experiencing accompanying side effects can easily lose control over their own emotions. While emotional imbalance can be a psychological consequence of disease and difficult treatment, it can also be caused by medication used in treatment. Child distress related to invasive medical procedures is well known (Salmon and Pereira 2002), but as Vatne et al. (2010) note, even noninvasive procedures may evoke negative emotions.

Vatne et al. (2012) found that during routine cardiac consultations, children did not openly express negative emotions frequently and were more likely to provide subtle cues of negative emotions, which were rarely recognized by the adults. When a child does express negative emotions, adults may consider using the opportunity to explore the child's emotional experience. There are many stress points for children during procedures related to diagnosis or intervention: in the case of cardiac catheterization and cardiovascular surgery, these include venipuncture, separation from parents at the time of transport to the operation room, anesthesia induction, and/or removal of chest tubes and intracardiac lines (LeRoy et al. 2003). Children undergoing procedures can benefit from comprehensive coping-skills training, which may include counseling and training in controlled breathing, progressive muscle relaxation, biofeedback, guided imagery, and cognitive reframing. These skills have been associated with a positive effect on stress-related behaviors in children both during and after hospitalization (Campbell et al. 1986).

A close interdisciplinary collaboration between professionals, including nurses, doctors, educators, psychologists, and social workers, is essential to provide comprehensive assistance to children with serious medical conditions and their families. All providers involved in a child's care should know the child's medical situation, the type of information the child has received, how the child seems to interpret and understand the information, and how the child reacted emotionally. It is important for care providers to explain the rationale for treatment and discuss its intended effects and possible side effects. The adults around the children must ensure that the information is interpreted and properly understood.

The Impact of Parent Involvement

Families' coping strategies and professionals' attitudes will further influence how children adapt. When a child is affected by serious disease, the interaction between the child and his or her parents may become disrupted, partly because of parental anxiety or depression. A fundamental question is, therefore, what do parents need so they can be present for their child and create a safe relationship. Parents need to be supervised and supported, and they need information about what to expect during their child's stay at the hospital, their own likely reactions, and how they can support their child. Information must be individualized based on parents' cultural and educational background. Preparation for a procedure therefore begins with child and family assessments. Important goals for procedure preparation include addressing parental concerns and needs so parents can be more emotionally available to their children. Before cardiac procedures such as catheterization or surgery, for example, parents have demonstrated significant levels of psychological distress and diminished coping abilities (Utens et al. 2000).

Parents may need guidance to understand their role in procedures. If their child does not cooperate, parents may feel responsible for the decision to go ahead with the procedure. This feeling of responsibility can increase stress in parents, who may then express negative feelings toward their child by saying things like "pull yourself together" rather than be supportive. Parents may verbalize their fear and anxiety directly or engage in behaviors that contribute to their children's anxiety (Salmon and Pereira 2002; Bush et al. 1986; Bevan et al. 1990). Parents can improve their children's coping abilities by engaging in humorous conversation or talking about topics unrelated to the procedure (LeRoy et al. 2003).

It is important for healthcare providers to establish healthy and trusting relationships with both children and their parents, so that parents feel a certain degree of security in connection with the medical treatment. Both parents and siblings may experience significant posttraumatic stress from a child's severe illness. It is therefore essential to take a family approach to care and to provide parents and family with psychological help when needed. Studies reveal that interventions addressing parental concerns regarding children's hospitalizations have been effective in reducing parental anxiety and enhancing child behavior outcomes (Campbell et al. 1992; Ferguson 1979).

Pre-procedure Evaluation: The Impact of Preparing the Child and Family

With advancements in medicine, more and more lifesaving procedures (e.g., bone marrow and other organ transplants, complex surgeries, etc.) will become available to children. These procedures may involve pain and other discomfort, prolonged separation from home and family, and significant risk for complications, especially if adherence were suboptimal. Pediatric consultation-liaison psychiatry practitioners have a key role in evaluating patients and families and providing multidisciplinary teams with important feedback, from a psychiatric perspective, on whether the patient is optimally ready for the procedure, whether anything else needs to be done to better prepare the patient and family, and what the balance is between risks and benefits in undergoing the procedure.

Table 11.1 Assessment and interventions regarding risky, stressful, and/or painful medical procedures

Acknowledge the child's pain, earlier/present experiences, response, and coping strategies
Acknowledge the parents' experience of their child's response
Go over the necessity, importance, and urgency of the procedure
Assess alternatives to the procedure
Provide adequate pain and distress treatment through:
Age-adjusted information and preparation
Opportunities to feel calm and experience predictability, sense of control, and overview of the situation
Active involvement of parents/caregivers in providing support and safety
Distraction and/or relaxation techniques, hypnotherapy
Private examination rooms
Calm and positive atmosphere
Pharmacotherapy as needed

In the pre-procedure evaluation, it is important to consider the timing of the procedure in terms of both child's and the family's well-being, as well as from a medical perspective. Is the child ready? Is the proposed treatment appropriate, or are other interventions necessary for optimal success? Information and preparation should always be adapted to the child's age, and parents should be present to actively support the child. Healthcare professionals should have the main responsibility for preparing the child (Table 11.1).

Psychoeducation is important, especially in helping to normalize symptoms, and can reduce both children's and parents' fears that something is wrong. Stress management is also very important, as children often struggle with anxiety related to medical procedures based on previous negative experiences. Sometimes children develop phobic anxiety for procedures. It is therefore important to create positive imagery and a "safe place." Breathing techniques, relaxation training, and self-hypnosis may also help (Gjems and Diseth 2011; Lindheim and Helgeland 2017; Huynh et al. 2008).

Case 11.2

As the pediatric consultation-liaison psychiatry fellow, you are asked by the multidisciplinary pediatric oncology team to evaluate Maria, "to provide input for the team as they consider surgical treatments for a new cancer and to provide support for patient and family."

Maria is in her room at the hospital together with her parents. One of her doctors and a nurse have just left the room after informing Maria about her new situation. You explain your role to Maria and her parents as a consultant for the team.

Maria openly shares her feelings with you: "I feel so terribly afraid. I have had cancer before, and now I have to start all over again. This is so unfair. Why does it have to happen to me again? Now the doctors told me that I have to go through an operation, but it can even be worse. I feel that I'm totally losing control over my life, I really don't know what to do."

Maria was diagnosed with cancer first time when she was 5 years old, and she went through treatment for about 2 years and was declared healthy when she was around 12 years old.

She is now 15 years old and has been diagnosed with a new type of cancer: a bone cancer in her leg. Maria seems adequately informed about the new cancer and about the nature of the proposed limb-salvaging surgery, which will require significant compliance with the rehabilitation regimen and which may involve significant pain. She understands that, in the worst-case scenario, she would require a leg amputation to save her life. She also understands that the surgery has approximately a "50/50" chance for success and may not lead to a cure. Maria feels extremely anxious; she recalls her previous experience with cancer treatment and she is terribly afraid.

You complete your assessment of the patient and family. Screening questions are negative for depression, anxiety, and other major psychiatric disorders. You review the patient and family's past experiences and coping with cancer and other medical illness. The parents also seem well-informed about the nature, risk, and implications of the proposed procedure, and, among the patient and her parents, there is no disagreement about the decision to proceed. There is no history of nonadherence, and the family seems to have a realistic plan (involving extended family) to care for the other two children and to ensure that one of the parents will be available to help Maria during the postsurgical rehabilitation. In your report for the team, you summarize your key findings and provide additional recommendations to optimally prepare Maria and her family for the procedure.

Based upon your recommendations, the multidisciplinary team aims to give Maria as much control and influence as possible and makes a schedule in collaboration with her. After establishing a safe and relaxing "safe place," the team psychologist has Maria imagine both outcomes: what life would be like if the surgery were successful and what it would be like to live with an amputation. Maria is also able to meet someone who went through the same procedure and needed an amputation.

Maria states, "I have to say that it helped me a lot to meet someone who had gone through an amputation and to see how that person managed to cope. Actually, she also had continued with some of the activities she used to do before." Maria sees and hears how that person had learned to cope with the situation, and therefore gains more hope and sense of predictability. In addition, Maria receives psychoeducation to help her normalize her feelings. Her parents receive systematic supervision to help them cope and optimally support their daughter.

In situations like Maria's, children need to know what they will have to go through during a procedure. It is important to create a plan and to give them choices and the opportunity to practice (gradual exposure). The plan should then be implemented calmly and with control, in conjunction with opportunities to practice coping mechanisms.

After the procedure, care providers should, through talking and playing, work through what the child experienced and observe the child's reactions: Does the child calm down quickly or is the child afraid and anxious? They should assess need for more additional follow-up and therapy. The child should also be rewarded. Children with complex trauma experiences will often need more focus on emotional and behavioral regulation than children with more limited trauma, and it will usually take longer to establish an alliance with such children. The timeframe should therefore be open and flexible (Cohen et al. 2006); a longer timeframe should also be accepted by the medical staff/administrators. Psychological interventions are further presented in the section below.

Anesthesia

Children below the age of 5 and patients with previous experience are known to be at higher risk of being stressed and uncooperative during the induction of anesthesia (Varughese et al. 2008). Some patients suffer from postoperative changes, such as sleep problems, weeks after surgery. The likelihood of such changes is higher when the child is anxious preoperatively (Kain et al. 1999; Goldschneider et al. 2014). Parents should be encouraged to ask the anesthesia team about available options for preinduction sedation and parental presence during induction of anesthesia, since such information can help them better to advocate for their child. Pediatricians should encourage adolescent patients to ask questions to make sure that they understand what is planned (Goldschneider et al. 2014). One cannot exclude the possibility that multiple exposures to anesthesia at an early age and years of painful, stressful, or even traumatic invasive treatment procedures may adversely affect childrens' neurodevelopment and psychological development with lasting and severe consequences. Recently, studies have reported possible negative neurodevelopmental effects of repeated exposure to anesthesia during surgery or treatment procedures before the age of 2 years (Sun 2010; Flick et al. 2011; Harmsen et al. 2016).

The long-term effects of anesthesia on the developing human brain are still unknown, but there is broad agreement that limiting exposure to general anesthesia in infants is a wise policy (Goldschneider et al. 2014).

Neuropsychological Assessment

The clinical course of a child whose disease, or its treatment, might influence brain functioning differently at different developmental stages needs to be established with a baseline evaluation and should also be monitored over time (Baron 2004) so that possible late effects of known risk factors can be identified and managed. These evaluations will also help families and schools have more realistic expectations for the child's functioning. At the same time, a neuropsychological evaluation makes it possible to focus not only on problems, deficits, and limitations but also on strengths. To determine what interventions are appropriate to help the child and to set realistic goals, it is important to point out what the child can do and to focus on available resources (Baron 2004).

Leukemia and CNS tumors, younger age at treatment, intrathecal chemotherapy, and cranial irradiation are all associated with adverse neurocognitive outcomes (Kahalley et al. 2013). Multiple meta-analyses demonstrate significant deficits in overall intellectual abilities, academic functioning, and specific cognitive skills, including attention, visual-motor functioning, processing speed, working memory (WM), and executive function (EF), among children with leukemia treated with intrathecal chemotherapy only and/or cranial irradiation (Kunin-Batson et al. 2011; Buizer et al. 2009; Campbell et al. 2007; Peterson et al. 2008; Walsh et al. 2015; Edelstein et al. 2011). Similar results are found among children with CNS tumors (de Ruiter et al. 2013; Robinson et al. 2010; Robinson et al. 2013; Saha et al. 2014). Importantly, impairment in these domains can impede children's ability to learn new information and to retain previously learned information. These impairments can lead to declines in cognitive functioning (Krull et al. 2008 Krull et al. 2013). Furthermore, they can also result in poor academic functioning, low self-esteem, and behavioral or emotional disorders (Zeltzer et al. 2009; Hutchinson et al. 2017) and can affect quality of life, particularly in the school environment (Butler and Copeland 2002).

Case 11.3

A 15-year-old patient states, "I really appreciate that I have been able to attend school again. For several years I missed a lot of school because of the brain tumor that I got when I was 8 years old. I am so thankful to my parents, who helped me a lot with school work. I am now 15 years old and I am thankful for surviving the disease and that I can go to school. At the same time, it is really hard to concentrate. I can be in the middle of a conversation and just 'fall out' and completely forget what we talked about. There is so much information to handle, and I think it is so difficult to ask over and over again. I don't have enough time to write down things that could help me. I always must read new information over and over again since I forget. When I get home from school, I don't have any energy left. I just need to sleep and go to bed early to be able to go to school the next day."

This adolescent girl shows a great ability to cope, and it is impressive that she is in school every day. At the same time, she also experiences several challenges related to her difficulties with short-term memory because of illness and treatment. These challenges can make it difficult for her to cope with many things in everyday life.

Because of the concerns, the team child psychiatrist convened a meeting involving the patient, the parents, the teacher, the school's special services coordinator, and the hospital team. In this meeting, it was decided that a new neuropsychological evaluation should be done since it had been many years since her first assessment at the time she was diagnosed with a brain tumor. The team also emphasized the importance of school accommodations. It was emphasized that she should have the opportunity to have as good a quality of life as possible and that she should have a balance that allows her to spend time in school and to still have enough energy to enjoy leisure/activities.

Specific neuropsychological tests are further discussed in the section below.

Psychological Interventions in Pediatric Psychosomatic Medicine

Several interventions have been developed to prepare children for different stressful, painful, or traumatic medical treatment procedures. These interventions include distraction and/or relaxation techniques, cognitive behavioral interventions, hypnotherapy and self-hypnosis, short-term play therapy, biofeedback, and eye movement desensitization and reprocessing (EMDR).

Distraction and/or Relaxation Techniques are frequently used to guide children's attention away from stressful stimuli to relaxing or entertaining stimuli. These techniques are most effective when adapted to the child's developmental level (Srouji et al. 2010; Vessey et al. 1994) and can be introduced by parents, nurses, medical doctors, child life specialists, and psychologists. Stimuli can be visual or auditory, including films/videos, cartoons, posters, bubbles, movement toys, books, video games, audio tapes (e.g., relaxation tapes), television, or conversation (Sander Wint et al. 2002). Previous research has shown that distraction can lead to a reduction in procedure times and in the number of staff required for the procedure (DeLoach Walworth 2005).

Cognitive Behavioral Interventions are the most commonly used interventions with older children and adolescents to minimize pain (Srouji et al. 2010) and have often been included in procedure preparation for children and adolescents with previous medical experiences. Cognitive interventions are mostly used to direct attention away from procedure-related pain and include listening to music, counting, and talking about things not related to the procedure (Uman et al. 2006). Specific examples include:

Preparation/Education/Information The procedure and feelings associated with the procedure are explained to the child in an age-appropriate way. The child is provided with instructions about what he or she will need to do during the procedure to help them understand what to expect (Tak and van Bon 2006).

Coping Statements The child is taught to repeat a set of positive thoughts such as "I can do this" or "this will be over soon" or "I know that I can lower my anxiety with my breathing" (LeRoy et al. 2003).

Imagery The child is asked to imagine an enjoyable item, experience, or safe place (e.g., being on the beach). During guided imagery, children learn to focus on a positive, relaxing picture or scene during times of stress. Trained health professionals help the child develop imagery and practice the intervention before the procedure. Active coaching during the procedure is usually needed (LeRoy et al. 2003).

Conscious Breathing Children are taught how to use controlled breathing techniques with slow, deep inhalation via abdominal muscles and slow, controlled exhalation (Jay et al. 1987). For younger children, it is common to have them blow bubbles (French et al. 1994).

Progressive Muscle Relaxation Children are taught how to use cue words to consciously and sequentially relax various muscle groups until they achieve total body relaxation (LeRoy et al. 2003).

Modeling Positive Coping Behaviors A child may watch another child or adult going through the procedure and rehearse the observed positive coping behaviors.

Desensitization This is a step-by-step approach to coping with the painful stimuli. It involves slowly introducing the procedure and tasks involved and effectively dealing with easier tasks before moving on to harder ones (Srouji et al. 2010).

Positive Reinforcement Children are rewarded with positive statements or gifts after a painful procedure (e.g., stickers, toys, games, small trophies).

LeRoy et al. (2003) emphasize that stress management programs that use a variety of the abovementioned techniques and that provide education and training have been most effective.

Hypnosis Hypnotherapy and self-hypnosis are tools used to assess for and develop protective factors and enhance positive adjustment. Meta-analyses and overviews have demonstrated the effectiveness of hypnotherapy for pediatric disorders like asthma, for chronic and acute pain, and for procedure-related distress (Huynh et al. 2008).

Play Therapy Short-term play therapy with an agreed upon, well-defined treatment focus, such as working on trauma after an operation or addressing what it means to die from cancer, has proved to be an effective method of presenting and exploring medical concepts and providing insight into children's understanding of their situation and how well they are coping. By using dolls to demonstrate, for example, the placement of intravenous lines, incisions, and chest tubes, the therapist can prepare children for medical procedures. During the play session, concrete simple explanations can be offered, and misperceptions can be corrected (LeRoy et al. 2003).

Biofeedback is a therapy that can assist children in managing a variety of health problems through muscle awareness and reeducation. It facilitates conscious relaxation and control of physiological processes through feedback, most often provided by physiological monitoring equipment (LeRoy et al. 2003). The method has been useful for patients with anxiety and stress, asthma, cystic fibrosis, bowel dysfunction, headaches, chronic pain, and sleep disorders. This type of training uses a specialized computer program and sensor connected to the child's body to measure breathing, heart rate, and skin temperature, which indicate sympathetic stimulation.

The tools learned in biofeedback help patients to better understand how their body works, so that they can apply techniques such as breathing exercises, muscle retraining, and lifestyle management to improve their well-being. This data graphically depicts physiological information such as muscle tension, skin temperature, and breathing patterns. Further, the information is analyzed and presented to the child to teach him/her how to control these processes. The child is taught to turn on the part of the nervous system that creates calm and that may decrease the awareness of pain. For example, when controlling breathing, children are taught to notice changes in how their body feels so that they can learn to create the same feeling on their own at home. Relaxation augmented by electromyographic biofeedback has been used successfully in a comprehensive stress management program for children undergoing cardiac catheterization (Campbell et al. 1986). The method requires a trained therapist and specialized equipment. A training period of 6 weeks may be needed to achieve optimal results (Richter 1984).

Eye Movement Desensitization and Reprocessing (EMDR) EMDR is an evidence-based treatment intervention, developed by Shapiro (Shapiro 2001). The clinical efficiency of EMDR for children has been demonstrated in a recent meta-analysis (Rodenburg et al. 2009) and other studies (Ahmad and Sundelin-Wahlsten 2008; Stallard 2006). EMDR therapy is an integrative psychotherapy approach that has been extensively researched and proven effective for the treatment of trauma. EMDR involves a set of standardized protocols that incorporates elements from many different treatment approaches (e.g., psychodynamic, cognitive, behavioral, client-centered) together with bilateral stimulation to dissipate the distress associated with an experience.

Psychological Screening and Pain Assessments

Several validated screening instruments have been developed to evaluate children's mental health, health-related quality of life, posttraumatic stress symptoms, and neuropsychological function, which are considered important in the pre-procedural phase.

Pain measurement tools have also been developed to estimate/evaluate the level of pain experienced before and after pre-procedures. Children as young as 3 years of age can quantify their pain when they are offered the right tools. Children between 3 and 5 years old can use the Faces scale, while children 10 and older can use the same numerical rating scale as adults (Zeltzer and Zeltzer 2016). Two pain measurements for children will be presented below.

Psychological and neuropsychological evaluation typically begins with an interview, in which parents detail their child's birth and development, social and emotional functioning, and school history and interests, as well as family history of educational and psychological functioning.

Screening of Mental Health

The strength and difficulties questionnaire (SDQ) is used to assess mental health in children and adolescents aged 11–17 years (Goodman 1997, 1999). The questionnaire has 25 items plus a supplement on the impact of difficulties on the child and the family. There are five subscales—emotional symptoms, conduct problems, hyperactivity, peer problems, and prosocial behavior—the first four of which are added to give a total difficulties score. There are similar versions for parents and teachers. The SDQ shows satisfactory reliability and validity (Goodman 1999; Heyerdahl 2003).

Screening of Health-Related Quality of Life (HRQOL)

The Pediatric Quality of Life Inventory (PedsQL™4.0) (Varni et al. 1999) measures health-related quality of life in children and adolescents. The 23-item PedsQL version 4.0 Generic Core Scales can be grouped into 4 domains of HRQOL: physical functioning (8 items), emotional functioning (5 items), social functioning (5 items), and school functioning (5 items). In addition to the 4 subscales, a total summary health score (23 items) can be computed. The PedsQL™4.0 Generic Core Scales are comprised of a self-report for children 5–18. The parent proxy report covers children ages 2–18 and assesses how parents perceive their child's HRQOL. The questions ask how much of a problem each item has been during the past month. The PedsQL™4.0 has demonstrated satisfactory psychometric properties (Varni et al. 2004; Reinfjell et al. 2006).

Screening of Posttraumatic Stress Symptoms

The Impact of Event Scale (IES) (Horowitz et al. 1979) is one of the most widely used self-report measures within the trauma literature (e.g. Weiss and Marmar 1997). The IES scale consist of 15 items, 7 of which measure intrusive symptoms (intrusive thoughts, nightmares, intrusive feelings, and imagery) and 8 of which measure avoidance symptoms (numbing of responsiveness, avoidance of feelings, situations, ideas). The combined score provides a total measure of subjective stress. All items of the IES are anchored to a specific event or stressor (Horowitz et al. 1979; Briere 1997). Respondents are asked to rate the items on a 4-point scale according to how often each has occurred in the past 7 days. The IES shows satisfactory reliability and validity (Corcoran and Foscher 1994).

Based on the IES, the CRIES-8/13 (Children's Revised Impact of Event Scale) is an 8/13-item instrument measuring traumatic stress in children. The child version of the instrument includes an 8-item version consisting of intrusion and avoidance items and a 13-item version containing additional hyperarousal items. The instruments are designed for use with children aged 8 years and above that are able to read independently. The CRIES is a good diagnostic screening tool for PTSD in children and is useful in identifying children requiring further assessment or intervention and those without need for further follow-up (Dow et al. 2012).

Case 11.4
A 10-year-old girl underwent mental health screening before an elective operation. The screening indicated symptoms of anxiety at a clinical level. Her parents offered the following explanation: "When our daughter was five years old, she fell into the water and nearly drowned; she continued to be extremely afraid of water, and we also remember that for her going to the dentist was very challenging. However, we thought it was a little better now since she is always coping well in school and has friends."

The psychiatric team at the hospital advised the surgery team to delay the operation until they could investigate the girl's anxiety and possible PTSD. They focused on gradually preparing her for the eventual surgery.

Testing of Neuropsychological Functioning

Neuropsychological assessment typically includes a multifaceted IQ test such as the Wechsler Intelligence Scale for Children (WISC), Fifth Edition (Wechsler 2014), which tests verbal comprehension, perceptual reasoning, working memory, and processing speed.

Depending on the child's age and ability level, various specific tests are used to assess different areas of function:

Executive Functioning can be evaluated using a number of different tests: the Wisconsin Card Sorting Test-64 (WCST-64) (Heaton et al. 1993) as a measure of abstract thinking and set-shifting/mental flexibility, the Color Word Interference Test (CWIT) from the Delis-Kaplan Executive Function System (D-KEFS) (Delis et al. 2001) as a measure of inhibition, the Verbal Fluency Test from the D-KEFS as a measure of verbal functioning, and Digit Span from the Wechsler Intelligence Scale for Children, Fifth Edition (WISC-V) (Wechsler 2014), as a measure of working memory.

Attention can be assessed using the Trail Making Test from the D-KEFS as a measure of psychomotor speed and divided attention and the Conners Continuous Performance Test 3rd Edition (CPT 3) (Conners 2014) as a measure of inattention, impulsivity, sustained attention, and vigilance.

Working Memory and Metacognitive Index can be evaluated using the Behavior Rating Inventory of Executive Function (BRIEF) (Gioia et al. 2000), a parent questionnaire consisting of 86 items rated as occurring never, sometimes, or often. All scaled scores are age and sex standardized, with a mean of 50 and standard deviation of 10.

Assessment of Pediatric Pain

Numeric Rating Scale (NRS) is a self-report consisting of sequential numbers from 0 to 10; it can also be used verbally. The scale is anchored by word descriptors with 0 meaning "no pain" and 10 meaning "most pain possible." The NRS requires numeric skills and is recommended for children and adolescents aged 8 years and older (Farrar et al. 2001).

The Faces Pain Scale – Revised (FPS-R) is a revised version of the scale developed by Bieri and Reeve. It consists of six gender-neutral line drawings of faces that are scored from 0 to 10; it has adequate psychometric properties and can be used for children ≥4 years (Bieri et al. 1990). For research use, the FPS-R has been recommended on the basis of utility and psychometric features (Tsze et al. 2013).

Preventing Long-Term Consequences

A biopsychosocial approach to illness emphasizes biological, psychological, and social factors in understanding what predisposes, provokes, and modifies or maintains disease (Diseth 2014; Gatchel et al. 2007). In working with children with severe medical disease, it is necessary to take a holistic approach to disease and to identify all possible stressors that may influence the illness situation (Frankel et al 2003; Kazak and Noll 2015). Relevant stressors should be captured early at the time of diagnosis and initiation of treatment (Stuber 1996; Kazak et al. 2006; Kassam-Adams 2006). Healthcare professional should emphasize the importance of preventing further traumatic experiences, identifying stress reactions, and helping parents to deal with the child's reactions (Diseth 2006; Kassam-Adams 2006; Stuber et al. 2006) (Table 11.2).

Conclusion

Children and adolescents coping with invasive medical conditions will face many physical and emotional challenges related to the pre-procedural phases of their care, which are often stressful. Children's ability to understand and adapt to severe disease, as well as to deal with treatment-related procedures, is dependent on their cognitive and emotional development, maturation, earlier concrete experiences of

Table 11.2 Preventing long-term consequences

Supervise/educate the medical staff	
	Acknowledge the risk of posttraumatic stress symptoms; *subjective* opinion > objective medical data
	Discuss how to *prevent* pain, stress, and traumatic experiences
Improve/change routines regarding the way stressful/painful or traumatic procedures are carried out	
	Create a higher degree of *predictability*, sense of *control*, and a better *overview* of the situation
	Provide the patient with adequate pain medication pre- and post-op (establish interdisciplinary teams that focus on pediatric pain)
Prepare and create a safe environment for the child; allot sufficient time for preparation	
	Teach coping skills/techniques including relaxation/breathing/distraction/externalization techniques
	Use hypnotherapy and cognitive behavioral therapy interventions
	Use toys and creative material, dolls, drawing materials, books
	Allow visits to the operating room; ensure stability in staff (nurses, doctors); create a daily agenda
Know how to face a chaotic situation	
	Quickly ensure physical presence/safety/care of a parent/caregiver
	Take the child from the examination room to his/her regular room
	Reestablish familiar, safe, and calm everyday routines; consider temporarily discharging from the hospital

Source: Adapted from Diseth (2006)

illness, and previous pain experiences, together with their family's coping skills and ability to assimilate information. Hospital personnel need increased knowledge of psychological consequences of serious disease in children so posttraumatic stress reactions can be optimally prevented.

References

Ahmad, A., & Sundelin-Wahlsten, V. (2008). Applying EMDR on children with PTSD. *European Child & Adolescent Psychiatry, 17*(3), 127–132.

Alderfer, M. A., Labay, L. E., & Kazak, A. E. (2003). Brief report: Does posttraumatic stress apply to siblings of childhood cancer survivors? *Journal of Pediatric Psychology, 28*(4), 281–286.

Baron, I. S. (2004). *Neuropsychological evaluation of the child.* New York: Oxford University Press.

Bevan, J. C., Johnston, C., Haig, M. J., Tousignant, G., Lucy, S., Kirnon, V., et al. (1990). Preoperative parental anxiety predicts behavioural and emotional responses to induction of anaesthesia in children. *Canadian Journal of Anaesthesia, 37*(2), 177–182.

Bibace, R., & Walsh, M. E. (1980). Development of children's concepts of illness. *Pediatrics, 66*(6), 912–917.

Bieri, D., Reeve, R. A., Champion, G. D., Addicoat, L., & Ziegler, J. B. (1990). The faces pain scale for the self-assessment of the severity of pain experienced by children: Development, initial validation, and preliminary investigation for ratio scale properties. *Pain, 41*(2), 139–150.

Brenner, E. M., & Salovey, P. (1997). Emotion regulation during childhood. Developmental, interpersonal and individual consideration. In ISDJS (Ed.), *Emotional development and emotional intelligence* (pp. 168–192). New York: Basic Books.

Brewster, A. B. (1982). Chronically ill hospitalized children's concepts of their illness. *Pediatrics, 69*(3), 355–362.

Briere, J. (1997). *Psychological assessment of adult post traumatic stress*. Washington, DC: American Psychological Association.

Buizer, A. I., de Sonneville, L. M., & Veerman, A. J. (2009). Effects of chemotherapy on neurocognitive function in children with acute lymphoblastic leukemia: A critical review of the literature. *Pediatric Blood & Cancer, 52*(4), 447–454.

Bush, J. P., Melamed, B. G., Sheras, P. L., & Greenbaum, P. E. (1986). Mother-child patterns of coping with anticipatory medical stress. *Health Psychology, 5*(2), 137–157.

Butler, R. W., & Copeland, D. R. (2002). Attentional processes and their remediation in children treated for cancer: A literature review and the development of a therapeutic approach. *Journal of the International Neuropsychological Society, 8*(1), 115–124.

Campbell, L., Clark, M., & Kirkpatrick, S. E. (1986). Stress management training for parents and their children undergoing cardiac catheterization. *The American Journal of Orthopsychiatry, 56*(2), 234–243.

Campbell, L. A., Kirkpatrick, S. E., Berry, C. C., Penn, N. E., Waldman, J. D., & Mathewson, J. W. (1992). Psychological preparation of mothers of preschool-children undergoing cardiac-catheterization. *Psychology & Health, 7*(3), 175–185.

Campbell, L. K., Scaduto, M., Sharp, W., Dufton, L., Van Slyke, D., Whitlock, J. A., et al. (2007). A meta-analysis of the neurocognitive sequelae of treatment for childhood acute lymphocytic leukemia. *Pediatric Blood & Cancer, 49*(1), 65–73.

Cohen, J., Mannarino, A. P., & Deblinger, E. (2006). *Treating trauma and traumatic grief in children and adolescents*. New York: Guildford Press.

Cohen, L. L., Lemanek, K., Blount, R. L., Dahlquist, L. M., Lim, C. S., Palermo, T. M., et al. (2008). Evidence-based assessment of pediatric pain. *Journal of Pediatric Psychology, 33*(9), 939–955. discussion 56–7.

Conners, C. K. (2014). *Conners continuous performance test 3rd edition (Conners CPT 3) & Conners continuous auditory test of attention (Conners CATA) – Technical manual*. New York/Toronto: MHS.

Corcoran, K., & Foscher, J. (1994). *Measures of clinical practice. A source book. 3rd adults*. New Yourk: The free press.

de Ruiter, M. A., van Mourik, R., Schouten-van Meeteren, A. Y., Grootenhuis, M. A., & Oosterlaan, J. (2013). Neurocognitive consequences of a paediatric brain tumour and its treatment: A meta-analysis. *Developmental Medicine and Child Neurology, 55*(5), 408–417.

Delis, D. C., Kaplan, E., & Kramer, J. H. (2001). *Dellis.Kaplan executive function system (D-KEFS). Examiner's manual*. San Antonio: The Psychological Corporation, Harcourt Assessment Company.

DeLoach Walworth, D. (2005). Procedural-support music therapy in the healthcare setting: A cost-effectiveness analysis. *Journal of Pediatric Nursing, 20*(4), 276–284.

Diseth, T. H. (2006). Dissociation following traumatic medical treatment procedures in childhood: A longitudinal follow-up. *Development and Psychopathology, 18*(1), 233–251.

Diseth, T. H. (2014). Kronisk somatisk sykdom og symptomatologi hos barn og unge. In A. A. Dahl, J. H. Loge, & T. F. Aarre (Eds.), *Psykiske reaksjoner ved somatisk sykdom* (pp. 674–694). Oslo: Cappelen Damm Akademisk.

Diseth, T. H., & Emblem, R. (2017). Long-term psychosocial consequences of surgical congenital malformations. *Seminars in Pediatric Surgery Accepted, 26*(5), 286–294.

Dow, B. L., Kenardy, J. A., Le Brocque, R. M., & Long, D. A. (2012). The utility of the Children's revised impact of event scale in screening for concurrent PTSD following admission to intensive care. *Journal of Traumatic Stress, 25*(5), 602–605.

Edelstein, K., D'Agostino, N., Bernstein, L. J., Nathan, P. C., Greenberg, M. L., Hodgson, D. C., et al. (2011). Long-term neurocognitive outcomes in young adult survivors of childhood acute lymphoblastic leukemia. *Journal of Pediatric Hematology/Oncology, 33*(6), 450–458.

Eiser, C. (1985). Changes in understanding of illness as the child grows. *Archives of Disease in Childhood, 60*(5), 489–492.

Eiser, C. (1998). Practitioner review: Long-term consequences of childhood cancer. *Journal of Child Psychology and Psychiatry, 39*(5), 621–633.

Farrar, J. T., Young, J. P., Jr., LaMoreaux, L., Werth, J. L., & Poole, R. M. (2001). Clinical importance of changes in chronic pain intensity measured on an 11-point numerical pain rating scale. *Pain, 94*(2), 149–158.

Ferguson, B. F. (1979). Preparing young children for hospitalization: A comparison of two methods. *Pediatrics, 64*(5), 656–664.

Flick, R. P., Katusic, S. K., Colligan, R. C., Wilder, R. T., Voigt, R. G., Olson, M. D., et al. (2011). Cognitive and behavioral outcomes after early exposure to anesthesia and surgery. *Pediatrics, 128*(5), e1053–e1061.

Frankel, R. M., Quill, T. E., & McDaniel, S. H. (2003). *The biopsychological approach: Past, present, future.* Rochester: University of Rochester Press.

French, G. M., Painter, E. C., & Coury, D. L. (1994). Blowing away shot pain: A technique for pain management during immunization. *Pediatrics, 93*(3), 384–388.

Gatchel, R. J., Peng, Y. B., Peters, M. L., Fuchs, P. N., & Turk, D. C. (2007). The biopsychosocial approach to chronic pain: Scientific advances and future directions. *Psychological Bulletin, 133*(4), 581–624.

Gioia, G. A., Isquith, P. K., Guy, S. C., & Kenworthy, L. (2000). *Behavior rating inventory of executive function (BRIEF): Professional manual.* Lutz: Psychological Assessment Resources.

Gjems, S., & Diseth, T. H. (2011). Somatic illness and psychological trauma in children: Prevention and treatment strategies. *Tidsskrift for Norsk Psykologforening, 48*, 857–862.

Goldschneider, K. R., Cravero, J. P., Anderson, C., Bannister, C., Hardy, C., Honkanen, A., et al. (2014). The Pediatrician's role in the evaluation and preparation of pediatric patients undergoing anesthesia. *Pediatrics, 134*(3), 634–641.

Goodman, R. (1997). The strengths and difficulties questionnaire: A research note. *Journal of Child Psychology and Psychiatry, 38*(5), 581–586.

Goodman, R. (1999). The extended version of the strengths and difficulties questionnaire as a guide to child psychiatric caseness and consequent burden. *Journal of Child Psychology and Psychiatry, 40*, 791–799.

Harmsen, W. J., Aarsen, F. J., van der Cammen-van Zijp, M. H., van Rosmalen, J. M., Wijnen, R. M., Tibboel, D., et al. (2016). Developmental problems in patients with oesophageal atresia: A longitudinal follow-up study. *Archives of Disease in Childhood. Fetal and Neonatal Edition, 102*(3), F214–F219.

Heaton, R. K., Chelune, G. J., Talley, J. L., Kay, G. G., & Curtiss, G. (1993). *Wisconsin card setting test manual: Revised and expanded.* Odessa: Psychological Assessment Resources.

Heyerdahl, S. (2003). SDQ – Strength and Difficulties Questionnaire: En orientering om et nytt spørreskjema for kartlegging av mental helse hos barn og unge, brukt i UNGHUBRO, OPPHED og TROFINN. *Norsk Epidemiologi, 13*(1), 127–135.

Horowitz, M., Wilner, N., & Alvarez, W. (1979). Impact of event scale: A measure of subjective stress. *Psychosomatic Medicine, 41*(3), 209–218.

Hutchinson, A. D., Pfeiffer, S. M., & Wilson, C. (2017). Cancer-related cognitive impairment in children. *Current Opinion in Supportive and Palliative Care, 11*(1), 70–75.

Huynh, M. E., Vandvik, I. H., & Diseth, T. H. (2008). Hypnotherapy in child psychiatry: The state of the art. *Clinical Child Psychology and Psychiatry, 13*(3), 377–393.

Jay, S. M., Elliott, C. H., Katz, E., & Siegel, S. E. (1987). Cognitive-behavioral and pharmacologic interventions for childrens' distress during painful medical procedures. *Journal of Consulting and Clinical Psychology, 55*(6), 860–865.

Kahalley, L. S., Conklin, H. M., Tyc, V. L., Hudson, M. M., Wilson, S. J., Wu, S., et al. (2013). Slower processing speed after treatment for pediatric brain tumor and acute lymphoblastic leukemia. *Psychooncology, 22*(9), 1979–1986.

Kain, Z. N., Wang, S. M., Mayes, L. C., Caramico, L. A., & Hofstadter, M. B. (1999). Distress during the induction of anesthesia and postoperative behavioral outcomes. *Anesthesia and Analgesia, 88*(5), 1042–1047.

Kassam-Adams, N. (2006). Introduction to the special issue: Posttraumatic stress related to pediatric illness and injury. *Journal of Pediatric Psychology, 31*(4), 337–342.

Kazak, A. E., & Noll, R. B. (2015). The integration of psychology in pediatric oncology research and practice: Collaboration to improve care and outcomes for children and families. *The American Psychologist, 70*(2), 146–158.

Kazak, A. E., Kassam-Adams, N., Schneider, S., Zelikovsky, N., Alderfer, M. A., & Rourke, M. (2006). An integrative model of pediatric medical traumatic stress. *Journal of Pediatric Psychology, 31*(4), 343–355.

Krull, K. R., Okcu, M. F., Potter, B., Jain, N., Dreyer, Z., Kamdar, K., et al. (2008). Screening for neurocognitive impairment in pediatric cancer long-term survivors. *Journal of Clinical Oncology, 26*(25), 4138–4143.

Krull, K. R., Brinkman, T. M., Li, C., Armstrong, G. T., Ness, K. K., Srivastava, D. K., et al. (2013). Neurocognitive outcomes decades after treatment for childhood acute lymphoblastic leukemia: A report from the St Jude lifetime cohort study. *Journal of Clinical Oncology, 31*(35), 4407–4415.

Kunin-Batson, A., Kadan-Lottick, N., Zhu, L., Cox, C., Bordes-Edgar, V., Srivastava, D. K., et al. (2011). Predictors of independent living status in adult survivors of childhood cancer: A report from the childhood Cancer Survivor Study. *Pediatric Blood & Cancer, 57*(7), 1197–1203.

LeRoy, S., Elixson, E. M., O'Brien, P., Tong, E., Turpin, S., Uzark, K., et al. (2003). Recommendations for preparing children and adolescents for invasive cardiac procedures: A statement from the American Heart Association Pediatric Nursing Subcommittee of the Council on cardiovascular nursing in collaboration with the Council on Cardiovascular Diseases of the Young. *Circulation, 108*(20), 2550–2564.

Lindheim, M. O., & Helgeland, H. (2017). Hypnosis training and education: Experiences with a Norwegian one-year education course in clinical hypnosis for children and adolescents. *The American Journal of Clinical Hypnosis, 59*(3), 282–291.

McGrath, P. J., & Frager, G. (1996). Psychological barriers to optimal pain management in infants and children. *The Clinical Journal of Pain, 12*(2), 135–141.

Morton, N. S. (1997). Pain assessment in children. *Paediatric Anaesthesia, 7*(4), 267–272.

Myant, K. A., & Williams, J. M. (2005). Children's concepts of health and illness: Understanding of contagious illnesses, non-contagious illnesses and injuries. *Journal of Health Psychology, 10*(6), 805–819.

Peterson, C. C., Johnson, C. E., Ramirez, L. Y., Huestis, S., Pai, A. L., Demaree, H. A., et al. (2008). A meta-analysis of the neuropsychological sequelae of chemotherapy-only treatment for pediatric acute lymphoblastic leukemia. *Pediatric Blood & Cancer, 51*(1), 99–104.

Reinfjell, T., Diseth, T. H., Veenstra, M., & Vikan, A. (2006). Measuring health-related quality of life in young adolescents: Reliability and validity in the Norwegian version of the Pediatric quality of life inventory 4.0 (PedsQL) generic core scales. *Health and Quality of Life Outcomes, 4*, 61.

Reinfjell, T., Diseth, T. H., & Vikan, A. (2007). Children and cancer: Children's adjustment to and understanding of their cancer. *Tidsskrift for Norsk Psykologforening, 44*, 724–734.

Richter, N. C. (1984). The efficacy of relaxation training with children. *Journal of Abnormal Child Psychology, 12*(2), 319–344.

Robinson, K. E., Kuttesch, J. F., Champion, J. E., Andreotti, C. F., Hipp, D. W., Bettis, A., et al. (2010). A quantitative meta-analysis of neurocognitive sequelae in survivors of pediatric brain tumors. *Pediatric Blood & Cancer, 55*(3), 525–531.

Robinson, K. E., Fraley, C. E., Pearson, M. M., Kuttesch, J. F., Jr., & Compas, B. E. (2013). Neurocognitive late effects of pediatric brain tumors of the posterior fossa: A quantitative review. *Journal of the International Neuropsychological Society, 19*(1), 44–53.

Rodenburg, R., Benjamin, A., de Roos, C., Meijer, A. M., & Stams, G. J. (2009). Efficacy of EMDR in children: A meta-analysis. *Clinical Psychology Review, 29*(7), 599–606.

Saha, A., Salley, C. G., Saigal, P., Rolnitzky, L., Goldberg, J., Scott, S., et al. (2014). Late effects in survivors of childhood CNS tumors treated on head start I and II protocols. *Pediatric Blood & Cancer, 61*(9), 1644–1652. quiz 53-72.

Salmon, K., & Pereira, J. K. (2002). Predicting children's response to an invasive medical investigation: The influence of effortful control and parent behavior. *Journal of Pediatric Psychology, 27*(3), 227–233.

Sander Wint, S., Eshelman, D., Steele, J., & Guzzetta, C. E. (2002). Effects of distraction using virtual reality glasses during lumbar punctures in adolescents with cancer. *Oncology Nursing Forum, 29*(1), E8–E15.

Shapiro, F. (2001). *Eye movement desensitization and reprocessing. Basic principles, protocols and procedures*. New York: Guilford Press.

Srouji, R., Ratnapalan, S., & Schneeweiss, S. (2010). Pain in children: Assessment and nonpharmacological management. *Int J Pediatr, 2010*, 1–11.

Stallard, P. (2006). Psychological interventions for post-traumatic reactions in children and young people: A review of randomised controlled trials. *Clinical Psychology Review, 26*(7), 895–911.

Stuber, M. L. (1996). Psychiatric sequelae in seriously ill children and their families. *The Psychiatric Clinics of North America, 19*(3), 481–493.

Stuber, M. L., Shemesh, E., & Saxe, G. N. (2003). Posttraumatic stress responses in children with life-threatening illnesses. *Child and Adolescent Psychiatric Clinics of North America, 12*(2), 195–209.

Stuber, M. L., Schneider, S., Kassam-Adams, N., Kazak, A. E., & Saxe, G. (2006). The medical traumatic stress toolkit. *CNS Spectrums, 11*(2), 137–142.

Sun, L. (2010). Early childhood general anaesthesia exposure and neurocognitive development. *British Journal of Anaesthesia, 105*(Suppl 1), i61–i68.

Tak, J. H., & van Bon, W. H. (2006). Pain- and distress-reducing interventions for venepuncture in children. *Child: Care, Health and Development, 32*(3), 257–268.

Tsze, D. S., von Baeyer, C. L., Bulloch, B., & Dayan, P. S. (2013). Validation of self-report pain scales in children. *Pediatrics, 132*(4), e971–e979.

Uman, L. S., Chambers, C. T., McGrath, P. J., & Kisely, S. (2006). Psychological interventions for needle-related procedural pain and distress in children and adolescents. *Cochrane Database of Systematic Reviews, 4*, CD005179.

Utens, E. M., Versluis-Den Bieman, H. J., Verhulst, F. C., Witsenburg, M., Bogers, A. J., & Hess, J. (2000). Psychological distress and styles of coping in parents of children awaiting elective cardiac surgery. *Cardiology in the Young, 10*(3), 239–244.

Varni, J. W., Seid, M., & Rode, C. A. (1999). The PedsQL: Measurement model for the pediatric quality of life inventory. *Medical Care, 37*(2), 126–139.

Varni, J. W., Burwinkle, T. M., Rapoff, M. A., Kamps, J. L., & Olson, N. (2004). The PedsQL in pediatric asthma: Reliability and validity of the pediatric quality of life inventory generic core scales and asthma module. *Journal of Behavioral Medicine, 27*(3), 297–318.

Varughese, A. M., Nick, T. G., Gunter, J., Wang, Y., & Kurth, C. D. (2008). Factors predictive of poor behavioral compliance during inhaled induction in children. *Anesthesia and Analgesia, 107*(2), 413–421.

Vatne, T. M., Slaugther, L., & Ruland, C. M. (2010). How children with cancer communicate and think about symptoms. *Journal of Pediatric Oncology Nursing, 27*(1), 24–32.

Vatne, T. M., Ruland, C. M., Ornes, K., & Finset, A. (2012). Children's expressions of negative emotions and adults' responses during routine cardiac consultations. *Journal of Pediatric Psychology, 37*(2), 232–240.

Vessey, J. A., Carlson, K. L., & McGill, J. (1994). Use of distraction with children during an acute pain experience. *Nursing Research, 43*(6), 369–372.

Vikan, A. (1988). Barns oppfatning av medisinske tiltak. In: P.E. Mjaavatn (Ed.). Barn. Nytt fra forskning om barn i Norge. Nr. 3. Norsk senter for barneforskning

Walsh, K. S., Paltin, I., Gioia, G. A., Isquith, P., Kadan-Lottick, N. S., Neglia, J. P., et al. (2015). Everyday executive function in standard-risk acute lymphoblastic leukemia survivors. *Child Neuropsychology, 21*(1), 78–89.

Wechsler, D. (2014). *Wechsler intelligence scale for children* (5th ed.). San Antonio: NCS Pearson.

Weiss, D., & Marmar, C. (1997). The impact of event scale – revised. In J. K. Wilson & T. M. Keane (Eds.), *Assessing psychological trauma and PTSD*. New York: Guilford.

Zeltzer, L. K., & Zeltzer, P. M. (2016). *Pain in children & young adults. The journey back to normal*. Encino: Shilysca Press.

Zeltzer, L. K., Recklitis, C., Buchbinder, D., Zebrack, B., Casillas, J., Tsao, J. C., et al. (2009). Psychological status in childhood cancer survivors: A report from the childhood Cancer Survivor Study. *Journal of Clinical Oncology, 27*(14), 2396–2404.

Chapter 12
Improving Adherence and Promoting Behavioral Change

Marisa Perez-Reisler

Definition and Impact of Adherence in Medical Settings

Treatment adherence consists of behaviors employed to follow recommendations by healthcare professionals with the goal of appropriate management or primary prevention of a disease state. Medication compliance is most commonly associated with treatment adherence. Other examples include lifestyle and behavior changes, such as following specific diet or exercise recommendations, complying with referrals to specialists and adhering to primary preventive practices like vaccinations. Identification of adherence problems is essential for medical providers as part of ongoing medical treatment and planning. Nonadherence can lead to significant medical repercussions and high medical costs (Brody 2017). Multiple factors contribute to treatment nonadherence. Among these factors are forgetfulness, cost, medication side effects, health-belief models, illness response and severity, as well as a myriad of intersecting psychosocial and healthcare system factors. Addressing these issues is a critical component to improving adherence.

Nonadherence in Adult Populations

Treatment nonadherence is common. One study showed adherence rates of approximately 50% for acute, short-term antibiotic administration in the treatment of respiratory tract infections. It is well-established that adherence rates decrease as dosing frequency increases in the adult population (Claxton et al. 2001). Table 12.1 shows

M. Perez-Reisler (✉)
Department of Psychiatry, University of Hawai'i John A. Burns School of Medicine, Honolulu, HI, USA
e-mail: marisape@hawaii.edu

A. P. S. Guerrero et al. (eds.), *Pediatric Consultation-Liaison Psychiatry*,
https://doi.org/10.1007/978-3-319-89488-1_12

Table 12.1 Adherence rates inversely related to dosing frequency of medication (adapted from Claxton et al 2001)

Dosing schedule	Adherence rates
Daily	79%
BID	69%
TID	65%
QID	51%

that daily dosing of a 5-day course of antibiotics has an adherence rate of 79%, which decreases in inverse proportion to the frequency of daily dosing, to 59% with four times daily dosing. In chronic medical conditions, which can involve prolonged or lifelong medication courses, multiple agents, and additional behavioral recommendations, adherence rates are lower, around 50% (Sabaté 2003). The morbidity and mortality associated with treatment nonadherence as well as the financial costs are large. These costs related to nonadherence are termed "healthcare waste" and account for 3–10% of total US healthcare costs (Iuga and McGuire 2014).

The remainder of this chapter will focus on nonadherence in pediatric medical care, where adherence rates for both acute and chronic illnesses are lower compared to adults. There are multiple contributing factors to the lower adherence rates in pediatrics, including the added variable of having both the patient and their family or caregiver involved and the medical provider needing to understand the developmental issues at stake for appropriate communication about illness education, treatment management, and anticipatory guidance and prevention. Discussion about modifiable targets of intervention will be illustrated utilizing case vignettes.

Nonadherence in Pediatric Populations

In pediatric populations, the nonadherence rates are even higher than for adults, with one study noting that 50–88% of children and adolescents do not adhere to their medication regimens (Logan et al. 2003). In acute pediatric illnesses such as otitis media and strep pharyngitis, adherence rates vary widely anywhere between 18 and 95% (Wu and Roberts 2008). In chronic pediatric illnesses, the adherence rate is less than 50% (Osterberg and Blaschke 2005). As healthcare professionals, how do we deal with this ubiquitous challenge, which is a significant contributor to worsened health outcomes and a large financial and public health burden? (McGrady and Hommel 2013).

It is vital for primary care and behavioral health providers, as well as other specialists working with child and adolescent populations, to understand factors involved with adherence and the impact on treatment outcomes. More specifically, we will be dealing with adherence for chronic pediatric illnesses including asthma, diabetes, juvenile rheumatoid arthritis (JRA), cystic fibrosis (CF), seizure disorders, obesity, solid organ transplants, bone marrow transplants, cardiac malformations, cerebral palsy (CP), human immunodeficiency virus (HIV), and congenital genetic and developmental disorders. Due to advances in healthcare, greater numbers of children survive acute lymphocytic leukemia (ALL), congenital heart conditions, and bone marrow or solid organ transplants. These patients' treatment adherence is vital for their survival and quality of life, despite studies showing that adherence rates for these chronic conditions are no better than in other pediatric populations (Rianthavorn et al. 2004).

Additionally, adherence rates in pediatrics are lower compared to adults in both low-risk illnesses, where health consequences are minimal or cumulative, and serious-risk illnesses, where medical treatment is mitigating the condition, but full remission is not expected (LaGreca and Bearman 2003). In the first case, many years need to pass for any manifestations of illness, and treatments may not show any demonstrable difference in outcome in the short term. For serious illnesses, patients and/or parents may believe that treatment would result in only limited impact on health outcomes and therefore may not be optimally compliant.

Barriers for Pediatric Patients

Adherence to treatment in pediatric patients is a complex dynamic. As medical providers, understanding barriers to address for patients and their families and educating about the challenges observed with specific illnesses are important to effectively engage patients and families and promote treatment adherence (Fig. 12.1).

Adherence barriers can be divided into categories: patient/family factors, illness factors, treatment factors, and healthcare system factors. These factors are all well-described in the literature. Patient/family factors include patient's developmental stage, cognitive skills, health-belief model, self-efficacy or self-management skills, psychosocial supports, environment, and patient/family psychological factors (DiMatteo 2004; LaGreca and Bearman 2003). Psychological factors include illness distress, underlying mood and anxiety or other psychiatric disorders, stress levels, history of trauma, communication and coping skills, as well as self-esteem and implicit and explicit bias. One significant psychological factor particularly present in chronic pediatric illnesses is "burnout" most notably found where treatment regimens require significant lifestyle changes and complex medication dosing over a long-term course. Patient and family burnout is a well-known factor associated with adherence problems (Warner and Hauer 2009).

Illness factors are specific to the type of illness and its symptom severity and other manifestations. Treatment factors include length of time required, frequency of dosing, effectiveness of treatment, invasiveness (difficulty of medication administration), and lifestyle changes including diet, exercise, and activity restrictions or modifications. The effect of treatment on illness and side effects are additional contributors to adherence rates. Healthcare systems can also promote or worsen adherence based on ease of enrolling in insurance coverage, copayments, as well as partnership with patients and providers and availability of other programs that might help with patient reminders or other system issues involved in adherence. Provider factors, including age, race/gender concordance or discordance, communication

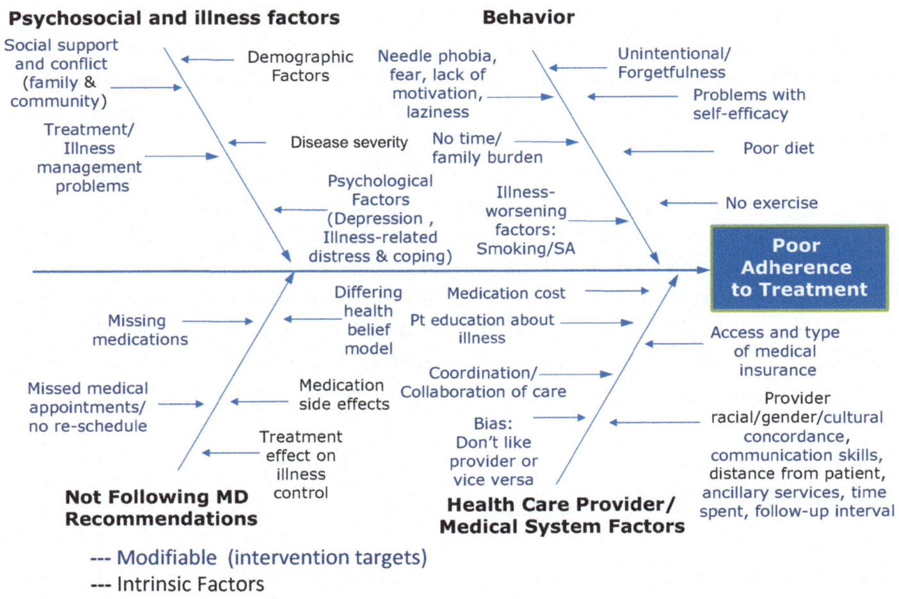

Fig. 12.1 Barriers to adherence. Fishbone diagram showing factors leading to poor adherence including: psychosocial and illness factors, behaviors and health care system factors

skills, explicit and implicit bias, and availability of ancillary help for education, medication administration, and appointment reminders, are additional factors that can affect a patient's adherence. Of the factors discussed above, while some are unmodifiable, many are modifiable factors that can be targets for intervention (see Table 12.2).

An emerging field of research into treatment adherence involves the concept of implicit bias and its effects on healthcare outcomes. Implicit bias is a largely unconscious and intrinsic automatic bias that every person, including physicians, has toward other people based on outward physical characteristics such as perception of age, race, skin color, gender, and class. It differs from explicit bias in that it is covert and typically unacknowledged. Implicit bias may be based on demographic and physical categories for provider and patient, including age, gender, race, cultural background, nationality, sexual orientation, socioeconomic class, and physical attributes (including weight, grooming, and dressing habits). Because adherence is a complex behavior, unconscious or implicit bias can be a dynamic factor due to the largely unacknowledged role it can exert in affecting both the patient and provider's attitudes, beliefs, and behaviors during and after treatment encounter. While the presence of implicit bias is well-established, its effects on adherence and healthcare outcomes have not been completely understood and are only recently being studied. A study by Blair et al. in 2014 did not find any significant effect of intrinsic bias either treatment changes or outcomes of patients with hypertension (Blair et al. 2014). A meta-analysis by FitzGerald and Hurst in 2017 showed that both healthcare profes-

Table 12.2 Adherence promotion interventions

Classification and intervention types
Educational
Behavioral
Parental monitoring
Cognitive behavioral therapy
Dialectical behavioral therapy
Operant-learning procedures
Self-management
Psychosocial
Family-based interventions
Parent guidance
Multi-systemic treatment
Cognitive behavioral therapy
Motivational interviewing
Dialectical behavioral therapy
Organizational approaches
Provider-driven: simplify regimen; use auto-delivery systems
Pharmacist driven
Reminder systems: text message, medication reminder applications
Case Manager
Multi-component interventions

sionals and patients have implicit bias and that these may correlate with a negative clinical interaction. This in turn may be postulated to have a detrimental effect on a patient's attitudes and behaviors toward their treatment plan, although a direct causal relationship has not been established (FitzGerald and Hurst 2017). Importantly, awareness of the existence of unconscious bias and self-awareness as patients and/or medical providers can help change attitudes and implement changes that can mitigate the disparities it can cause when otherwise it would not be identified and addressed. Additionally, perspective-taking or understanding a patient's viewpoint and individuation, taking in account the patient's characteristics rather than that of their identified group, may minimize the impact of intrinsic bias (Chapman et al. 2013).

Understanding the Metrics

In the medical literature, metrics employed to quantify adherence rates vary among studies, making it somewhat difficult to make direct comparisons. For example, in some studies, pharmacy refills are used to quantify medication compliance, but since these tallies are devoid of clinical context, medication intolerance due to side effects is measured as noncompliance. To account for other ways to measure adherence, other studies utilize questionnaires or direct data, including blood levels, glucometer readings, and electronic measurements that may avoid this potential miscount but have their own inherent metric errors. Use of at least two metric systems can help improve the correlation for errors inherent in each system (Bhatia et al. 2017) as currently there is no "gold standard" measure for adherence.

Role of Consultation-Liaison Psychiatry

In primary care settings, behavioral noncompliance constitutes the largest reason for psychiatric consultation (16.2%), and on inpatient wards it is the second highest concern for consultation (13%) (Campbell and Cardona 2007). Additionally, depression is a known risk factor for adherence problems, with depressed patients being three times as likely to be nonadherent as compared to nondepressed patients (DiMatteo et al. 2000). Consultation-liaison psychiatrists and other behavioral health specialists can be valuable team members identifying and recommending a plan to address adherence barriers, including psychiatric illnesses, in patients and/or their parents. Other common psychiatric symptoms and disorders that can negatively impact adherence include anxiety, posttraumatic stress disorder, and substance abuse. Identifying a depressed patient (or caregiver/family) and screening for comorbid disorders with treatment recommendations could significantly improve a patient's adherence rate. Depending on one's scope of practice, a consulting psychiatrist could potentially provide short- or long-term direct follow-up care, possibly in the same medical facility as the referring provider. This arrangement can optimize continuity of care and collaborative treatment.

Case Vignette 12.1

Joey is a 7-year-old boy with eczema, allergic rhinosinusitis, and mild persistent asthma with several emergency department visits this winter for asthma exacerbations, usually triggered by viral upper respiratory infections. He lives with his mother, grandparents, baby brother, and pet dog. His grandfather is a smoker. He takes a short-acting beta-agonist (SABA) as needed for asthma exacerbations, fluticasone nasal spray, and inhaled corticosteroid (ICS) twice daily. Recently, his mother lost her job and medical insurance coverage and was unable to buy his daily inhaled steroids and fluticasone, so she has been giving him his medication only when he is symptomatic. He has stopped playing soccer, as he feels too tired, and has missed several school days over the winter due to asthma flares. He wishes he could play soccer again and feels he is "not as good" as his other friends who still play, causing him to feel sad sometimes. Joey's case is discussed in a collaborative primary care/integrated behavioral health team meeting where you are present as a consultant.

Improving Adherence in Pediatric Asthma

Like in other chronic illnesses, adherence rates in pediatric asthma fluctuate between 30 and 70%, averaging approximately 50% (Bender 2002). In addition to added direct costs for controlling asthma flares, nonadherence may lead to medication dose escalations or switching medications especially when nonadherence is not identified and mislabeled a medication failure (Bender and Bender 2005). These changes can lead to worsened outcomes, as the patient may be inadvertently given a higher dose than needed with resultant side effects, as well as higher resource utilization. Monitoring treatment adherence is an essential component of good medical care. Multiple strategies have been identified to improve adherence for asthma and are listed in Table 12.3 (Lemanek et al. 2001). In the case example, asthma education includes identifying Joey's asthma triggers, particularly modifiable ones, and the steps the family must take to minimize his exposure to them. It is important to understand this family's health-belief model, including their knowledge about the asthma regimen medications and the need to take them daily, and to insure communication with the provider if barriers do not allow them to continue this plan. Shared treatment decision-making, which addresses barriers to treatment, has been shown to improve adherence (Wilson et al. 2009). Poor control of asthma has resulted in Joey participating less in extracurricular sports. Determining methods to improve his symptom control can be framed in relation to his daily goals for school and sports participation. Determining whether he is allergic to his pet dog, or at least reducing his contact with the pet while investigating this association, can be an initial goal for the provider to address with the family. Additionally, helping his grandfather with a referral for smoking cessation could also be identified as another modifiable factor for symptom control. Another alternative would include advice on risk reduction for his exposure to secondhand smoke, especially while his grandfather is working on decreasing or discontinuing cigarette smoking. Referral for assistance in applying for publicly funded medical insurance, in finding cheaper alternatives for his daily medications, and in accessing resources to aid in pick-up

Table 12.3 Empirically supported treatments (ESTs) in pediatrics

Illness and intervention types
Asthma
Organizational approaches
Educational strategies
Behavioral strategies or combination
Multi-component treatment[a]
JRA
Behavioral strategies
Educational strategies
Diabetes
Operant-learning procedures
Multi-component treatment/ self-management training
Cognitive behavioral/self-regulation procedures

Adapted from Lemanek et al. 2001
[a]Future research needed to determine efficacy

of medications could be a key way for the provider to improve Joey's asthma control. The family had managed his asthma successfully when the medications were available, so organizational strategies can be discussed for review, but are unlikely to make significant changes in his case. Addressing another modifiable risk factor for worsened asthma control, assessment of comorbid depression, or anxiety affecting Joey or his caretakers can also help improve treatment adherence. In this case, Joey's asthma symptoms directly affect his ability to participate in sports but also lead to self-esteem changes as he compares himself to his peers. If his asthma symptoms do not improve, the negative effects on his self-esteem can lead to more significant mood and anxiety symptoms. Developmentally appropriate illness education that includes anticipatory guidance and prevention geared toward both the family and patient is key to encouraging his autonomy and feeling of self-control. Also, inquiring about the effect of his mother's job loss on the family and its effect on his treatment may yield additional ways to optimize his care. For asthma of greater severity, multicomponent treatment is a helpful tool. For adolescent children with text message capability, use of text reminders can be a powerful aid for improving treatment adherence (Petrie et al. 2012).

Case Vignette 12.2

Emma is a 13-year-old female with Type 1 diabetes mellitus (T1DM) diagnosed at age 6 and a recent hospitalization for diabetic ketoacidosis last month. Her most recent hemoglobin A1C level of 11 is elevated. You were asked to consult for concern of possible depression and treatment adherence issues impacting her diabetes care. Upon chart review and interview of the patient, you learn the following:

Emma lives at home with both her parents. She explains she is struggling with her 8th grade coursework and "feels stupid" since she is in danger of failing this year. She is tearful, recently having superficially scratched her wrists after an argument with her parents. She denied any suicidality, but sometimes feels she does not have a good reason to be alive. She reports that for several weeks to months, she rarely checks her finger-stick glucose level at school and only occasionally at home. Prior to the start of the school year, she was able to independently manage her diabetes, with her parents needing to supervise her only on rare occasions. Since summertime, her parents noted she was more withdrawn or angry at home, and they had more difficulty communicating with her. This change coincided with the family moving neighborhoods and schools and complaints that she did not have any friends at her new school.

In this case example, we are being asked to identify barriers to Emma's adherence to her diabetes care. T1DM is a complex medical illness where multiple components, including glucometer monitoring, sliding scale insulin administration, dietary routines, exercise, and self-care, are necessary for optimal control (LaGreca and Mackey 2009). In addition to information about her specific treatment recommendations, other factors for the consultant to consider are age, gender, family dynamics and conflicts, socioeconomic level, comorbid illnesses and disease severity, as well as response of disease to treatment. In her specific example, we would also get information about her level of functioning at home and school, her ability to self-monitor her treatment, and her level of parental supervision. The family health-belief model is an additional important factor in our assessment. Some factors associated with better health and glycemic control include increased frequency of blood glucose monitoring, lower family conflict around diabetes, and better self-management (Rohan 2015). All three of these factors are problematic in Emma's case and can be targets for behavioral intervention.

Despite Emma having become self-sufficient with her diabetes care in the past, the recent stressors have triggered depressive symptoms, impairing her ability to independently manage her healthcare needs. Having either Type 1 or Type 2 diabetes mellitus doubles the risk (in comparison to the general population) for depression (Lustman and Clouse 2005). Concomitant depression, through lack of motivation, guilt about burdening others, or hopelessness, can hamper youths' ability to communicate effectively with family members or to request additional help from school staff. Poor glucose control can also worsen mood, energy, and cognitive abilities (Sommerfield et al. 2004). As a young teenager, Emma is also in a developmental stage where acquiring self-sufficiency in caring for her own needs, including some of her diabetes management, is expected by her family and healthcare professionals. This transition toward increased self-reliance is a vulnerable period for adherence in adolescents (Warner and Hauer 2009). This vulnerability is in part because her treatment requires constant adjustment of her daily activities and schedule during a developmental phase where having diabetes may become a conflict for typical adolescent goals, such as "fitting in" and developing strong peer relationships. Mindful of the significant intervention required for successful diabetes care, the consultant should explore with her and her family what treatment component she can initiate responsibility for and should help the family to ensure that all aspects of her medical care are prioritized. Brief or occasional vacation periods, similar to a respite period, where a caregiver can become the central administrator of her medical treatment, can also be used to minimize burnout from the constant vigilance necessary for diabetic treatment (Warner and Hauer 2009). Reinforcing her self-efficacy skills for components of treatment she is managing may include providing additional positive encouragement and illness education. Additionally, indirectly assessing compliance and addressing questions or barriers that arise would have significant payoffs in improving her adherence rate. Monitoring her adherence more closely, by increasing office visits or more facilitating outreach and communication with her healthcare provider for blood glucose monitoring, would be indicated given the developmental transitions of adolescence (Taddeo et al. 2008).

Screening for eating disorders or disordered eating is important in adolescent girls with T1DM because disturbed eating patterns are frequently observed, although eating disorder rates are not higher than in the general population (LaGreca and Mackey 2009). In some cases, nonadherence, particularly when related to insulin, can be due to reluctance to gain weight (LaGreca and Mackey 2009). Nonadherence or misuse of insulin also must be closely monitored and considered a type of self-harming behavior, particularly if depressive symptoms including suicidal ideation are present. For self-harming behavior, dialectical behavioral therapy strategies, to improve affective regulation, distress tolerance, and interpersonal effectiveness, can be useful for improving adherence. In this case example, use of a mood diary card can be a helpful technique for monitoring the frequency of compliance with finger sticks and insulin injections. Ensuring a good therapist-patient relationship by maintaining an optimistic yet pragmatic problem-solving approach is important for the patient to acquire further self-efficacy skills. In other cases, motivational interviewing can be utilized to further elucidate the patient's understanding of and commitment to the medical treatment plan. Especially for adolescents managing their diabetes for several years, maintaining consistency and motivation to adhere to their treatment regimen can become problematic, and motivational interviewing allows use of techniques to further engage and motivate patients to participate or address gaps in coping and adaptation to self-care with family members. Motivational interviewing strategies include a nonjudgmental stance and exploration of underlying motivations or problem areas leading to poor adherence.

Emma can also benefit from a multicomponent intervention and operant learning procedures to address adherence problems, as both have shown efficacy as interventions (Hood et al. 2010; Kahana et al. 2008; Lemanek et al. 2001; Taddeo et al. 2008). Operant learning that involves reinforcements such as token incentives that are accumulated on a weekly basis when diabetes treatment goals are met has been shown to improve adherence in adolescents (Lemanek et al. 2001). Referral to a psychologist and/or psychiatrist for evaluation for depressive symptoms, ideally with possibility of collaborative care with the medical provider, will further address adherence barriers related to mood and behavior that are impacting diabetes self-care in her case. Including both an individual- and family-based approach has shown good evidence for improving family conflict and treatment adherence in adolescents (Berg et al. 2008; Wysocki et al. 2008). Education to reinforce both her individual and family's knowledge related to diabetes and illness management can address both the knowledge-based and communication barriers within her family system (Whittemore et al. 2010 and Rohan 2015). Some important points to discuss with Emma and her family is that being female and having recently gone through puberty are two known risk factors for future diabetes-related complications (Rohan 2015). Having a diagnosis of T1DM for a longer period is also associated with worsening self-management (Hood et al. 2010). If no improvement occurs, or for high-risk individuals, multisystemic therapy is a more intensive intervention shown to improve diabetes adherence (Ellis et al. 2005). Identifying some of the modifiable risk factors involved in Emma's diabetes adherence problem can prove useful to develop individually tailored brief questionnaires that can help her provider understand how to prioritize resources associated with improving her diabetes adherence. These assessments can include self-efficacy screens and mood screens, along with her finger-stick glucose and follow-up hemoglobin A1C levels, to determine progress on treatment adherence. Facilitation of data collection and follow-up information by a diabetic nurse educator, social worker, or nurse practitioner can greatly aid endocrinologists or pediatricians managing these follow-up visits.

In T1DM, operant learning procedures, multicomponent treatments, self-regulation, and CBT have established efficacy and are mainstay therapies that the mental health provider can utilize (Kahana et al. 2008; Lemanek et al. 2001) for addressing adherence barriers. Additionally, some components of dialectical behavioral therapy (DBT) or motivational interviewing (MI) are other evidence-based therapies that may prove be helpful for behavioral activation (LaGreca and Bearman 2003).

Improving Adherence in Acute Lymphocytic Leukemia

Besides diabetes and asthma, another well-studied chronic illness in the pediatric population is acute lymphocytic leukemia (ALL). A recent study by Bhatia et al (2017) revealed that adherence rates for a 2-year course of once-daily 6-mercaptopurine (6MP) are over-reported in ALL patients enrolled in their study. For effective treatment, 95% of doses must be taken. The study used patient and parent self-questionnaires and employed electronic microchips on pill bottles for correlation between questionnaires and actual dose-taking. They found that up to 84% of patients were over-reporting their medication compliance on self-reports, with 23.6% of the patients who were over-reporting medication doses taken having the highest noncompliance rates in the study. This finding is concerning due to risk of relapse and highlights the need for oncologists and pediatricians to actively monitor treatment adherence with measures other than self-report. Forgetfulness was identified as the primary barrier to medication adherence. Since this study was completed, oncologists at the medical center are using text message reminders and requesting texts back from parents to improve parent vigilance methods (Fitzmaurice 2017).

Use of New Technology to Monitor and Promote Adherence

Both eHealth and mHealth are terms used to describe new technologies used in healthcare delivery. Examples include electronic monitoring; short message service (i.e., text messaging); Internet-based, mobile medical applications; and illness-specific devices (Wu and Hommel 2014). Diabetes care can include continuous insulin monitoring and administration (insulin pump) as a treatment consideration. There is also a specific glucometer, iBGStar, that connects to a smartphone application for communication between the patient/family and their doctor (Wu and Hommel 2014). While these technologies are very promising, barriers to implementation still exist, including patient and provider access to these platforms or devices as well as ability to engage in use of a new system.

Healthcare System Changes and Financial Costs of Nonadherence

In addition, US healthcare reform proposes a payment schedule based on outcome results, emphasizing even more the role of healthcare professionals in the responsibility of our patient's behaviors toward treatment. This type of proposed insurance system also can create additional incentives as well as barriers in adherence outcomes. For example, reimbursements or financial incentives that can improve care coordination, improvements in data sharing across EHRs, and patient incentives can all facilitate adherence monitoring and rates (Cutler and Everett 2010). Further research is needed to find out how the bundling of insurance payments via accountable care organizations and capitated costs might affect adherence. On the one hand, providers are incentivized to monitor and improve patient's adherence to treatment. On the other hand, these changes might create a system where healthcare providers and organizations refuse to take patients with more serious health conditions.

Conclusion

Pediatric medical practitioners are at the front lines in managing patients' illnesses. It is imperative to remember that nonadherence is a common and significant problem. Furthermore, developing an approach to screen for adherence issues with any recommended medical treatment is critical. Even in the earliest phases of care, education, anticipation of difficulties, and open communication lines are important for patients and families to develop confidence in exploring and reporting any problems that could affect the treatment. Understanding the developmental phases of childhood and adolescence, family health-belief models, the existence of bias, both implicit and explicit, and current family functioning in regard to the child's illness and treatment is vital for maintaining family-centered care that addresses potential adherence barriers. Collaboration with ancillary staff and mental health professionals when needed is also a helpful intervention.

Follow-up visits should consistently include methods to monitor for adherence as well as a depression screen. Given the over-reporting of adherence on self-reports, practitioners should consider having two types of data to better correlate their patient's adherence rates. In the case of diabetes, a diary and the glucometer readings would provide good backup on reliability of the reporting patient and family. Other emerging technologies, including medication reminder apps or text message systems, can be used with self-report or retrospective reporting.

Importantly, awareness of adherence patterns in our pediatric populations allows us to implement developmentally appropriate family-centered interventions.

References

Bender, B. G. (2002). Overcoming barriers to nonadherence in asthma treatment. *The Journal of Allergy and Clinical Immunology, 109*, S554–S559.

Bender, B. G., & Bender, S. E. (2005). Patient-identified barriers to asthma treatment adherence: Responses to interviews, focus groups, and questionnaires. *Immunology and Allergy Clinics of North America, 25*(1), 107–130.

Berg, C. A., et al. (2008). Role of parental monitoring in understanding the benefits of parental acceptance on adolescent adherence and metabolic control of type 1 diabetes. *Diabetes Care, 31*(4), 678–683. https://doi.org/10.2337/dc07-1678.

Bhatia, S., et al. (2017). Comparison of self-report and electronic monitoring of 6MP intake in childhood ALL: A children's oncology group study. *Blood, 129*(14), 1919–1926. https://doi.org/10.1182/blood-2016-07-726893.

Blair, I. V., Steiner, J. F., Hanratty, R., et al. (2014). An investigation of associations between clinicians' ethnic or racial bias and hypertension treatment, medication adherence and blood pressure control. *Journal of General Internal Medicine, 29*(7), 987–995. https://doi.org/10.1007/s11606-014-2795-z.

Brody. (2017). The cost of not taking your medicine. *NY Times*. https://nyti.ms/2psUF6a. Accessed 17 Apr 2017.

Campbell, J., & Cardona, L. (2007). The consultation and liaison processes to pediatrics. In A. Martin & F. Volkmar (Eds.), *Lewis's child and adolescent psychiatry: A comprehensive textbook* (4th ed., pp. 912–920). Philadelphia: Lippinkott Williams & Wilkins.

Chapman, E. N., Kaatz, A., & Carnes, M. (2013). Physicians and implicit bias: How doctors may unwittingly perpetuate health care disparities. *Journal of General Internal Medicine, 28*, 1504. https://doi.org/10.1007/s11606-013-2441-1.

Claxton, A. J., Cramer, J., & Pierce, C. (2001). A systematic review of the association between dose regimens and medication compliance. *Clinical Therapeutics, 23*, 1296–1310.

Cutler, D. M., & Everett, W. (2010). Thinking outside the pillbox – medication adherence as a priority for healthcare reform. *NEJM, 362*(17), 1553–1555.

DiMatteo, M. R. (2004). Social support and patient adherence to medical treatment: A meta-analysis. *Health Psychology, 23*(2), 207–218. https://doi.org/10.1037/0278-6133.23.2.207.

DiMatteo, M. R., Lepper, H. S., & Croghan, T. W. (2000). Depression is a risk factor for noncompliance with medical treatment meta-analysis of the effects of anxiety and depression on patient adherence. *Archives of Internal Medicine, 160*(14), 2101–2107. https://doi.org/10.1001/archinte.160.14.2101.

Ellis, D. A., et al. (2005). Use of multisystemic therapy to improve regimen adherence among adolescents with type 1 diabetes in chronic poor metabolic control a randomized controlled trial. *Diabetes Care, 28*(7), 1604–1610. https://doi.org/10.2337/diacare.28.7.1604.

FitzGerald, C., & Hurst, S. (2017). Implicit bias in healthcare professionals: A systematic review. *BMC Medical Ethics, 18*, 19. https://doi.org/10.1186/s12910-017-0179-8.

Fitzmaurice, S. (2017, February 2). *Study: Children, parents over-report leukemia treatment adherence American Society of Hematology*. Accessed on 1 Dec 2017 from http://www.hematology.org/Newsroom/Press-Releases/2017/7045.aspx

Hood, K. K., et al. (2010). Interventions with adherence-promoting components in pediatric type 1 diabetes meta-analysis of their impact on glycemic control. *Diabetes Care, 33*(7), 1658–1664. https://doi.org/10.2337/dc09-2268.

Iuga, A., & McGuire, M. (2014). Adherence and health care costs. *Risk Manag Healthc Policy, 7*, 35–44. https://doi.org/10.2147/RMHP.S19801.

Kahana, S., Drotar, D., & Frazier, T. (2008). Meta-analysis of psychological interventions to promote adherence to treatment in pediatric chronic health conditions. *Pediatr Psychol, 33*(6), 590–611. https://doi.org/10.1093/jpepsy/jsm128.

LaGreca, A. M., & Bearman, K. J. (2003). Adherence to pediatric treatment regimens. In M. C. Roberts (Ed.), *Handbook of pediatric psychology* (3rd ed., pp. 119–140). New York: Guilford Press.

LaGreca, A. M., & Mackey, E. R. (2009). Type I diabetes mellitus. In Donahue & Woodward (Eds.), *Behavioral approaches to chronic illness in adolescents: An integrative approach* (pp. 85–100). New York: Springer. https://doi.org/10.1007/978-0-387-87687-0.

Lemanek, K. L., Kamps, J., & Chung, N. B. (2001). Empirically supported treatments in pediatric psychology: Regimen adherence. *Journal of Pediatric Psychology, 26*(5), 253–275. https://doi.org/10.1093/jpepsy/26.5.253.

Logan, D., et al. (2003). The illness management survey: Identifying adolescents' perceptions of barriers to adherence. *Journal of Pediatric Psychology, 28*(6), 383–392. https://doi.org/10.1093/jpepsy/jsg028.

Lustman, P. J., & Clouse, R. E. (2005). Depression in diabetic patients: The relationship between mood and glycemic control. *Journal of Diabetes and its Complications, 19*(2), 113–122.

McGrady, M. E., & Hommel, K. A. (2013). Medication adherence and health care utilization in pediatric chronic illness: A systematic review. *Pediatrics, 132*(4), 730–740. https://doi.org/10.1542/peds.2013-1451.

Osterberg, L., & Blaschke, T. (2005). Adherence to medication. *The New England Journal of Medicine, 353*, 487–497. https://doi.org/10.1056/NEJMra050100.

Petrie, K. J., Perry, K., Broadbent, E., & Weinman, J. (2012). A text message programme designed to modify patients' illness and treatment beliefs improves self-reported adherence to asthma preventer medication. *British Journal of Health Psychology, 17*, 74–84. https://doi.org/10.1111/j.2044-8287.2011.02033.x.

Rianthavorn, P., Ettenger, R. B., Malekzadeh, M., Marik, J. L., & Struber, M. (2004). Noncompliance with immonsuppressive medications in pediatric and adolescent patients receiving solid-organ transplants. *Transplantation, 77*, 778–782.

Rohan, J. M. (2015). Predicting health resilience in pediatric type 1 diabetes: A test of the resilience model framework. *Journal of Pediatric Psychology, 40*(9), 956–967. https://doi.org/10.1093/jpepsy/jsv061.

Sabaté, E. (Ed.). (2003). *Adherence to long-term therapies: Evidence for action*. Geneva: World Health Organization.

Sommerfield, A. J., Deary, I. J., & Frier, B. M. (2004). Acute hyperglycemia alters mood state and impairs cognitive performance in people with type 2 diabetes. *Diabetes Care, 27*(10), 2335–2340. https://doi.org/10.2337/diacare.27.10.2335.

Taddeo, D., Egedy, M., & Frappier, Y. J. (2008). Adherence to treatment in adolescents. *Paediatrics & Child Health, 13*(1), 19–24.

Warner, & Hauer. (2009). Unique considerations when using treating adolescents with chronic illness. In Donahue & Woodward (Eds.), *Behavioral approaches to chronic illness in adolescents: An integrative approach* (pp. 15–81). New York: Springer. https://doi.org/10.1007/978-0-387-87687-0.

Whittemore, R., Jaser, S., & Jia, G. (2010). A conceptual model of childhood adaptation to type 1 diabetes. *Nursing Outlook, 58*(5), 242–251.

Wilson, et al. (2009). Shared treatment decision making improves adherence and outcomes in poorly controlled asthma. *American Journal of Respiratory and Critical Care Medicine, 181*, 566. https://doi.org/10.1164/rccm.200906-0907OC.

Wu, Y. P., & Hommel, K. A. (2014). Using technology to assess and promote adherence to medical regimens in pediatric chronic illness. *The Journal of Pediatrics, 164*(4), 922–927.

Wu, Y. P., & Roberts, M. C. (2008). A meta-analysis of interventions to increase adherence to medication regimens for pediatric otitis media and streptococcal pharyngitis. *Journal of Pediatric Psychology, 33*(7), 789–796. https://doi.org/10.1093/jpepsy/jsn009.

Wysocki, et al. (2008). Randomized, controlled trial of behavioral family systems therapy for diabetes: Maintenance and generalization of effects on parent-adolescent communication. *Behavior Therapy, 39*(1), 33–46.

Chapter 13
Identifying and Managing Brain and Behavior Conditions

Serena A. Fernandes, Kevin K. Tsang, and Patricia Ibeziako

Introduction

The central nervous system (CNS) controls cognition, affect, and behavior, and CNS disorders often present with psychiatric symptoms and have great psychosocial impact. Neuropsychiatry involves the comprehensive evaluation and management of children with complex neurobehavioral problems associated with a range of CNS disorders, including neurodegenerative diseases, developmental disorders, seizure disorders, stroke, brain tumors, and inflammatory and infectious CNS diseases, among others. This chapter will review several childhood CNS disorders and highlight the neuropsychiatric considerations in their presentation, assessment, and treatment.

Seizures

Vignette A

A 12-year-old girl presents to her pediatrician after her parents notice that, for the past 6 weeks, she has had unusual involuntary hand and body movements. At first, her right hand would occasionally clench a few times and then relax. Over the next few weeks, the muscles in her right arm would also jerk, and she would experience anxiety and fear before these movements. Her parents report that, after her arm movements, she would appear to "zone out" and not be herself for some time afterward.

S. A. Fernandes (✉) · K. K. Tsang · P. Ibeziako
Department of Psychiatry, Boston Children's Hospital/Harvard Medical School, Boston, MA, USA
e-mail: serena.fernandes@childrens.harvard.edu

A. P. S. Guerrero et al. (eds.), *Pediatric Consultation-Liaison Psychiatry*,
https://doi.org/10.1007/978-3-319-89488-1_13

Table 13.1 Types of seizures

Generalized seizures: occurring throughout the cortex	Partial seizures: localized in one area of the brain
Tonic-clonic (grand mal): Sudden loss of consciousness, followed by a tonic phase with contraction of muscles and then a clonic phase with symmetric rhythmic contraction of the extremities	*Simple*: Consciousness is unaffected
Absence (petit mal): Brief alterations in consciousness with motionless staring	*Complex*: Consciousness is altered
Myoclonic: Brief and sudden muscle contractions	
Atonic (akinetic, "drop"): Sudden loss of muscle tone	

While in the office, her right hand and arm begin moving, and a few seconds later, her head and neck turn to the right. She then extends both arms, lets out a cry, and slumps down onto the floor. She then has symmetrical rhythmical movement of all her extremities for 30 s.

Epilepsy or seizure disorders are the most common childhood neurological disorder, affecting about 1% of children between birth and 17 years of age (Williams et al. 2016). Seizures are abnormal paroxysmal electrical discharges in the brain that result in changes in motor function, sensation, or consciousness and are further subclassified into various seizure types (Table 13.1)(Huffman et al. 2010).

The young girl in vignette A initially had simple partial seizures (hand movements without change in consciousness), which then progressed to complex partial seizures (arm movements with altered consciousness), which then progressed to a generalized seizure (tonic-clonic movements with loss of consciousness).

It can be challenging to differentiate neuropsychiatric phenomena that occur during (ictal), before or after (peri-ictal), or between (interictal) seizures from primary psychiatric symptoms. Broadly, seizure-related psychiatric symptoms often have abrupt onset and offset, occur with other stereotyped manifestations of seizures (i.e., automatisms), and are frequently short-lived (i.e., few minutes), with possibly altered consciousness, poor recall of the event, and almost always an abnormal electroencephalogram (EEG). When psychotic symptoms are present, they usually involve olfactory, gustatory, or tactile hallucinations. Primary psychiatric symptoms, in contrast, usually have a more gradual onset, absence of stereotyped movements, absence of altered consciousness or recall, and a normal EEG. When psychotic symptoms are present, they usually involve paranoia or auditory hallucinations (Huffman et al. 2010). Complex partial seizures, especially those with a temporal lobe focus, are commonly associated with neuropsychiatric phenomena including sensory, affective, perceptual, behavioral, or cognitive symptoms, such as the young girl's premonitory anxiety and fear. Complex partial seizures risk being missed as they often lack tonic-clonic activity, and the electroencephalogram (EEG) may even appear normal (Huffman et al. 2010).

Cortical insults, whether acute, as in concussion, infection, or bleeding, or chronic, as in intracranial tumors, poststroke cortical damage, or neurodegenerative disease, can result in seizures. In the pediatric population, seizure disorders often co-occur with autism spectrum disorder, cerebral palsy, Down syndrome, intellectual disability (Jones et al. 2008), and syndromes involving cortical malformations, such as lissencephaly, Sturge-Weber syndrome, tuberous sclerosis, and focal cortical dysplasia (Wilfong 2016). Certain pediatric genetic and metabolic disorders are also associated with seizures and include the various epilepsy syndromes, such as Lennox-Gastaut syndrome, Landau-Kleffner syndrome, and juvenile myoclonic epilepsy (Wilfong 2016).

Psychiatric and behavioral comorbidities are estimated to affect 20–60% of children with chronic epilepsy and most commonly include attention-deficit/hyperactivity, depressive, and anxiety disorders and, less frequently, psychotic disorders (Jones et al. 2008). Behavioral issues include hyperactivity, inattention, and oppositional defiant and conduct problems and appear to be more prevalent in conditions with structural brain abnormalities (Jones et al. 2007). Psychiatric disorders are thought to develop from multiple factors, including the underlying neurobiological abnormalities preceding and consequent to the epilepsy, family and social stresses secondary to epilepsy, and medication-related effects (Jones et al. 2008).

Attention-deficit hyperactivity disorder (ADHD) is the most common comorbid psychiatric disorder, affecting an estimated 20–50% of children with epilepsy. Attention problems can be adversely influenced by epileptiform activity, irrespective of seizure type, cause, or severity; structural abnormalities; medication effects; and earlier age of seizure onset, which is associated with greater cognitive deficits (Williams et al. 2016; Jones et al. 2008). Medication management includes cautiously selecting appropriate antiepileptic drugs (AEDs), as some may worsen ADHD symptoms. For example, topiramate is associated with cognitive slowing and worsened concentration, while barbiturates are associated with inattention and hyperactivity (Jones et al. 2008). Because of the various risks involved with ADHD medications, ADHD treatment should maximize behavioral and parental interventions. ADHD treatment involving stimulant or alpha-adrenergic medication often raises concern for reducing seizure threshold, but the benefits of improved academic and behavioral performance may outweigh the minimal risk of increase in seizure frequency if families are adequately informed and patients are closely monitored (Williams et al. 2016). In children with comorbid epilepsy and ADHD, methylphenidate is largely effective, while amphetamines and atomoxetine are less effective. Alpha-adrenergic agents are less effective than stimulants but should be considered when stimulants are inefficacious or have intolerable side effects or when patients have comorbid emotional conditions. Other alternatives include tricyclic antidepressant and bupropion, but these medications present greater concerns about lowered seizure threshold and have not been studied with comorbid epilepsy in the pediatric population (Williams et al. 2016).

Vignette A Continued

The young girl is started on carbamazepine at 100 mg twice daily for treatment of the complex partial seizure disorder with secondary generalization. She responds well without further seizures. A few weeks later, she and her parents return to the pediatrician and report that she has been spending more time isolating herself in her room, is sad and tearful, has decreased energy and motivation, and recently revealed thoughts of wanting to die. Her pediatrician suspects that she is depressed, in part because of the recent diagnosis of a seizure disorder, and starts her on fluoxetine 10 mg daily. About 1 week after starting the fluoxetine, she presents to the hospital with nausea, vomiting, dizziness, and trouble with motor coordination. On testing, her serum carbamazepine level is found to be toxic.

Population-based studies suggest that depression and anxiety symptoms are more prevalent among children and adolescents with epilepsy than among the general population or among peers with other chronic medical conditions. Unfortunately, these symptoms are underdiagnosed and undertreated. Depressive symptom prevalence rates can range from 10% to 30%, and, while depressive symptoms often present as they do in the general population, they may also be temporally associated with seizures, which may often go unrecognized. Untreated depression in children and adolescents with epilepsy can have serious consequences, including psychosocial impairment and suicidality, which occurs at a higher rate than in the general population (Reilly et al. 2011). It is therefore important to carefully screen for and aggressively treat depression in youth with epilepsy. Temporal lobe foci, a negative attitude toward seizures, and a negative assessment of family relationships present a higher risk for depression, while seizure type does not. Study results are mixed as to whether frequency, severity, age of onset, degree of control, and family history of seizures are correlated (Reilly et al. 2011). AEDs, many with known behavioral side effects, can alter mood and anxiety when initiated as well as when discontinued, and multiple studies have found polytherapy to be associated with increased symptom severity (Reilly et al. 2011). Treatment of depression generally follows that of children who do not have epilepsy and emphasizes psychological therapies and pharmacological management if necessary. Psychotherapy can include group and individual cognitive behavioral therapy (CBT), interpersonal therapy, and family therapy (Reilly et al. 2011). Selective serotonin reuptake inhibitors (SSRIs) are first-line antidepressants as they have fewer adverse effects, are less likely to lower the seizure threshold, and have minimal overdose risk (Reilly et al. 2011). Tricyclic antidepressants and monoamine oxidase inhibitors are not recommended due to risk of lowering the seizure threshold, cardiac side effects, and risk in overdose. Bupropion immediate release (IR) is not recommended due to risk of lowering the seizure threshold and risk of seizure in overdose (Bujoreanu et al. 2011). It is important to monitor for interactions between AEDs and antidepressants. For example, SSRIs such as fluoxetine may inhibit certain CYP450 enzymes and raise AED levels, while some AEDs such as carbamazepine induce CYP450 enzymes and reduce the levels and efficacy of certain SSRIs (Jones et al. 2008). In our case, the young girl's depressive symptoms and suicidality may represent a reaction to her chronic illness, an endogenous depression, or a side effect of her anticonvulsant, carbamazepine. In addition, fluoxetine inhibits certain CYP450 enzymes and thereby decreases metabolism of carbamazepine. The increased serum concentrations, in turn, produce toxic side effects. In our case, there may be a need to change the anticonvulsant regimen.

Anxiety symptoms are also common in children and adolescents with epilepsy. As with depression, it is helpful to identify symptoms temporally related to seizures. Some anxiety symptoms may arise from fear of having a seizure while away from parents and may resemble separation anxiety. It is also important to differentiate panic attacks from complex partial seizures. Management includes psychotherapy and medications such as SSRIs. AEDs should be carefully evaluated, as some have been associated with anxiety as a side effect, while others may induce anxiety upon discontinuation (Reilly et al. 2011).

Bipolar spectrum disorder is often a diagnostic challenge. This diagnosis excludes causation by another medical illness such as epilepsy and is difficult to differentiate from mood changes that may be seizure related. Medication management using AED monotherapy for epilepsy and bipolar disorder is appropriate (Bujoreanu et al. 2011).

Seizure-related psychotic symptoms are categorized based on their relationship to the seizure itself: ictal, postictal, or interictal psychosis. Postictal psychosis is the most common, may occur after a prolonged seizure or cluster of seizures, can last several days, and usually resolves spontaneously. Children experiencing seizure-related psychosis – unlike psychosis from primary psychotic disorders – generally cannot recall the content of the hallucinations (Jones et al. 2008; Bujoreanu et al. 2011). Medication management should include assessing AEDs for potential risk of precipitating psychotic symptoms and assessing antipsychotic medications for risk of interactions with AEDs and for risk of lowering seizure threshold. Clozapine and chlorpromazine are generally avoided due to greater risk – compared to other antipsychotics – of lowering seizure threshold. Clinicians should also carefully consider the longer-term metabolic risk of second-generation antipsychotics (Jones et al. 2008, Bujoreanu et al. 2011).

Stroke

Vignette B

A 9-year-old African-American boy presents to the emergency room 30 min after having a 2-min seizure that was witnessed by his parents, who found that he was subsequently unable to speak or move his right arm or leg. On exam, he is drooling from the right side of his mouth, and his right arm and leg are flaccid and immobile. He has hyperactive deep tendon reflexes and a positive Babinski sign on the right. His medical history is notable for sickle cell anemia. Two days ago, he was seen in the emergency room because of a headache accompanied by right-sided facial weakness that was diagnosed as a complicated migraine after negative imaging and resolution of symptoms within an hour.

Pediatric stroke or cerebral vascular accidents (CVAs) are neurological injuries secondary to cerebral blood vessel occlusion or rupture that result in compromised function of brain areas and that are classified into ischemic and hemorrhagic subtypes. Ischemic strokes are secondary to arterial occlusion or, less commonly, occlusion of cerebral veins or sinuses, while hemorrhagic strokes are secondary to bleeding from cerebral artery rupture or to bleeding in an ischemic area. They are generally rare events. Ischemic and hemorrhagic CVAs have an incidence of 1.2–13 cases per 100,000 children below age 18 years (Tsze and Valente 2011). In western counties, arterial ischemic stroke (AIS) accounts for about half of all strokes in children (Tsze and Valente 2011) and is notable for a higher incidence – 1 per 4000 live births – during the perinatal and neonatal period (Jeong et al. 2015). Stroke is more common in boys than girls and in black children than children of other ethnicities, even after accounting for sickle cell disease as a risk factor (Tsze and Valente 2011).

Ischemic stroke usually presents as a focal neurological deficit, and the acute onset of any focal neurological deficit in children should be managed as a stroke until proven otherwise. Common focal manifestations include hemiplegia, occurring in up to 94% of cases, as well as diplopia, dysarthria, vertigo, and ataxia. Hemorrhagic strokes commonly present as headaches and altered level of consciousness and are more commonly associated with vomiting than ischemic strokes (Jeong et al. 2015). At the onset of the stroke, seizures of various types occur in up to 50% of children experiencing either type of stroke (Tsze and Valente 2011). Stroke presentation often varies based on age. Younger children demonstrate more non-specific symptoms, such as seizures, irritability, lethargy, sleep changes, poor feeding, vomiting, or sepsis-like features, and are less likely to have focal deficits, while older children, like adults, demonstrate more specific neurological deficits, such as hemiparesis and language and speech difficulties. Specific types of stroke can also present differently in each age group. Venous sinus thrombosis and subarachnoid hemorrhage in infants can present with bulging fontanelles while in older children can present with signs of increased intracranial pressure (ICP) and meningismus (Tsze and Valente 2011). In vignette B, the boy has several presenting symptoms that raise concern for a left-sided stroke: acute-onset neurological deficits (aphasia, right hemiparesis, and right lower facial weakness) and a seizure at the time of onset of neurological deficits. In addition, he has individual risk factors of male gender, African-American ethnicity, and sickle cell disease.

Retrospective studies suggest that more than a third of children with arterial strokes had preceding transient ischemic attacks (TIAs), which are brief episodes of neurovascular compromise with symptom resolution within 24 hours and which are often undiagnosed (Tsze and Valente 2011). Misdiagnosis of strokes is also frequent, given that many other diseases can mimic a stroke: complex migraines, which can cause focal, quickly resolving neurological symptoms; metabolic abnormalities, such as hypoglycemia; intracranial neoplasms; infections such as meningitis and herpes simplex encephalitis; and even somatic symptom disorders.

Partial seizures can result in transient postictal hemiparesis (Todd's paralysis), but if the duration of the deficit is greater than the duration of the seizure, stroke should be considered. Rarer mimics include alternating hemiplegia and metabolic disorders such as MELAS (mitochondrial myopathy, encephalopathy, lactic acidosis, and stroke) (Tsze and Valente 2011). In retrospect, the vignette B patient's previously diagnosed complex migraine (focal right-sided facial weakness, without neuroimaging abnormalities and with quick resolution) was likely a TIA. His second presentation clearly warranted another stroke investigation because of additional focal deficits and duration (30 min) greater than seizure length (2 min).

The International Pediatric Stroke Study (IPSS) and other stroke studies identify the following major etiologies: cardiac, hematologic, infectious, vascular, syndromic and metabolic, vasculitic, oncologic, traumatic, and drug-related (Jeong et al. 2015). A patient's risk factors can vary by geography, ethnicity, age at presentation, and availability of medical resources to survive other illnesses that can increase stroke risk. For example, hemoglobinopathies, including sickle cell disease, are a common cause of stroke in children of Mediterranean and African heritage; moyamoya disease (involving blocked arteries in the base of the brain and tiny artery tangles formed to compensate for the blockage) is a relatively more common cause of stroke in children of Japanese heritage; and coagulation disorders are a relatively more common cause of stroke in children of European heritage (Jeong et al. 2015; Lynch and Han 2005).

Management of pediatric stroke is based on small nonrandomized trials, case series, consensus or individual expert opinions, or adult stroke studies. Generally, children with stroke require immediate attention, stabilization through supportive care, and treatment of acute complications such as infection, seizures, increased ICP, and increased blood pressure. If possible, they should be transferred to an institution with pediatric neurovascular expertise (Lynch and Han 2005). Further treatment depends on the stroke type and etiology and can involve acute surgical and medical management such as surgical evacuation, shunt placement, embolization, thrombolytic agent administration, and short- and long-term anticoagulation.

Pediatric ischemic stroke leads to significant morbidity and mortality: 10–25% of children die from the stroke; up to 25% experience recurrence; and up to 66% experience persistent neurological deficits or sequelae, including motor problems, epilepsy, cognitive and learning disorders, or developmental problems (Tsze and Valente 2011). Poorer outcomes are associated with decreased consciousness and seizures during presentation, presence of an underlying causative disease, middle cerebral artery origin, and infarction volumes greater than 10% of intracranial volumes (Lynch and Han 2005).

Pediatric hemorrhagic stroke also leads to significant morbidity and mortality: 25% of children die from the stroke; about 30% experience seizures or cognitive or motor problems; and about 40% of children are neurologically normal (Lynch and Han 2005). Predictors of poorer outcomes and death include age less than 3 years, decreased consciousness on presentation, infratentorial location, and underlying blood disorder or vascular malformation. The highest risk of recurrent hemorrhagic stroke is within the first year and usually in children who do not receive intervention for underlying vascular anomalies; hence, aggressive treatment involving embolization or surgical excision is usually pursued (Lynch and Han 2005).

Childhood stroke results in significant long-term cognitive, language, and psychiatric impairment, likely due to underlying neural network damage that impairs already developed skills and thwarts the development of emerging skills (Greenham et al. 2017). It is difficult, because of stroke heterogeneity, to identify risk factors associated with poor outcomes. Little association has been found between outcomes and age at stroke or lesion location. On the other hand, poststroke epilepsy and greater neurological deficits appear associated with poorer cognitive and psychosocial outcomes (Greenham et al. 2017; O'Keeffe et al. 2014). Arterial ischemic stroke has been associated with deficits in intelligence, memory, language, processing speed, and executive function, which involves attention, cognitive flexibility, and planning (Lynch and Han 2005; O'Keeffe et al. 2014). Children with ischemic stroke are reported to have poststroke psychiatric and behavioral issues, including ADHD, anxiety disorders, mood disorders, personality changes (Lynch and Han 2005), and externalizing behaviors such as aggression, hyperactivity, and emotional lability (Greenham et al. 2017). Hemorrhagic stroke has been associated with deficits in intelligence, memory, speech and language, learning, and behavior (Lynch and Han 2005). One element of interest is the debate around the role of neuronal plasticity in children with stroke. Some studies associate younger age with poorer functional outcome and more severe neurological disability, while others suggest some support for a theory of early brain plasticity, with better outcomes in children between age 1 and 6 years (O'Keeffe et al. 2014).

In both vignettes presented thus far, a combined neurology-psychiatry service could be very effective in following up the patients, in addressing long-term rehabilitative needs, and in supportively screening for and intervening upon any behavioral symptoms that may emerge – either from the previous neurological insult or from the neurological condition's psychosocial impact on the patient and the family. In the next several sections, we present other neurological conditions that are potentially associated with behavioral sequela and that may be optimally managed through a collaboration between neurology and consultation-liaison psychiatry.

Brain Tumors

CNS tumors are the second most common pediatric cancer, making up about 20% of all pediatric cancers and having a 5-year survival rate approaching 60–70% for primary malignant tumors (Shah et al. 2015). Treatment regimens are tailored to tumor histology and generally involve a combination of surgery, radiation, and chemotherapy. Children may experience both acute and chronic cognitive, psychiatric, and behavioral changes from the direct effects of tumors, from cell-destroying treatments given to a developing brain, from medication side effects such as corticosteroids, and from other posttreatment complications such as endocrine disorders, secondary malignancies, strokes, seizures, moyamoya disease, and motor dysfunction. Factors affecting cognitive and psychiatric outcomes include tumor type, location, size, and presence of metastases; patient age, sex, prior neurodevelopmental state, and psychological adjustment; family socioeconomic status, values, and adjustment; and various aspects of treatment including involvement of intracranial surgery, chemotherapy, and cranial radiation of a certain field and at a certain dose (Turner et al. 2009). Studies of long-term psychiatric sequelae in children are limited, but studies of adult survivors of pediatric brain cancer suggest that rates of depression, anxiety, suicidal ideation, psychotic disorders, and other behavioral problems are higher in the survivor population than the normal adult population. Female sex, astrocytomas, and glial tumors are associated with psychiatric side effects of treatment; craniospinal radiotherapy is associated with depression, anxiety, and schizophrenia; surgical treatment is associated with suicidality; and cerebellar vermis damage is associated with behavioral abnormalities (Shah et al. 2015).

Posterior fossa tumors, which include astrocytomas, medulloblastomas, and ependymomas, account for up to 60% of all pediatric brain tumors and often present with symptoms of hydrocephalus and raised ICP. These symptoms may include nausea, vomiting, lethargy, and irritability. Tumor-related damage to the cerebellum and other brain structures, hydrocephalus, damage related to treatment (resection, chemotherapy, or radiotherapy), endocrine complications, or tumor recurrence (Lassaletta et al. 2015) may impact cognitive and neuropsychiatric outcomes. Cerebellar damage is linked to decreased intellectual function; impairment in executive function, spatial cognition, attention, and working memory; personality changes; linguistic difficulties; and behavioral disturbances ranging from irritability to autism-like behaviors. Posterior fossa syndrome (cerebellar mutism syndrome) can occur 1–2 days after resection in up to one third of children following damage to the cerebellum and involves reduced or entirely absent speech, dysarthria, emotional lability, personality/behavioral change, disinhibition or inappropriate behavior, and apathy. While symptoms tend to improve with time, up to two thirds of these patients might have speech and language dysfunction 1 year later (Lassaletta et al. 2015).

Craniopharyngiomas are rare, benign, slow-growing tumors that are typically located in the sellar and/or suprasellar region and have high survival rates greater than 90%. The tumor frequently invades critical neurovascular structures such as the frontal lobes, cranial nerves, hypothalamus, and pituitary and often results in vision loss, panhypopituitarism, and diabetes insipidus. Given the location, complete resection is often infeasible; therefore, treatment usually involves adjunctive radiation therapy, which is associated with a high risk of tumor recurrence. Factors thought to negatively impact outcome include degree of hypothalamic involvement; hormonal manifestations, including diabetes insipidus and low growth hormone; hydrocephalus; younger age at onset; time since treatment; tumor size; retrochiasmatic location; recurrence; repeated surgeries; and frontal lobe dysfunction from surgical and radiation treatments. Intelligence, attention, and verbal memory are relatively preserved, but there are often deficits in executive function and spatial working memory and notable social-behavioral difficulties, including depression, anxiety, emotional dysregulation, impulsivity, and aggressiveness. Social functioning is often greatly impacted; difficulties may include social isolation and self-perceived unattractive appearance as a result of hormonal disorders (Zada et al. 2013).

Radiotherapy is often an integral part of treatment of brain tumors, especially when the tumor location or type limits efficacy of resection or chemotherapy, but it has both acute and chronic cognitive and behavioral effects. Cranial radiation in children is associated with declines in intelligence, memory, attention, and cognitive processing; behavioral and language disturbances; and hypothalamic-pituitary deficiency. Contributing factors are thought to be radiation-induced focal necrosis and white matter changes (demyelination and reactive gliosis), and, consequently, greater injury is seen with higher radiation doses, larger radiation field, increased time from radiotherapy, and younger age at treatment. Radiation necrosis of cerebral arteries can result in small cerebral strokes, which can result in further cognitive impact and other neuropsychiatric sequelae seen in strokes (Lassaletta et al. 2015; Nejad et al. 2010).

Chemotherapy can also contribute to neurocognitive decline, although it appears to be less severe than that secondary to radiation therapy and may involve specific areas in attention, visual processing, and visual-motor functioning. Some chemotherapy agents are known to be neurotoxic. Methotrexate can result in a short-term delirium as well as white matter injury and associated cognitive impairments (Roddy and Mueller 2016; Kaufman 2007).

Other medications that are used in pediatric cancer treatment and that are associated with mental status changes include AEDs; antiemetics, which may precipitate dystonia and Parkinsonian side effects through dopamine blockade; and antihistamines, opioids, benzodiazepines, and sedative-hypnotics, which are frequently used for pain, pruritus, anxiety, and insomnia but which can result in delirium. Corticosteroids are also well-known to induce insomnia, irritability, mood lability, and psychosis. Psychosis is usually managed symptomatically with antipsychotics (Nejad et al. 2010).

In a cohort of survivors of childhood brain tumor or acute lymphocytic leukemia (ALL), methylphenidate has been used to improve attention/concentration, social functioning, and academic performance (Lassaletta et al. 2015). A small pilot study utilizing donepezil in survivors of childhood brain tumors found improvement in memory and executive function (Roddy and Mueller 2016).

Hydrocephalus

Pediatric hydrocephalus is one of the most common birth defects and involves excessive cerebrospinal fluid that leads to ventricular enlargement, displacement of adjacent brain structures, and increased ICP (Lacy et al. 2012). The most common etiologies are myelomeningocele and associated Chiari malformation, aqueductal stenosis, intraventricular hemorrhage, and Dandy-Walker syndrome. Hydrocephalus may also be a complication of meningitis, traumatic brain injury, tumors, and infectious diseases (Martini 2010). Management is primarily through surgical shunting procedures to relieve elevated ICP (Lacy et al. 2012).

Hydrocephalus within the first year of life exerts pressure and alters blood flow in the cortex and other brain structures, impacts neuronal development across gray and white matter regions and developing circuits, and ultimately impacts the development of cognitive processes (Lacy et al. 2008). Children with hydrocephalus show deficits in verbal and nonverbal intellectual functioning (Lacy et al. 2008) and in executive functioning, including planning, working memory, and attention (Lacy et al. 2012). They also have a higher prevalence of behavioral and emotional challenges, including difficulties with self-regulation and emotional control (Lacy et al. 2012), anxiety, and somatic symptoms such as headache and stomachache (Lindquist et al. 2006).

Hydrocephalus with concurrent learning disabilities appears to strongly increase the risk of behavioral difficulties, disruptive behavior, and anxiety. Comorbid cerebral palsy and epilepsy further increase the risk of behavioral issues. Notably, the prevalence of autism among children with hydrocephalus is much higher than in the normal population. Furthermore, the prevalence of autism is up to five times higher in children with comorbid epilepsy or cerebral palsy compared to children with only hydrocephalus. (Lindquist et al. 2006). Shunt failure may present with signs of ICP. The signs may include headache, vomiting, lethargy, and papilledema or vague signs such as behavior change and decreased school performance (Martini 2010).

Spina Bifida

Spina bifida is a congenital neural tube defect and includes three main types:

1. Spina bifida occulta, in which some vertebrae are not completely closed, but the spinal cord and meninges are maintained without any neurological compromise.
2. Meningocele, in which the meninges herniate between incomplete vertebrae, but the spinal cord and, hence, neurological function is generally not affected.
3. Spina bifida myelomeningocele (SBM), the most severe form, in which the meninges, spinal cord, and nerve roots protrude through the spine and in which there is altered spinal function and brain development.

Common cerebral changes in SBM include cortical malformations of the posterior cortex and white matter, midbrain, cerebellum, and corpus callosum and hydrocephalus (Vinck et al. 2009). Spinal lesions, depending on location, may result in differing levels of motor functioning, ranging from ambulating with assistance to needing a wheelchair, and may also affect urological functioning (Martini 2010).

Cognitive abilities in children with SBM can range from normal to more severe impairment. In children with SBM and hydrocephalus, intellectual functioning is generally in the average to low average range, and there are often deficits in visual perception, motor skills, and memory. Also, despite often good verbal skills, there may be more subtle difficulties with verbal memory, speech fluency and articulation, executive functioning, and attention (Vinck et al. 2009).

Systemic Lupus Erythematosus

Vignette C

A 12-year-old girl of Asian Indian heritage is brought by her parents to her pediatrician because of mood and behavioral changes. For the past 3 months, parents have noted increased anxiety and depression, which they attributed to their daughter struggling to keep up with classwork. In the past month, her mood and behavior have worsened, with irritability, unprovoked anger outbursts, and physical aggressiveness. Yesterday, she reported being afraid of a threatening black figure in her room despite knowing that there was nothing present. Her pediatrician elicits that she has also experienced headache, increased fatigue, muscle aches/pains, joint stiffness, and decreased appetite. On exam, the pediatrician notes a light purplish rash across the bridge of her nose, swollen joints, and newly diagnosed hypertension.

The patient is admitted to the local hospital. Brain MRI shows multiple lesions in both cerebral hemispheres, and immunological testing shows positive antinuclear antibody and anti-double-stranded DNA (anti-ds DNA) antibodies.

Systemic lupus erythematosus (SLE) is a chronic autoimmune disease that affects multiple organ systems and that has varied symptom presentations and degrees of severity, ranging from rash and joint pain to life-threatening organ failure. Prevalence is about 3–8 per 100,000 children (Benseler and Silverman 2007). There is a higher prevalence in females and in Hispanic, African, North American First Nation, and Southeast and South Asian populations (Soybilgic 2015). The average age of onset is 13 years. The etiology is unknown but thought to be multifactorial with genetic, hormonal, and environmental components (Soybilgic 2015). Childhood-onset SLE, in comparison to adult-onset SLE, demonstrates greater disease activity at presentation and over time (Kohut et al. 2013).

Neuropsychiatric SLE (NPSLE) manifestations are classified by the American College of Rheumatology into 19 separate clinical syndromes (Table 13.2), covering CNS and peripheral nervous system manifestations as well as neurological and psychiatric symptoms. In the pediatric SLE population, prevalence of NPSLE symptoms is estimated at 22–95% (Ferraria et al. 2013), with about 70% of children having one or more symptoms within 1 year of SLE onset (Benseler and Silverman 2007). The etiology likely involves autoantibody-mediated CNS damage involving inflammation and neuronal cell death (Levy et al. 2009). It appears to be more aggressive and early-onset in children compared to in adults and results in higher rates of organ damage (Ferraria et al. 2013).

NPSLE should be considered in the differential diagnosis for new-onset severe neurologic or psychiatric disease in a child or adolescent (Soybilgic 2015).

Table 13.2 Neuropsychiatric lupus syndromes

Central nervous system
Headaches
Seizure disorders
Cerebrovascular disease
Demylinating syndrome
Myelopathy
Movement disorder
Aseptic meningitis
Cognitive dysfunction
Acute confusional state
Mood disorder
Anxiety disorder
Psychosis
Peripheral nervous system
Mononeuropathy, single/multiplex
Polyneuropathy
Cranial neuropathy
Acute inflammatory demyelinating polyneuropathy
Plexopathy
Mysasthenia gravis

Adapted from The American College of Rheumatology

Depression and anxiety (which were the presenting symptoms in vignette C) may result from direct CNS effects of the disease, from the impact of another NPSLE symptom (i.e., neurocognitive impairment and poor academic performance), from effects on other systems (i.e., pulmonary hypertension and fatigue), from complications of treatment (i.e., corticosteroids and mood effects), or from stress from having a chronic illness with various clinical sequelae (i.e., facial skin rashes, weight gain from steroid treatment, etc.) (Kohut et al. 2013).

NPSLE psychiatric manifestations include mood disorders, anxiety disorders, acute confusional states, psychosis, and potentially neurocognitive dysfunction (Benseler and Silverman 2007). In Sibbitt el al.'s study (2002), the most common pediatric neuropsychiatric manifestations were mood disorders (57%), cognitive dysfunction (55%), acute confusional states (35%), and psychosis (12%). Neurocognitive impairment can occur without other SLE disease symptoms or other NPSLE manifestations; is seen in nearly 50–65% of the pediatric SLE population; and involves difficulties in complex problem-solving, working and verbal memory, processing speed, attention, visuospatial learning, and visuomotor integration (Levy et al. 2009).

Depression impacts approximately 15–55% of the pediatric SLE population (Knight et al. 2014). Unlike adult SLE, pediatric SLE does not appear to be a significant risk factor for primary depression. Because physical symptoms of depression, such as fatigue, sleep disturbances, and poor appetite, often overlap with SLE symptoms, it is helpful for the clinician evaluating a child with SLE for possible depression to screen carefully for affective mood symptoms, such as negative mood and poor self-esteem. Notably, among pediatric patients with SLE, up to 34% report suicidal ideation (Knight et al. 2014), and 15–20% experience anxiety. Among patients with pediatric NPSLE, 12–40% have psychotic symptoms, which classically involve visual hallucinations and sometimes auditory or tactile hallucinations. Unlike in primary psychotic disorders, insight is usually preserved (Benseler and Silverman 2007). Mania and bipolar disorder are relatively uncommon in pediatric SLE (Benseler and Silverman 2007).

Treatment of pediatric SLE varies depending on the nature of the underlying process (i.e., inflammatory or thrombotic) and is focused on minimizing organ damage, reducing the duration and severity of flares, and symptomatically managing sequelae. NPSLE management lacks specific protocols, but for significant CNS disease, immunosuppressive therapy usually involves corticosteroids alone or in combination with other agents such as azathioprine, mycophenolate mofetil, or cyclophosphamide. In refractory or life-threatening cases, plasma exchange, intravenous immunoglobulin, and rituximab have been used (Soybilgic 2015). Treatment for affective and psychotic manifestations includes antidepressants and antipsychotics (Soybilgic 2015). For children, psychological support and educational interventions to maximize function are also helpful (Levy et al. 2009). Overall, greater than 90% of patients survive, and 80–95% enter remission (Soybilgic 2015). However, pediatric NPSLE patients who manifested seizures or cerebrovascular disease or who had severe disease activity are at risk for long-term sequelae, including persistent seizures or persistent cognitive impairment (Benseler and Silverman 2007; Soybilgic 2015).

Encephalitis and Meningitis

Meningitis, an inflammation of the meninges, and encephalitis, an inflammation of the brain parenchyma, can result in both acute and chronic neuropsychiatric symptoms. The most common causes of meningitis and encephalitis are bacterial, viral, fungal, or parasitic infections and noninfectious etiologies such as autoimmune diseases, malignancies, and medication side effects (Parmar and Ibrahim 2012). Acute presentations can include delirium, psychosis, mania, depression, anxiety, agitation, catatonia, or other behavioral changes (Nejad et al. 2010). Long-term cognitive and behavioral changes can vary depending on the cause, severity, length of illness, and success of treatment.

Congenital infections can have long-term brain effects depending on fetal age at the time of infection. Insults in the first or second trimesters often result in CNS malformations such as microcephaly, while later infections often result in destructive lesions such as aqueductal stenosis, hydrocephalus, calcifications, demyelination, and atrophy (Parmar and Ibrahim 2012).

Bacterial meningitis is a serious and often fatal infection in many parts of the world despite antibiotic treatment and relative availability of preventative vaccines. The risk of mortality or developing neurocognitive and behavioral complications is related to age, causative pathogen, severity of illness at time of presentation, and time of initiation of antibiotic therapy. About half of long-term survivors experience some sequelae, which include cognitive delay with low IQ and intellectual disability, learning disabilities, speech and language deficits, hearing and vision loss, emotional and behavioral including ADHD-like symptoms, motor delay/impairment, and seizures (Chandran et al. 2011; Ramakrishnan et al. 2009). Tuberculosis meningitis often presents with delirium (Nejad et al. 2010), and its complications include hydrocephalus and seizures. Prognosis is related to early diagnosis and treatment, and long-term deficits include visual and hearing loss and cognitive impairment (Wood 2012). Treatment relies on antibiotics and potentially corticosteroids for patients with cerebral edema or high levels of bacteria in the CSF (Nejad et al. 2010).

Syphilis is a common infection worldwide, and its infection of the central nervous system, termed neurosyphilis, can occur early or late in the disease and includes syphilitic meningitis and parenchymatous neurosyphilis (tabes dorsalis (also known as demyelination of the dorsal columns of the spinal cord) and general paresis). Neurosyphilis is well-known to mimic many other neuropsychiatric disorders and can present with symptoms of dementia, delirium, psychosis, hallucinations (usually auditory), depression, mania, anxiety, paranoia delusions (usually persecutory), bizarre or violent behavior, or personality changes Cognitive changes include poor concentration and memory, executive dysfunction, irritability, and loss of higher cortical functions (Beauchemin and Laforce 2014). Congenital syphilis, acquired in utero or at the time of delivery, is a major cause of stillbirth and newborn mortality. It can result in acute syphilitic meningitis, which presents similarly to bacterial meningitis and which can involve increased intracranial pressure. Congenital syphilis can also result in chronic meningovascular syphilis, which presents with progressive hydrocephalus, neurodevelopmental regression, and seizures. If untreated, neurosyphilis can develop into syphilitic endarteritis, which can lead to cerebral infarction, significant developmental delay, and pituitary involvement (Triemstra et al. 2017).

Viral meningitis rarely involves the brain parenchyma, and when signs of brain dysfunction such as seizures are present, it is usually indicative of encephalitis. Treatment is largely supportive, and while most children make a complete recovery, early life viral meningitis may increase the risk of longer-term cognitive effects and seizure disorders, hydrocephalus, learning disabilities, lower intelligence, and behavior disorders (Norris et al. 1999).

The human immunodeficiency virus (HIV) can impact children and adolescents' neurological, cognitive, and psychiatric functioning in various ways, depending on means and timing of acquisition of the infection, primary CNS effects of the HIV infection, presence of opportunistic infections, and medication side effects (Nejad et al. 2010). HIV infects CNS microglia and macrophages and triggers immune-mediated and inflammatory changes that cause neuronal cell damage and death. In the pediatric population, the late effects of neuronal cell damage result in two types of HIV encephalopathy: a progressive encephalopathy with acquired microcephaly, loss of previously acquired skills, and corticospinal tract abnormalities and a static encephalopathy with cognitive and motor delays, but without a loss of acquired skills or neurological deficits (Benton 2011). Use of highly active antiretroviral therapy (HAART) has been found to reduce the incidence of progressive encephalopathy (Benton 2011). Cognitive changes in HIV-infected children include deficits in general intellectual functioning, executive functioning, processing speed, working memory, planning/reasoning, attention, visual-spatial ability, and visual memory (Phillips et al. 2016). Compared to non-infected peers, HIV-infected youth evidence higher rates of depression, anxiety, ADHD, behavioral issues, and substance abuse (Benton 2011). Through viral load suppression during infancy or early childhood, combination antiretroviral therapy has resulted in a dramatic decrease in incidence of severe neurocognitive impairment (Crowell et al. 2015).

HIV meningitis presents with fever, headache, acute confusional state, meningeal irritation, and cranial nerve palsies; often occurs at time of seroconversion; and improves with supportive care. CNS opportunistic infections can result in complications of meningitis, encephalitis, and abscesses (Nejad et al. 2010). With progression of HIV to acquired immunodeficiency syndrome (AIDS), children are at risk for progressive multifocal leukoencephalopathy from acquisition or reactivation of the JC polyomavirus. This condition, which is managed with HAART, involves CNS demyelination, which results in hemiparesis, ataxia, and dysarthria (Schwenk et al. 2014).

The autoimmune encephalitides are a new field of active investigation, as these autoimmune disorders often present with neurological and psychiatric manifestations. One of the best studied types is anti-N-methyl-D-aspartate (anti-NMDA) receptor encephalitis, an autoimmune disorder in which antibodies attack the NMDA glutamate receptor and cause a distinct course of illness marked by an initial period of about 1 week with viral illness-like prodrome with lethargy, headache, myalgia, and fever, followed by a 1–3-week period of behavioral changes including delusions, hallucinations, disorganized thoughts and behaviors, anxiety, agitation, paranoia, mood lability and bizarre behaviors, and personality change. Children and adolescents often present with mania-like symptoms, including irritability, behavioral outbursts, sleep dysfunction, hyperactivity, and hypersexuality. Children and adolescents may also experience cognitive changes, including short-term memory deficits, confusion, altered speech (i.e., echolalia, perseveration, mutism), and subsequently neurological involvement with abnormal movements (i.e., orofacial dyskinesias, dystonia, and chorea), autonomic instability, and seizures, which may also occur during earlier stages. This condition, although most commonly affecting young adult women, can affect males and females of all ages ranging from infancy to old age. Diagnosis requires a positive serum or cerebrospinal fluid (CSF) antibody titer, but the diagnosis is often made based on clinical symptoms, abnormal CSF studies (showing pleocytosis or oliogoclonal bands), and EEG (usually abnormal, showing slow, disorganized delta/theta activity, and sometimes seizures). Imaging can be variable and sometimes show mild enhancement. Treatment is becoming increasingly standardized with a focus on immune therapy, including "first-line" treatments of corticosteroids and intravenous immunoglobulin, "second-line" treatments of rituximab and cyclophosphamide, treatment of any underlying identified tumor, and significant supportive care. During the illness, psychiatric symptoms and agitation are often managed with AEDs, anticholinergics, benzodiazepines, and antipsychotics, including sedating antipsychotics given that patients appear to be sensitive to dopamine antagonism and at high risk for extrapyramidal symptoms with high-potency antipsychotics (Kayser and Dalmau 2011). Cognitive and psychiatric symptoms are slowest to improve, and current follow-up studies suggest that longer-lasting cognitive deficits in memory and executive dysfunction may occur in almost 90% of patients (Moura et al. 2016).

Conclusion

Children and adolescents with neurological disorders are an especially vulnerable population. For all the conditions described in this chapter, an astute and informed psychiatrist can play essential roles in the healthcare team, during the acute inpatient and outpatient follow-up phases. In either of these contexts, a team-integrated pediatric consultation-liaison psychiatrist can assist with recognizing and diagnosing psychiatric manifestations; managing the emotional and behavioral effects of the illness and its treatment; and managing the long-term cognitive, psychiatric, and behavioral impacts on the developing brain.

References

Beauchemin, P., & Laforce, R., Jr. (2014). Neurocognitive changes in tertiary neurosyphilis: A retrospective chart review. *The Canadian Journal of Neurological Sciences, 41*(4), 452–458.

Benseler, S. M., & Silverman, E. D. (2007). Systemic lupus erythematosus. *Rheumatic Diseases Clinics of North America, 33*(3), 471–498. vi.

Benton, T. D. (2011). Psychiatric considerations in children and adolescents with HIV/AIDS. *Pediatric Clinics of North America, 58*(4), 989–1002.

Bujoreanu, I. S., Ibeziako, P., & Demaso, D. R. (2011). Psychiatric concerns in pediatric epilepsy. *Pediatric Clinics of North America, 58*(4), 973–988.

Chandran, A., Herbert, H., Misurski, D., & Santosham, M. (2011). Long-term sequelae of childhood bacterial meningitis: an underappreciated problem. *The Pediatric Infectious Disease Journal, 30*(1), 3–6.

Crowell, C. S., Huo, Y., Tassiopoulos, K., Malee, K. M., Yogev, R., Hazra, R., Rutstein, R. M., Nichols, S. L., Smith, R. A., Williams, P. L., & Oleske, J. (2015). Muller WJ; PACTG 219C study team and the pediatric HIVAIDS cohort study (PHACS). Early viral suppression improves neurocognitive outcomes in HIV-infected children. *AIDS, 29*(3), 295–304.

Ferraria, N., Rocha, S., Fernandes, V. S., Correia, T., & Gonçalves, E. (2013). Juvenile systemic lupus erythematosus with primary neuropsychiatric presentation. *BMJ Case Reports, 2013*, bcr2012008270.

Greenham, M., Anderson, V., Hearps, S., Ditchfield, M., Coleman, L., Mackay, M. T., Monagle, P., & Gordon, A. L. (2017). Psychosocial function in the first year after childhood stroke. *Developmental Medicine & Child Neurology, 59*, 1027–1033.

Huffman, J. C., Brennan, M. M., Smith, F. A., & Stern, T. A. (2010). Patients with neurologic conditions I. Seizure disorders (including Nonepileptic Seizures), cerebrovascular disease, and traumatic brain injury. In T. A. Stern, G. L. Fricchione, N. H. Cassem, M. S. Jellinek, & J. F. Rosenbaum (Eds.), *Massachusetts general hospital handbook of general hospital psychiatry* (pp. 237–253). Philadelphia: Saunders Elsevier, Inc.

Jeong, G., Lim, B. C., & Chae, J. H. (2015). Pediatric Stroke. *Journal of Korean Neurosurgical Association, 57*(6), 396–400.

Jones, J. E., Watson, R., Sheth, R., Caplan, R., Koehn, M., Seidenberg, M., & Hermann, B. (2007). Psychiatric comorbidity in children with new onset epilepsy. *Developmental Medicine and Child Neurology, 49*(7), 493–497.

Jones, J. E., Austin, J. K., Caplan, R., Dunn, D., Plioplys, S., & Salpekar, J. A. (2008). Psychiatric disorders in children and adolescents who have epilepsy. *Pediatrics in Review, 29*(2), e9–e14

Kaufman, D. M. (2007). Brain tumors and metastatic cancer. In *Clinical neurology for psychiatrists* (6th ed., pp. 465–484). Philadelphia: Saunders Elsevier, Inc.

Kayser, M. S., & Dalmau, J. (2011). Anti-NMDA receptor encephalitis in psychiatry. *Current Psychiatry Reviews, 7*(3), 189–193.

Knight, A., Weiss, P., Morales, K., Gerdes, M., Gutstein, A., Vickery, M., & Keren, R. (2014). Depression and anxiety and their association with healthcare utilization in pediatric lupus and mixed connective tissue disease patients: a cross-sectional study. *Pediatric Rheumatology Online Journal, 12*, 42.

Kohut, S. A., Williams, T. S., Jayanthikumar, J., Landolt-Marticorena, C., Lefebvre, A., Silverman, E., & Levy, D. M. (2013). Depressive symptoms are prevalent in childhood-onset systemic lupus erythematosus (cSLE). *Lupus, 22*(7), 712–720. https://doi.org/10.1177/0961203313488840.

Lacy, M., Pyykkonen, B. A., Hunter, S. J., Do, T., Oliveira, M., Austria, E., Mottlow, D., Larson, E., & Frim, D. (2008). Intellectual functioning in children with early shunted posthemorrhagic hydrocephalus. *Pediatric Neurosurgery, 44*(5), 376–381.

Lacy, M., Baldassarre, M., Nader, T., & Frim, D. (2012). Parent ratings of executive functioning in children with shunted hydrocephalus. *Pediatric Neurosurgery, 48*(2), 73–79.

Lassaletta, A., Bouffet, E., Mabbott, D., & Kulkarni, A. V. (2015). Functional and neuropsychological late outcomes in posterior fossa tumors in children. *Child's Nervous System, 31*(10), 1877–1890.

Levy, D. M., Ardoin, S. P., & Schanberg, L. E. (2009). Neurocognitive impairment in children and adolescents with systemic lupus erythematosus. *Nature Clinical Practice. Rheumatology, 5*(2), 106–114.

Lindquist, B., Carlsson, G., Persson, E. K., & Uvebrant, P. (2006). Behavioural problems and autism in children with hydrocephalus : a population-based study. *European Child & Adolescent Psychiatry, 15*(4), 214–219.

Lynch, J. K., & Han, C. J. (2005). Pediatric stroke: what do we know and what do we need to know? *Seminars in Neurology, 25*(4), 410–423.

Martini, D. R. (2010). Neurological disease. In R. J. Shaw & D. R. DeMaso (Eds.), *Textbook of pediatric psychosomatic medicine* (pp. 33–45). Washington, DC: American Psychiatric Publishing, Inc.

Moura, M., Silva-Dos-Santos, A., Afonso, J., & Talina, M. (2016). First-episode psychosis in a 15 year-old female with clinical presentation of anti-NMDA receptor encephalitis: A case report and review of the literature. *BMC Research Notes, 9*, 374.

Nejad, S. H., Roffman, J. L., Kueppenbender, K., Smith, F. A., Huffman, J. C., & Stern, T. A. (2010). Patients with neurologic conditions II. Movement disorders, multiple sclerosis, and other neurologic conditions. In T. A. Stern, G. L. Fricchione, N. H. Cassem, M. S. Jellinek, & J. F. Rosenbaum (Eds.), *Massachusetts general hospital handbook of general hospital psychiatry* (pp. 255–272). Philadelphia: Saunders Elsevier, Inc.

Norris, C. M., Danis, P. G., & Gardner, T. D. (1999). Aseptic meningitis in the newborn and young infant. *American Family Physician, 59*(10), 2761–2770.

O'Keeffe, F., Liégeois, F., Eve, M., Ganesan, V., King, J., & Murphy, T. (2014). Neuropsychological and neurobehavioral outcome following childhood arterial ischemic stroke: attention deficits, emotional dysregulation, and executive dysfunction. *Child Neuropsychology, 20*(5), 557–582.

Parmar, H., & Ibrahim, M. (2012). Pediatric intracranial infections. *Neuroimaging Clinics of North America, 22*(4), 707–725.

Phillips, N., Amos, T., Kuo, C., Hoare, J., Ipser, J., Thomas, K. G., & Stein, D. J. (2016). HIV-associated cognitive impairment in perinatally infected children: A meta-analysis. *Pediatrics, 138*(5), e20160893.

Ramakrishnan, M., Ulland, A. J., Steinhardt, L. C., Moïsi, J. C., Were, F., & Levine, O. S. (2009). Sequelae due to bacterial meningitis among African children: a systematic literature review. *BMC Medicine, 7*, 47.

Reilly, C., Agnew, R., & Neville, B. G. (2011). Depression and anxiety in childhood epilepsy: A review. *Seizure, 20*(8), 589–597.

Roddy, E., & Mueller, S. (2016). Late effects of treatment of pediatric central nervous system tumors. *Journal of Child Neurology, 31*(2), 237–254.

Schwenk, H., Ramirez-Avila, L., Sheu, S. H., Wuthrich, C., Waugh, J., Was, A., Degirolami, U., Burchett, S., Koralnik, I. J., & Ahmed, A. (2014). Progressive multifocal leukoencephalopathy in pediatric patients: Case report and literature review. *The Pediatric Infectious Disease Journal, 33*(4), e99–e105.

Shah, S. S., Dellarole, A., Peterson, E. C., Bregy, A., Komotar, R., Harvey, P. D., & Elhammady, M. S. (2015). Long-term psychiatric outcomes in pediatric brain tumor survivors. *Child's Nervous System, 31*(5), 653–663.

Sibbitt, W. L., Jr., Brandt, J. R., Johnson, C. R., Maldonado, M. E., Patel, S. R., Ford, C. C., Bankhurst, A. D., & Brooks, W. M. (2002). The incidence and prevalence of neuropsychiatric syndromes in pediatric onset systemic lupus erythematosus. *The Journal of Rheumatology, 29*(7), 1536–1542.

Soybilgic, A. (2015). Neuropsychiatric Systemic Lupus Erythematosus in Children. *Pediatric Annals, 44*(6), e153–e158.

Triemstra, J., Reno, K., Chohlas-Wood, R., & Nash, C. (2017). A brief resolved unexplained event and congenital neurosyphilis. *Pediatric Annals, 46*(2), e61–e64.

Tsze, D. S., & Valente, J. H. (2011). Pediatric stroke: A review. *Emergency Medicine International, 2011*, 734506.

Turner, C. D., Rey-Casserly, C., Liptak, C. C., & Chordas, C. (2009). Late effects of therapy for pediatric brain tumor survivors. *Journal of Child Neurology, 24*(11), 1455–1463.

Vinck, A., Mullaart, R., Rotteveel, J., & Maassen, B. (2009). Neuropsychological assessment of attention in children with spina bifida. *Cerebrospinal Fluid Research, 6*, 6.

Wilfong, A. (2016). *Seizures and epilepsy in children: Classification, etiology and clinical features*. UpToDate. Wolters Kluwer. Updated: September, 2016.

Williams, A. E., Giust, J. M., Kronenberger, W. G., & Dunn, D. W. (2016). Epilepsy and attention-deficit hyperactivity disorder: links, risks, and challenges. *Neuropsychiatric Disease and Treatment, 12*, 287–296.

Wood, K. (2012). Tuberculosis meningitis. *Hospital Pediatrics, 2*(2), 111–114.

Zada, G., Kintz, N., Pulido, M., & Amezcua, L. (2013). Prevalence of neurobehavioral, social, and emotional dysfunction in patients treated for childhood craniopharyngioma: A systematic literature review. *PLoS One, 8*(11), e76562.

Chapter 14
Genetics in Pediatric Consultation-Liaison Psychiatry and Multidisciplinary Management of Complex Conditions

Branko Aleksic, Itzel Bustos Villalobos, Hideki Kasuya, and Anthony P. S. Guerrero

Complex Conditions and Situations in Medicine and the Role of the Pediatric Consultation-Liaison Psychiatrist

Pediatric consultation-liaison psychiatrists play important roles in helping health-care teams to optimally manage complex conditions. These roles can include: helping pediatric colleagues to consider genetic and other medical etiologies for behavioral symptoms, leading and/or optimizing multidisciplinary teams in managing complex conditions, and helping families to cope with illnesses with significant impacts on well-being. In this chapter, we explore some of these roles and provide an overview of the specialized topic of psychiatric genetics, which is the topic of interest to both contemporary psychiatry and pediatrics yet often not always specifically covered in standard references for consultation-liaison psychiatry.

B. Aleksic (✉)
Office of international affairs, Nagoya University, Graduate School of Medicine, Nagoya, Aichi, Japan
e-mail: Branko@med.nagoya-u.ac.jp

I. B. Villalobos · H. Kasuya
Office of international affairs, Nagoya University, Graduate School of Medicine, Nagoya, Aichi, Japan

Department of Psychiatry, University of Hawai'i John A. Burns School of Medicine, Honolulu, USA

A. P. S. Guerrero
Department of Psychiatry, University of Hawai'i John A. Burns School of Medicine, Honolulu, USA
e-mail: GuerreroA@dop.hawaii.edu

A. P. S. Guerrero et al. (eds.), *Pediatric Consultation-Liaison Psychiatry*,
https://doi.org/10.1007/978-3-319-89488-1_14

Vignette

The first-year pediatric resident at a medium-sized community-based children's hospital refers a 5-year-old girl to the pediatric consultation-liaison psychiatry team. She is currently admitted for an exacerbation of persistent asthma. The chief concern is that "every time she's here, she's a terror to manage. She hits the staff, tries to pull out her intravenous line and her nasal cannula, and needs to be wrestled to have procedures done. It wasn't so bad when she was little, but now that she's big, we're worried that she may hurt one of the staff. Would it be possible to transfer her to your psychiatric service?"

This is the first time that the pediatric consultation-liaison team is involved. You learn from the pediatric team that the patient has a history of language and motor delays, but has never been formally tested because "the family is so disorganized and can't seem to manage to get her enrolled in school." They note that the mother herself and several other relatives have had a history of learning difficulties.

In many hospitals worldwide, healthcare staff on general medical units may express discomfort with managing patients with acute behavioral symptoms; however, most psychiatric units are neither safe nor appropriate for managing the acute symptoms that necessitated the pediatric hospitalization. In such cases, the pediatric consultation-liaison psychiatrist plays an essential role in insuring that patients are managed safely and that staff feel supported.

In addition to trying to address the most pressing of the presenting concerns, notably the destructive behavior, the effective consultant, in such situations of medical and psychosocial complexity, should also take the time to insure an adequate differential diagnosis and biopsychosocial formulation and to consider how to effectively manage the high emotions triggered among the staff and the impact of these emotions on medical decision-making.

Your evaluation finds that there are likely multiple factors involved in the "why now" of the patient's acute agitation. There is physical discomfort from the difficulty breathing, difficulty communicating her needs and desires in an unfamiliar setting, and a tendency of both the parent and staff to manage disobedience using inconsistent methods and with an overreliance on yelling and shaming. Your plan includes interventions geared toward each of these factors.

In addressing the issue of why the patient is recurrently ill and needing hospitalizations, you identify additional factors: the patient and the mother both may have developmental delays and/or learning difficulties that impact upon adherence to recommended treatment; and the healthcare providers, for whatever reason, appear to view the child as simply being "bad" and the parent as simply being "overwhelmed."

You communicate with both the hospital-based team as well as the primary care team. You provide both support and education about the child and family's needs. You offer suggestions about how to communicate in simple, clear language and to have clear behavioral expectations – with associated rewards and consequences.

Following current guidelines for evaluation of children with intellectual disability, you suggest that the team order a chromosome microarray and Fragile X test.

The child's asthma and behavior improve. After the discharge, you learn from the primary care physician that Fragile X testing was positive on both the patient and the mother, and further testing is being done on other relatives. With improved understanding of the conditions faced by both patient and mother, the primary care team can provide more effective overall healthcare, and there are no further hospitalizations for asthma.

The vignette above describes a case of Fragile X syndrome (FXS), an X-linked disorder that is the leading cause of inherited intellectual disability. It is estimated that FXS affects approximately 1 in 2500–5000 boys and 1 in 4000–6000 girls. FXS is caused by mutations in the *FMR1* gene, which is located on the X chromosome, and specifically at Xq27.3, which coincides with the folate-sensitive fragile site. Cytogenetic methods used in the past to diagnose FXS have been replaced by molecular diagnosis of *FMR1* DNA using PCR (Richter et al. 2015).

A diagnosis of FXS is often made in children that show delayed or absent speech by approximately 3 years of age. Hypotonia, delayed motor milestones, hand flapping, poor eye contact, and irritability may occur in children before 2 years of age. Boys with FXS may typically have attention deficit hyperactivity disorder, with significant impulsivity and anxiety, as well as repetitive language, hand biting, hand stereotypies, rocking, and sometimes head banging. The diagnosis of autism spectrum disorder is often made before the diagnosis of FXS because the problems described are often combined with social and language deficits. Approximately 30% of boys with FXS meet the diagnostic criteria for autism and these children have the lowest developmental and adaptive behavior scores of those with FXS. Other clinical observations may reveal the FXS phenotype in the family. Sometimes a family history of intellectual disability, autism spectrum disorder, neurological problems, or early menopause will be strong indication for the clinician to diagnose FXS in the family.

In this case, the pediatric consultation-liaison psychiatrist's knowledge of genetics enabled the team to not only make an accurate medical diagnosis but to also receive accurate information that significantly improved the dynamics of the interaction between the child, parent, and healthcare team. At this point, we believe that a brief overview of basic genetics, followed by a more specific discussion of psychiatric genetics, is in order.

Basic Genetics

Genetics is the study of how heritable traits are transmitted from one generation to another. It has been known that traits are often very similar in families. It was only less than 200 years ago that the importance of genetic inheritance and its impact on human health were recognized.

Natural Selection

Darwin and Wallace observed the tendency in populations to produce more offspring than required to sustain the population's present number. Consequently, because of the abundance of offspring, the population could collapse from competition for resources. On the other hand, within populations, there are natural variations that are the source of natural selection. These variations impact an individual organism's competitiveness and ultimately its chances of reproducing offspring who would inherit advantageous variations. The following sections discuss the sources of these variations.

Inheritance of Traits

Sexual reproduction, involving the mixing of genes once every generation, evolved as a mechanism that increased a species' variation and presumably its chances for survival.

Among animals, when sex cells unite at conception, the resulting offspring will have at least two factors (alleles) for each trait. The laws of probability are important when the gametes are formed, and it is a matter of chance which factor for a given trait is going to be incorporated into a specific gamete. It is known that so-called Mendelian laws cannot explain all traits. In cases of codominance, both variants of the trait are expressed (Bamshad et al. 2011). Incomplete dominance results in a mixture of traits. In cases of multiple alleles, there are more than just two possible ways a given gene can be expressed. It is important to note that most expressed traits, such as height, intelligence, or skin color, are influenced by many genes all acting on the same apparent trait. In addition, each gene that acts on the trait may have multiple alleles. Environmental factors can influence and modify the expression of genetic information and create more variation, and sexual reproduction is the largest and most important factor related to genetic variation among individuals in population.

Mutation

It is important to recognize that each time cells divide to create new cells, this huge DNA molecule must replicate so that the new cells have the information required to function. Subsequently, each time the DNA is copied, there are small changes due to replication errors. Most of them are identified and repaired immediately. However, if such change or mutation is not corrected, it may result in a slightly different protein. These so-called mutated proteins may not function normally and may be cause of genetic disorders. Conversely, not very often, the altered protein may function better than the original or result in a trait that results in an advantage. Such beneficial mutations are one source of the so-called physiological genetic variation.

Gene Flow

Another source of genetic variation is gene flow, which is the introduction of new alleles to any population. Often, the reason for this is migration, when new individuals of the same species enter a population. Environmental conditions in the previous habitat may have selected different forms of traits (e.g., skin color). Alleles for these traits would be different from the alleles present in the new population. Subsequently, there will be interbreeding that will eventually introduce new variants of the genes responsible for several traits, and advantageous alleles will become more frequent in the population.

Genetic Drift

Genetic drift can be defined as change in allele frequency that is random and not related to selection pressures. Alleles are randomly allocated into sex cells. As it is a matter of chance, it may be possible that both parents transmit the same allele for a specific trait to all offspring. When the offspring reproduce, they can transmit only one allele of the trait that they inherited from their parents. Genetic drift can result in significant changes in a population in only a few generations if the population is not very large. Genetic drift may result in reduced genetic variability in a specific population. In a population with limited genetic diversity, there is a relative large probability that environmental factors may reduce or extinguish the population.

Psychiatric Genetics

It is known that many conditions and diseases have a genetic component. Some disorders, such as sickle cell disease and cystic fibrosis, are caused by mutation in a single gene. The causes of many other disorders, however, are much more complex. Common medical problems, such as psychiatric disorders, diabetes, and obesity, are associated with the effects of multiple genes in combination with lifestyle and environmental factors. Conditions caused by many contributing factors are called complex or multifactorial disorders (Uher 2014). Although complex disorders often cluster in families, they do not have a very straightforward pattern of inheritance. Consequently, it is complicated to calculate risk of inheriting these disorders. Complex disorders are also difficult to study and treat because the specific factors that cause most of these disorders have not yet been determined. However, researchers continue to look for major contributing genes for many common complex disorders.

As behavior is a complex phenomenon, the genetic background of psychiatric disorders is notoriously complicated. For example, no Mendelian forms of psychiatric disorders have been described, but rare and high-risk structural variants (such as copy number variants [CNVs]) may be related to schizophrenia onset in a relatively small number of cases (Gelernter 2015). These rare variants are not completely penetrant, and they are rarely specific (i.e., pleiotropic effect), and risk is increased for schizophrenia, autism spectrum disorder, developmental delay, intellectual disability, and other neurodevelopmental syndromes. Most of CNVs are relatively large and generally nonrandom distributed, typically clustering around so-called hot spots. Several rare CNVs affect single genes, enabling researchers to perform functional studies that may give us insight into the disease mechanism. The strongest signal or number of putative genes was found in the major histocompatibility complex region, and it is thought that neurodevelopmental abnormalities due intrauterine infection may be related to increased risk for psychiatric disorders. Another signal for schizophrenia was found in microRNA-137, an important regulator of neuronal development influencing neurogenesis and maturation and specifically expressed at synapses in the cortex and hippocampus. Future studies of networks regulated by microRNA-137 may provide some insights into schizophrenia pathophysiology (O'Donovan and Owen 2016). There has been some controversy related to the nature of the genetic contribution to individual susceptibility to common complex diseases such as cancer, systemic lupus erythematosus, or Crohn's disease. The so-called "common disease-common variant (CDCV)" hypothesis states that genetic variations with relatively high frequency (>5%) in the population, but relatively small effect size (probability that carrier will be affected), are the main contributors to genetic susceptibility to common diseases. The "common disease-rare variant (CDRV)" hypothesis, conversely, holds that multiple rare DNA sequence variations, each with relatively large effect size, are the main contributors to genetic susceptibility to common diseases. Both hypotheses seem to be valid based on available empirical evidence.

Common Disease-Common Variant Hypothesis

The CDCV hypothesis has its foundation in a relatively large number of studies, but one of the most prominent, by Reich and Lander, considered what they termed as "allelic spectrum of disease" and used empirical data to analyze the aforementioned spectrum (Reich and Lander 2001). This spectrum is the complete set of variations that contribute to a disease, including low-risk, high-risk, common (i.e., having a frequency of greater than 5% in the population), and rare (i.e., having a frequency less than 1%) variations. The theory explains well the genetic architecture of diseases where the genetic etiology is well understood but also has some ramifications on the common disease-common variant (CDCV) hypothesis. Although not fully supporting the CDCV hypothesis, Lander and Reich concluded that, based on the present empirical data, the CDCV is probably compatible with many diseases.

Common Disease-Rare Variant Hypothesis

A number of scientists expressed their doubts regarding the CDCV hypothesis and, as a substitute, offered the CDRV hypothesis (Pritchard 2001). For example, evolutionary processes that led to emergence of *H. sapiens* would be more congruent with the existence of multiple rare variations contributing to disease instead of common variations. Basically, random processes would result in a relatively low frequency of mutations. These random processes have influenced the genetic background of the human population, have resulted in mildly deleterious disease-related variations, and are subsequently present in quite high total frequency with extensive allelic heterogeneity. For example, common variations are likely to be older and hence have been subjected to selective pressure over time. By reaching a relatively high frequency, these variants probably have not been subjected to negative selection. Conversely, rare variants are either likely to be recent and not under negative selection for a long time or at low frequency because they are under strong negative selection due to their deleterious effect. Therefore, it may be interesting that recent reports on the frequency of human alleles and their likely "biologically relevant effects" suggest that less frequent variations are more likely to be functional than common variations, which is in line with the expected positive or negative selective forces that are influencing the frequency of variants.

The common disease-rare variant model is sometimes referred to as the "Anna Karenina principle" (McClellan and King 2010), because the consequence of the common disease-rare variant model is that there must be a large number of variants that would be individually very rare (most of time family specific) but collectively are the main genetic risk factor responsible for a common disease. The sentence of Tolstoy's Anna Karenina ("Every unhappy family is unhappy in its own way") reflects this corollary.

Helping Multidisciplinary Teams and Families Around Complex Conditions (Other Illustrative Examples)

Case Vignette

You are the consultant in a psychiatric practice integrated within a rural primary care clinic. In your weekly meetings with the primary care team, a family doctor presents a case of a young girl, currently 28 months of age, who is being monitored for delayed language and motor skills and failed screening tests (administered at 18 and 24 months) for autism.

She had normal growth and development until 16 months of age. However, at 25 months, she was noted to have slower head growth, and she had progressive loss of expressive and receptive language and motor skills. She developed hand wringing by 29 months. No other family members had any neurological disease, and there was no consanguinity in the family.

You commend your primary care colleague for (1) routinely screening for and accurately identifying developmental delays, (2) routinely screening specifically for autism, and (3) identifying certain "red flags" for a progressive neurological condition including loss of developmental milestones and abnormal head growth. Based on the presenting symptoms, you concur with the primary care physician's decision to order specific testing for Rett syndrome.

Rett syndrome (RS) is a severe neurodevelopmental disorder primarily affecting females and has an incidence of 1:10,000 female births by the age of 12 years making it one of the most common genetic causes of severe mental impairment in females. It is characterized by apparently normal development for the first 6–18 months and is followed by the loss of acquired motor skills and the ability to engage in social interaction and the development of stereotypic hand movements. There is wide variability in the rate of progression and severity of the disease. In addition to the classical form of RS, there are several recognized variants, which do not fit a typical presentation. Although it was initially believed that the recognizable features of RS appear after an apparently normal prenatal, perinatal, and early infancy period, more recent studies have clearly shown that, in the first 6 months of life, the female RS infant may show some very subtle abnormalities, particularly those that are related to behavior. A general delay of development is followed by the loss of fine and gross motor skills, social interaction, and intellectual capacity. A more definitive clinical picture evolves in stages over several years, culminating in motor deterioration and death.

Testing for mutations in the X-chromosome-linked methyl-CpG-binding protein 2 (MECP2) gene confirmed the diagnosis of Rett Syndrome. The primary care physician appropriately informs the family and refers the patient for appropriate rehabilitative and specialist services.

Several months later, your primary care colleague asks if you might be able to sit in on a session with the parents, who wish to talk about medication options "to improve muscle strength and overall behavior" for their daughter. At first, you wonder if such questions may be better answered by the neurological or genetics consultant, but because you trust your colleague's judgment in appropriately engaging your expertise, you agree to your colleague's request. In preparation, you extensively review the latest literature.

The parents are very grateful to meet you, together with their primary care provider. They express their wish that there were some medications to help slow down the deterioration, but they fully understand that the evidence for the use of medications is very limited. There is currently no history of seizures or seizure-like activity.

The parents greatly appreciate the opportunity to discuss their emotions as they face the diagnosis of a life-shortening illness in their daughter. They initially believed that the prognosis would be relatively positive for a straightforward case of an autism spectrum disorder, and they are still grieving over the loss of the hopes and dreams they had for their daughter, who is the only girl among their three offspring. They describe their sleep deprivation and exhaustion and the financial and other practical impacts of the significant attention needed by their daughter. Based on screening questions and observations, you are concerned that one of the parents may have symptoms of a major depression.

You work with the primary care physician on identifying further community resources and referrals. The parents are happy that the primary care physician will continue to meet regularly with them to provide monitoring and support.

The case above illustrates the important roles that the pediatric consultation-liaison psychiatrist can play in: helping families to cope with a less-than-ideal prognosis, screening families for the need for other mental health services, and overall empowering the primary care team to incorporate these elements of care in longitudinal treatment. Additionally, if the consultant in the above vignette were only focused on the question of "possible medications" without addressing these other psychosocial priorities (explicitly presented or otherwise), then there could have been the risk of exposing the child to treatments with the potential for more harm than benefit.

Case Vignette

The patient, a 9-year old boy, is admitted to a small rural hospital for extended observation following a tonsillectomy and adenoidectomy for obstructive sleep apnea. The team, already frustrated that the family does not yet feel he is "well enough yet" to go home, consults you "urgently" with the concern that he may once again return with breathing trouble if "his behavior isn't fixed." They also wonder what to do about his "psych meds" now that he is staying in the hospital longer than one day.

You carefully review the medical history. The patient was born at term following an uncomplicated pregnancy. Cardiac decelerations occurred during labor, prompting an emergency cesarean section. Birth weight was 2.73 kg with Apgar scores of 6 and 7 at 1 min and 5 min, respectively. At birth, he was noted to be markedly hypotonic, and he fed poorly. There was no muscle weakness or wasting, and tendon reflexes were brisk. The testes were undescended, and the scrotum was underdeveloped; otherwise, there were no obvious dysmorphic features.

Family history was negative for neonatal hypotonia, neuromuscular disease, and developmental delay. The baby's feeding ability gradually improved to the point of allowing him to be discharged from the hospital. The working diagnosis at that time was central hypotonia of undetermined etiology.

The patient was referred to a developmental treatment program and had a carefully supervised eating routine. At the age of 6 years, he was significantly delayed from language and cognitive standpoints, functioning, in general, at about a 3–3.5-year-old level. Although his height was in the 98th percentile at 4 years of age, there was a subsequent gradual deceleration in growth velocity. Subsequently, his weight increased significantly and disproportionately to his height.

At this point, you query the team on if the patient had ever been formally tested for Prader-Willi syndrome.

Prader-Willi syndrome (PWS) is the most common genetic cause of obesity with an estimated incidence of 1:15,000 – 1:25,000 live births. The reported prevalence varies, but both sexes appear to be equally affected. PWS is the first human syndrome shown to be associated with genetic imprinting. The original descriptions of this syndrome included short stature, hypotonia, hypogonadism, and mental impairment. As child grows to 2–4 years, failure to thrive related, at least in part, to poor muscle tone and poor suck are replaced by increased appetite and food intake resulting in obesity and its comorbidities. This aspect is important when assessing the child with suspected PWS. Infants with Prader-Willi syndrome are usually diagnosed with neonatal hypotonia, hypoplasia of the clitoris/labia minora in girls and small penis and undescended testes in boys. The hypotonia is associated with poor suck and feeding, followed, in many cases, by failure to thrive. Mothers may report decreased fetal activity, and infants are often found in the breech position at the time of delivery. Clinical features include increased neonatal head to chest circumference ratio, narrow bifrontal diameter, almond-shaped eyes, downturned angles of the mouth with abundant and thick saliva, and small hands and feet with straight borders of the ulnar side of the hands and inner side of the legs. The presence of some of these features associated with neonatal hypotonia should prompt physicians to make an early diagnosis of PWS during infancy. These features may become more prominent by age 2–3 years. Excessive eating and obsession with food generally begins in the preschool age group and will lead to morbid obesity if not controlled (Butler et al. 2016).

As these individuals grow older, manifestations such as obesity, short stature, hypogonadism, skin picking, and psychiatric problems become more obvious. Holm et al. first established consensus criteria for the clinical diagnosis of PWS in 1993, and these criteria were used until the introduction of the highly sensitive genetic testing (Holm et al. 1993). Currently, these criteria are used as a screening tool for determining the need for further PWS specific genetic testing. It is important to note that, in many infants, poor cry and unexplained hypotonia may be the only clear clinical manifestations and indication for genetic testing. Therefore, it is important to be vigilant of these symptoms as they may be important when considering practical aspects of consultation-liaison regarding suspected PSW.

You meet with the patient and the mother. You empathize with the mother's sources of frustration: that he seems "so sleepy" and not likely to function well at home, that "no one has really given me answers about why my son keeps having problems," and that "I still hear him breathing loud even though they tell me that they took out his tonsils."

You learn that the patient had previously seen an outpatient psychiatrist for "ADHD" and "conduct disorder." He is noted to "run away from the classroom" and to become "very violent" mostly in the context of having his access to food restricted. He had been tried on various medications, including serotonin-selective reuptake inhibitors. His current regimen – initiated by the previous psychiatrist (who has since relocated) and continued by the primary care physician – includes a relatively high dose of a long-acting stimulant for ADHD and a relatively low dose of a sedating atypical antipsychotic agent.

Following your visit with the patient and his mother at bedside, you are almost immediately surrounded by the nurse, the charge nurse, the hospital case manager, and the attending physician, asking what the "verdict" is on whether they can "send him out today."

At first, you seem taken aback over being asked to play a role that ordinarily should belong to the attending physician. Resisting the temptations to run away to the office or to engage your colleagues in a potentially complex and emotional discussion in a less-than-private location, you take this feeling of discomfort as a prompt to meaningfully engage with the team and to carefully gather (without feeling rushed) more information to guide your recommendations.

You walk toward an available conference room and offer to arrange a sit-down meeting with the team members. You are grateful for their agreement that this is a good idea. You ask everyone to introduce themselves and to state their role in the patient's care and goals for the meeting. You encourage the attending physician to summarize the patient's current situation and to take leadership in the decision on next steps. You listen empathically as the colleagues discuss their concerns. You also share what you know about the patient and convey the mother's various concerns. In doing so, you share your perspectives: that the current psychiatric medication regimen should be currently held (in view of the apparent sedation) and potentially reevaluated (in view of the potential risk of weight gain for one of the medications), that there may be a genetic diagnosis that might be important to further evaluate, and that (as a next step) the team should meet directly with the mother to hear and discuss her concerns.

Following this intervention, the mother is grateful for everyone's care and agreeable to discharge with close follow-up with the primary care physician. Prior to discharge, and following your recommendations, the team ordered array CGH and fragile X DNA testing.

This vignette illustrates the important role that well-functioning teams play in optimizing a patient's care. If either the consultation-liaison psychiatrist or primary team members made decisions rashly or simply in response to patients' or colleagues' heightened emotions triggered by complex medical and psychosocial situations, then poor decisions and outcomes may occur.

In the vignettes discussed in this chapter, the consultation-liaison psychiatrist played a role in decisions to perform genetic testing, intended to provide valuable information about prognosis (which is essential for the consultant to understand) and other aspects of management. The next section, continuing the same vignette, discusses aspects of genetic testing that are important for the consultation-liaison psychiatrist to understand.

Genetic Testing and Genetic Counseling

You hear an update from the primary care physician, with whom you communicated and who is very grateful for your involvement: although the fragile X test was negative, array CGH detected one deletion on 22q11.2, which was thought to be pathogenic, and a relatively short duplication on 18q12.1, which was of uncertain clinical significance. Parental testing showed that the phenotypically healthy father had the 18q12.1 duplication and that the 22q11.2 deletion was de novo. *The family was advised that the 22q11.2 deletion was likely to be cause of child's neurodevelopmental problems and duplication on 18q12.1 was benign.*

Genetic testing is the analysis of human DNA, RNA, chromosomes, or proteins used to detect abnormalities related to an inherited disorder. Tests can directly examine the DNA or RNA that make up a gene (direct testing), look at markers that are co-segregated with a disease-causing gene (linkage testing), examine the protein products of genes (biochemical testing), or examine the entire chromosome (cytogenetic testing). Although the tests themselves generally require only easily obtained blood specimens, decisions around genetic testing involve special considerations (Demkow and Wolanczyk 2017).

The Internet provides a vast amount of readily available information. As a result, it is common for patients, guided by what they read on the Internet, to request a specific drug or laboratory test from their physicians. However, the request may be based on a less-than-comprehensive search of the Internet or on information given by an acquaintance. The request for a test is sometimes based on a misunderstanding of the patient's symptoms, family condition, or other risk factors or on a newly reported scientific discovery.

When considering genetic testing, medical specialists need to be aware of the difference between clinically available tests and "research only" tests. Although testing is available for hundreds of inherited diseases, molecular genetic testing is still in its infancy and promises to become a larger part of primary care practice. Physicians must be familiar with the appropriate uses of genetic testing for their patients and with current resources that will allow them to convey reliable information. For each patient with an inherited disease, the practitioner must be able to define his or her own role and that of the genetics professional by becoming familiar with the elements of a genetic consultation.

There are several types of genetic testing. Diagnostic testing is genetic testing that is done on a person with symptoms of a genetic condition (either approved or not approved for testing). Predictive testing is a type of testing performed on healthy relatives who are at high-risk for a monogenic disorder with later onset. Susceptibility testing, or sometimes referred to as a risk profiling, is a genetic test of one or more genetic markers intended to identify risk (either increased or decreased) for multifactorial conditions in a healthy person. Pharmacogenetic testing is testing for genetic susceptibility to noxious reactions to drugs or other drug effects influenced by certain genotypes. Carrier testing is a genetic test that can detect a gene mutation that commonly has no adverse effects on an individual's health but that could have adverse effects on other family members inheriting the mutation. Prenatal testing is a genetic test on a pregnant person, suspected by genetic counselors to have a fetus with increased risk for a certain condition. Preimplantation genetic diagnosis is testing of one or two cells of in the blastocyst to detect point mutations and chromosomal rearrangements in the context of a positive family history of Mendelian or chromosomal disorders, in order to select the unaffected embryos to be implanted. Genetic screening is offering testing to individuals and families who are not at high-risk.

Ethical issues are of great importance in medical genetics. Due to the advances in medical genetics and innovations in genetic diagnostic methods, awareness of the human genome is increasing, and new genes associated with human diseases are discovered. These discoveries entail new responsibilities and raise legal and ethical issues. Individuals are concerned with the exposure of their genetic information, which increases the possibility of abuse and threatens sense of security. In other words, experts in medical genetics play key roles: in balancing the patients' and families' needs, in insuring access to and benefit from advances in diagnostic and therapeutic procedures, and in ensuring safety and privacy by keeping medical information confidential. Nevertheless, medical genetics is not able to appropriately answer ethical issues and dilemmas alone, and challenges will be encountered in different societies with different cultures, beliefs, and religions (Appelbaum and Benston 2017). Dialogue and collaboration among multiple disciplines, including child and adolescent psychiatrists and other behavioral healthcare providers, are important when helping families facing such challenges. Although advances in genetic testing have benefited patients, novel approaches to education and counseling are needed to provide patients with a complete and balanced report on their options and on the ramifications of any results from genetic testing.

The primary care physician requests your input on how the outpatient team, including the genetic counselor, can most effectively convey to the family the results of the genetic testing. You meet with the team and review some of the potential concerns related to prognosis, treatability of the behavioral symptoms, and potential heritability of this or other genetic conditions in the family. They let you know that the family is planning another pregnancy. You offer to be present for the family meeting, which proves to be successful and much appreciated by all.

Summary

It is important for the child and adolescent psychiatrist, particularly when caring for children with medical illness, to recognize signs and symptoms of a potential genetic diagnosis, as these conditions have implications for treatment and counseling. It is also important for child and adolescent psychiatrists, in caring for children with potentially complex conditions with significant impacts on prognosis and family well-being, to employ consultation and liaison skills to help optimize overall healthcare.

Patients with genetic conditions may have unusual psychiatric symptoms or other unusual history and physical findings. In addition, child and adolescent psychiatrists should think about genetic possibilities and collaborate with the primary medical team to make referrals for genetic evaluation when appropriate. Recognition of the importance of genetic diagnoses in child and adolescent may stimulate further research into the prevalence of genetic disease, effective methods of screening and diagnosis, and strategies for treatment and management.

References

Appelbaum, P. S., & Benston, S. (2017). Anticipating the ethical challenges of psychiatric genetic testing. *Current Psychiatry Reports, 19*(7), 39.

Bamshad, M. J., Ng, S. B., Bigham, A. W., Tabor, H. K., Emond, M. J., Nickerson, D. A., & Shendure, J. (2011). Exome sequencing as a tool for Mendelian disease gene discovery. *Nature Reviews. Genetics, 12*(11), 745–755.

Butler, M. G., Manzardo, A. M., & Forster, J. L. (2016). Prader-Willi syndrome: Clinical genetics and diagnostic aspects with treatment approaches. *Current Pediatric Reviews, 12*(2), 136–166.

Demkow, U., & Wolanczyk, T. (2017). Genetic tests in major psychiatric disorders-integrating molecular medicine with clinical psychiatry-why is it so difficult? *Translational Psychiatry, 7*(6), e1151.

Gelernter, J. (2015). Genetics of complex traits in psychiatry. *Biological Psychiatry, 77*(1), 36–42.

Holm, V. A., Cassidy, S. B., Butler, M. G., Hanchett, J. M., Greenswag, L. R., Whitman, B. Y., & Greenberg, F. (1993). Prader-Willi syndrome: Consensus diagnostic criteria. *Pediatrics, 91*(2), 398–402.

McClellan, J., & King, M. C. (2010). Genetic heterogeneity in human disease. *Cell, 141*(2), 210–217.

O'Donovan, M. C., & Owen, M. J. (2016). The implications of the shared genetics of psychiatric disorders. *Nature Medicine, 22*(11), 1214–1219.

Pritchard, J. K. (2001). Are rare variants responsible for susceptibility to complex diseases? *American Journal of Human Genetics, 69*(1), 124–137.

Reich, D. E., & Lander, E. S. (2001). On the allelic spectrum of human disease. *Trends in Genetics, 17*(9), 502–510.

Richter, J. D., Bassell, G. J., & Klann, E. (2015). Dysregulation and restoration of translational homeostasis in fragile X syndrome. *Nature Reviews Neuroscience, 16*(10), 595–605.

Uher, R. (2014). Gene-environment interactions in common mental disorders: An update and strategy for a genome-wide search. *Social Psychiatry and Psychiatric Epidemiology, 49*(1), 3–14.

Chapter 15
Interfacing with Palliative and End-of-Life Care and Ethical Decisions

Anna C. Muriel, Chase Samsel, and Maryland Pao

Background

The psychiatric care of youth with serious medical illness involves thoughtful interaction with a wide range of medical specialties, including the relatively young field of pediatric palliative care (PPC). This growing subspecialty is devoted to improving quality of life for children with serious illness and their families through pain and symptom management, skilled communication about priorities, and well-coordinated care throughout the disease trajectory. As in adult palliative care, the focus is on symptom management and achieving goal concordant care rather than the cure of disease (www.capc.org/topics/pediatric-palliative-care/ 2017). The field of palliative care grew out of a British movement spearheaded by Dame Cicely Saunders who founded St. Christopher's Hospice in London in 1967. Trained as a nurse, social worker, and physician, she asserted the importance of dignity, compassion, and respect for dying people. She was known to pay close attention to the narratives of patients and articulated the concept of "total pain" that encompassed physical, emotional, and spiritual distress (Richmond 2005).

PPC has grown since the 1980s to encompass medical, psychosocial, and spiritual care that extends into the early stages of serious and chronic illness for children and that may be offered alongside treatment with curative intent (Temel et al. 2010). PPC has been shown to improve physical symptoms and end-of-life communication for children and their families by helping parents and children to identify and imple-

A. C. Muriel · C. Samsel
Dana-Farber Cancer Institute and Boston Children's Hospital, Boston, MA, USA
e-mail: anna_muriel@dfci.harvard.edu; chase_samsel@dfci.harvard.edu

M. Pao (✉)
National Institute of Mental Health, NIH, Bethesda, MD, USA
e-mail: paom@mail.nih.gov

A. P. S. Guerrero et al. (eds.), *Pediatric Consultation-Liaison Psychiatry*,
https://doi.org/10.1007/978-3-319-89488-1_15

ment their care goals, as well as enhance health-related quality of life, strength, and resilience in the face of serious illness (Wolfe et al. 2008; Hays et al. 2006; Himelstein et al. 2004).

PPC is usually practiced in interdisciplinary teams that may include physicians from a range of specialties (e.g., primary care, intensive care, hospitalist medicine, oncology, neonatology, etc.), advanced practice nurses, social workers, and sometimes psychologists, chaplains, art therapists, and child life specialists in primarily inpatient settings. In 2013, 69% of the 162 children's hospitals in the United States had a PPC team; the structure and consultation patterns vary depending on the institution (Feudtner et al. 2013). It is critical for pediatric psychosomatic medicine clinicians to understand the principles underlying PPC and how best to collaborate with palliative care teams in the complex system of care for seriously ill children.

Overlap Between Child Psychiatry and Pediatric Palliative Care

Pediatric consultation-liaison (CL) psychiatry focused on the psychological coping and adaptation of medically ill children from the 1950s through the 1990s and was renamed pediatric psychosomatic medicine in the mid-2000s. General child psychiatry, on the other hand, moved into outpatient settings and emphasized disorders such as attention-deficit/hyperactivity disorder, mood and anxiety disorders, conduct disorder, eating disorders, and other behavioral disorders without comorbid medical illness. During the 1990s, psychotropic medication treatment trials in children advanced rapidly, as did medical technological advances that made many previously life-threatening illnesses become chronic medical conditions. Today, many children survive what once were lethal disorders, but still may experience delayed physical and emotional development in the context of complicated medical procedures and treatments. These youths must engage in complex medical decision-making and may also experience comorbid psychiatric conditions into young adulthood and survivorship. Given their in-depth training in child development, family systems, psychological coping, and risk factors for psychopathology, child psychiatrists have much to contribute to an understanding of youth's experiences of serious illness and death (Buxton 2015, Muriel et al. 2016).

The field of PPC shares many tenets of psychosocial practice with psychiatry, including an emphasis on the importance of doctor-patient communication and the exploration of the values and priorities of young patients and their families (Bartell and Kissane 2005). Figure 15.1 describes both the distinct and overlapping areas of expertise of these two fields (Muriel et al. 2016). PPC clinicians, however, are not mental health providers and have limited training in the assessment and treatment of complex psychopathology, including assessment of suicidal ideation, which does occur in youth with serious illness (Brinkman et al. 2014). Medical teams, including PPC, therefore still rely on psychiatric consultation when faced with comorbid med-

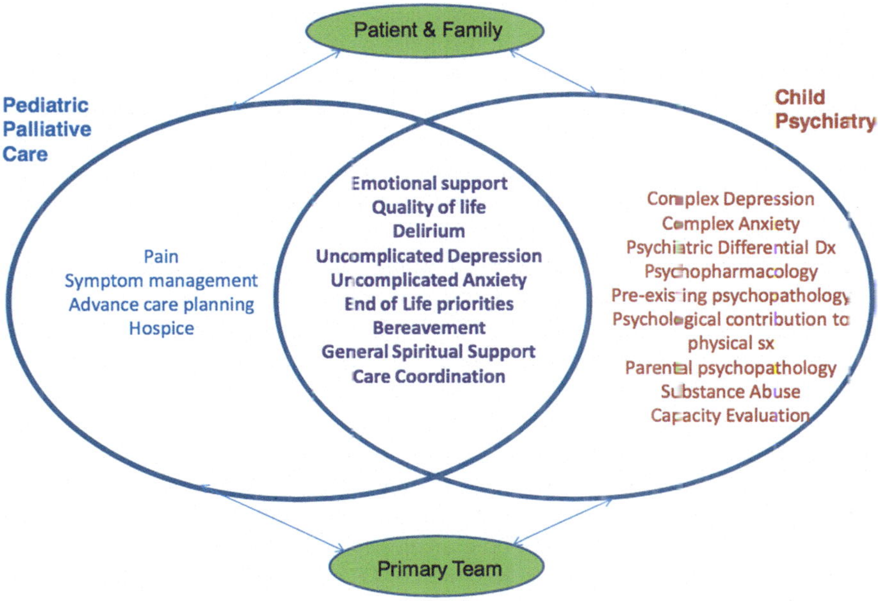

Fig. 15.1 Overlapping and distinct expertise

ical and psychiatric illness or when mental health issues impact ethical dilemmas in the care of seriously ill children. PPC and psychiatry services both serve as consultants to the primary medical team, as well as to the patient and family, and definition of clinical roles and good communication between the services is essential. The specific areas of interaction may vary depending on the availability of each service in an institution. Certain subspecialties such as oncology or solid organ transplant may have embedded child psychiatrists, and palliative care teams may have different capacities to work with children across the trajectory of illness. In addition, both PPC and child psychiatrists may work on multidisciplinary teams alongside social workers, psychologists, chaplains, and child life specialists.

Psychiatric Syndromes in Children at End of Life

The general approaches for consultation psychiatry with medically ill children apply to those with advanced or terminal illness as well, with some specific considerations for children and adolescents closer to the end of life. As addressed in other chapters, the differential diagnosis for depression and anxiety symptoms must take into account physical symptoms such as pain, physical deconditioning, dyspnea, nausea, anorexia, constipation, or malnutrition. At end of life, metabolic and endocrine function may also become dysregulated, further affecting mood and anxiety symptoms. Social withdrawal and energy conservation may occur as part of the dying process, making children look apathetic or depressed. Psychological issues such as anticipatory grief and loss, fear of death, and communication challenges can also contribute to worsening mood and may not be addressed by medication. PPC clinicians may need assistance from psychiatrists in distinguishing depressive syndromes that may respond to antidepressants or stimulants from those that may need to be addressed with therapeutic or communication interventions or simply tolerated as a part of grief and the end-of-life experience.

Children may have been taking psychotropic medications earlier in their illness to manage depression, anxiety, or mood and behavioral dysregulation. Many of these may be continued until the end of a child's life to avoid discontinuation syndromes or return of symptoms. However, tablet formulations may need to be converted to liquid, sublingual, or transdermal preparations as ease of intake by mouth sometimes changes. Compounding pharmacies and hospice programs may be helpful in finding good alternatives. On the other hand, medications for pain or other physical symptoms like dyspnea or hypertension may also address psychiatric symptoms such as anxiety or insomnia, allowing the team to simplify medication regimens and discontinue psychotropic medications. In other cases, potential side effects such as metabolic changes, sedation, or QTc prolongation may be less concerning at end of life, allowing for more liberal use of antipsychotics for delirium or stimulants for fatigue or sedation due to analgesics.

Ethics, Palliative Care, and Pediatric Consultation-Liaison Psychiatry

Ethics committees in pediatric care were developed in the 1980s and were focused around decisions to withhold or withdraw life-sustaining treatment in newborns with serious medical conditions. This development led the American Academy of Pediatrics to create specific guidelines for infant bioethics committees (1984). As medical progress provides life-prolonging treatment in many situations, the field of bioethics has established widely accepted guidelines for making decisions about end-of-life care. Ethics committees are usually consulted when there is conflict about decisions (1) between the patient and family, (2) between the patient/family and clinicians, (3) among different members of the team, or (4) when there are legal or policy issues. The most common areas of conflict include withholding or withdrawing care, sometimes discussed as redirecting efforts from curative to supportive care and using sedating analgesic medications that may also have the "double effect" of hastening death.

The framework for bioethical consultation may include considerations of medical indication, patient preferences, quality of life, and external factors (Jonsen et al. 2015). Table 15.1 outlines another framework described by McCullough and Ashton

Table 15.1 Framework for ethics consultation (Mccullough and Ashton 1994)

1.	What are the facts of the case?
2.	What are our obligations to the patient?
3.	What are our obligations to third parties?
4.	Do our obligations converge or conflict?
5.	What is the strongest objection that could be made to a convergence of obligations? How can this objection be effectively countered?
6.	Could the ethical conflict have been prevented?

(Mccullough and Ashton 1994). Psychiatry may also be consulted in ethically challenging cases when parental mental health concerns impact medical decision-making or when the child has significant psychiatric or developmental disabilities that affect the assessment of quality of life.

Youth with progressive neurologic illnesses have to address and plan for a shortened lifespan and the balance between quality and quantity of life. Psychiatrists may be called upon to assess for depression or capacity for medical decision-making in the context of progressive symptoms.

Case 15.1

An urgent capacity evaluation is requested for an 18-year-old young man with Duchenne's muscular dystrophy after he reports to his social worker that he is refusing oral or gastrostomy tube nutrition due to a desire to "die faster."

While any licensed medical professional may do a capacity assessment, psychiatric consultation-liaison physicians have unique expertise. Furthermore, hospital staff may consult psychiatry if they do not agree with the results of a capacity assessment from a nonmental health clinician.

Case 15.2

The team is concerned about depression and suicidal ideation as the patient has also told staff he no longer wants a planned tracheostomy to address increasing respiratory failure. His family and team feel conflicted as the patient has Do Not Resuscitate (DNR) (in some states Allow Natural Death "AND") and Medical Orders for Life-Sustaining Treatment (MOLST) forms delineating no cardiopulmonary resuscitation, but they feel at odds around his choice to forego nutrition or the potentially life-extending tracheostomy, to which he previously consented. His palliative care team wonders if he is too depressed to have capacity to make such choices.

Capacity consults for refusal of care in individuals with life-limiting illnesses, even with legal advanced directives to forego treatment, are not uncommon, usually because of systemic issues including staff moral distress, misunderstanding about advance directives, and concerns about change in decision-making due to altered mental states. The reasoning behind capacity consults can often contain explicit and implicit ethical questions in addition to the request for assessment of mental status.

Case 15.3

His family has been giving him hydration through his gastrostomy tube despite his wishes not to receive it, and his weakness makes him unable to resist. His parents feel conflicted about going against his wishes (as does his palliative care team) especially given that he is now legally an adult, but they feel that he is not behaving like himself. He is refusing to speak with his family about his decision.

Family distress may contribute to staff moral distress, and thus it is often social workers and palliative care clinicians who advocate for psychiatric involvement. A history from parents regarding patients as behaving or thinking differently from their baseline warrants a differential diagnosis of delirium, depression, anxiety, traumatic stress, psychosis, and other psychiatric conditions.

Case 15.4

On interview, this young man is frustrated and states people cannot hydrate him against his will. As the psychiatrist explains her role and desire to understand his symptoms and suffering and help him advocate for his needs, he relates how depressed he feels about his situation. He is upset with his family and team's refusal to consider his decisions and continuing to hydrate him against his will.

Psychiatric consultation for capacity in individuals with life-limiting illness requires alliance-building, clear delineation of role, and gradual discussion and questioning around capacity, to ease defensiveness and facilitate shared problem-solving. This patient benefits from the psychiatric presence and approach. Beginning with a discussion of his mood and circumstances, history-taking, dialogue, and patient advocacy follow. Were the patient refusing to talk, he would be informed that the team must assume he does not have capacity to make decisions. Angry or desperate patients may then be motivated to engage in the interview and dialogue regardless of their capacity. In this case, rapport-building and a collaborative approach was sufficient. This style and approach allows for a calm and productive exploration around the reasons for the consult, risk assessment, and solutions.

Case 15.5

The patient goes on to describe his limited quality of life as he has decreased use of his hands and is disappointed about turning 18 and becoming an adult, but feeling less autonomous. He is not enjoying reading or watching his preferred TV series and has been more isolated from friends on social media. Upon reflection on his mood and thought process, he states he does not feel like his usual self and admits to feeling depressed and hopeless. His sleep has been more disrupted than usual, with early morning awakening and nighttime ruminations.

As in many capacity consults, the psychiatrist can "find out what is really going on" with the patient's mental state and decision-making. Skillful history-taking and consideration of differential diagnosis allow for many vectors of intervention. Most patients with life-limiting illnesses, chronic feelings of helplessness, and loss of agency benefit from being empowered with choices about preferred activities and which ones they are most invested in doing. These may not always be the activities that the medical team or their parents prioritize.

Case 15.6

When given options to improve his mood, he states he would be interested in relief from his negative emotions and consents to a trial of a rapid-acting agent for depression.

Collaborative problem-solving around psychiatric symptoms and interventions is validating to patients whose capacity is being questioned and can lead to further engagement around the initial capacity and medical care concerns. Psychiatrists should gauge how much time is needed before a decision must be made regarding a capacity concern and utilize as much flexibility as possible to come to an agreeable outcome for patients, families, and staff. Staff may be frustrated that the initial consult question is not being immediately answered, but they may not have other options, and hopefully they can come to understand the effectiveness of this patient-centered approach over time.

Case 15.7

The consultant initiates methylphenidate 5 mg once daily and titrates to twice-a-day dosing. The patient can feel a significant improvement in his mood, energy and ability to enjoy things in the first few days of treatment. With increased energy and motivation, he agrees to restart tube feedings. They ultimately settle on 10 mg long-acting methylphenidate every morning.

With successful psychiatric treatment, the tension points for the family, staff, and patient are relieved without having to hydrate or treat against the patient's will. He had some impairment in his decision-making and exhibited maladaptive coping at the time, but it was resolved without a binary, black-or-white capacity determination. There may be a false dichotomy in many capacity consults unless the patient is actively suicidal, delirious, manic, and/or psychotic.

Case 15.8

The patient eventually engages in decision-making about options for more sensitive hand remote controls for his wheelchair and video games. The palliative care team helps to find a technology company that charitably donates equipment to the patient and family. The patient sustains his improved mood with meaning-centered psychotherapy and ultimately decides to undergo the tracheostomy for mechanical ventilation in the next few weeks without any further discussion of his capacity.

The involvement of the psychiatrist does not end at the agreement to restart tube feeds, as many psychiatric issues were identified that impaired the patient's quality of life. The patient, family, and medical team members may find value in the psychiatrist continuing to be involved to provide ongoing mental status assessments and serve as an advocate for the patient's interests once capacity concerns are resolved. Improved agency and engagement in pleasurable activities improve the patient's mood further and result in making life-extending treatment decisions.

The role of depression in impairing quality of life and contributing to patients' foregoing life-sustaining therapies in a passively suicidal way is an important phenomenon that warrants involvement and exploration from psychosomatic medicine and palliative care clinicians.

The assessment and treatment of delirium is a mainstay in the practice of pediatric psychosomatic medicine and may also bring consultants into collaboration with palliative care specialists. There is growing attention to delirium in very young children, with increasing evidence about how to assess the neuropsychiatric functioning of infants and provide effective treatments to enhance their quality of life and capacity for meaningful engagement with caregivers (Traube et al. 2017). As neonatal care advances and more infants with complex conditions survive, psychiatrists may be engaged in assessment and treatment of the very young. Neonatal pediatric palliative care is also a developing field that informs practice in this area.

Case 15.9
An ex-28-week preemie, now 4 months old, with hypoxic-ischemic encephalopathy and seizure disorder on anticonvulsants, short gut after necrotizing enterocolitis, central apnea on caffeine, oxygen-dependent chronic lung disease, and DNR orders, is referred for evaluation of a change in mental status. A psychiatrist on the consultation service has recently given pediatric grand rounds on delirium in infants with multiple risk factors.

Given the variance from "typical" developmental milestones, assessment must be based on changes from the child's individual baseline status, with an eye toward immediate priorities and goals of care. Bedside nurses can use standardized assessment tools such as the Cornell Assessment of Pediatric Delirium (CAPD) to document mental status over time (Silver et al. 2015).

Case 15.10
The nursing staff reports that the infant previously responded to caregivers by tracking faces, grasping fingers, and reaching for objects. Since having an increase in his oxygen requirement, he responds to physical handling only intermittently and, although awake, does not look at caregivers or have any purposeful movement. His sleep is disrupted, with no regular naps and sleep-wake pattern reversal. Other than tachypnea, he has no vital sign changes or other changes to baseline. On exam, he is a very small infant who appears irritable and unresponsive to soothing. The family and team agree on the goal of improved quality of life, with an understanding that his lung disease is likely to progress further.

Emerging data on the treatment of infant delirium informs a thoughtful multimodal approach that can include antipsychotic medication. In end-of-life care, the potential long-term side effects are less relevant than balancing immediate symptom relief with the immediate safety and side effect profile. Although choice of low-dose antipsychotic use may vary based on regional practices, quetiapine has been used safely and effectively in research populations (Groves et al. 2016; Joyce et al. 2015).

Case 15.11
The psychiatry consultant diagnoses delirium and considers treatment with an antipsychotic medication to improve his mental clarity and ability to interact with his family. After discussion regarding a possible risk of lowering seizure threshold, the team and family agree to a trial of quetiapine (0.5 mg/ kg starting at HS). The infant sleeps at night, but remains irritable and less responsive during the day. Quetiapine

is changed to twice-a-day dosing, resulting in the infant having a calmer demeanor and improved engagement with caregivers. He ultimately dies a few weeks later after a profound apneic episode and is not resuscitated per family's wishes and DNR order. Staff and family are appreciative of more quality time with their child.

Palliative Sedation

There are times when children with life-threatening illness have severe and refractory physical or emotional suffering that is not relieved with the usual palliative interventions. In these cases with very short life expectancy, palliative sedation may be considered to relieve symptoms that are otherwise not treatable. Examples of such refractory symptoms that may also be the focus of psychiatric consultation include anxiety associated with dyspnea, delirium, or agitation. Psychiatrists may be called upon to consider all possible treatments, including antipsychotics, before the team may consider palliative sedation. While the goal of psychotropic intervention is to relieve symptoms and minimize sedation, this is not always possible. Palliative sedation may therefore be considered and involve higher-dose benzodiazepines or other anesthetics such as pentobarbital, dexmedetomidine, or propofol (Anghelescu et al. 2012). The distinction between palliative sedation and euthanasia is the intent of the clinicians. The aim of palliative sedation is relief of suffering, not shortening of life (de Graeff and Dean 2007). Although euthanasia or assisted death for adults is legal in some states, it is not available for children in the United States.

Advance Care Planning

Childhood cancer affects children and adolescents worldwide and is the second leading cause of death in youth 5–14 years and among the top 10 causes of death among aged 10–24 years (Kochanek et al. 2016). There are 300,000 new cases of childhood cancer diagnosed worldwide each year: 215,000 in children under the age of 14 years and 85,000 in adolescents between the ages of 15 and 19 years (2016) http://www.acco.org/blog/iccd-2017-info-graphics/

While the number of new childhood cancer cases continues to grow, the number of available treatments for childhood cancer globally does not. Survival rates for the most common forms of childhood cancer can range from as low as 10% in low- and middle-income countries to as high as 84% in high-income countries. Cultural differences, access to health care, basic socioeconomic disparities, and these differences in survival impact the practice of advance care planning and palliative care globally.

In 2004, Himelstein delineated four components of advance planning for life-limiting illnesses: (1) identification of the decision-makers; (2) clarification of patient and parents' understanding of the illness and prognosis; (3) establishment of care goals –curative, uncertain, or comfort care; and (4) joint decision-making regarding use or nonuse of life-sustaining medical interventions such as mechanical ventilation, intravenous hydration, or phase I chemotherapy (Himelstein et al. 2004). Over the past decade, as family and medical caregivers recognize that adolescents and young adults (AYA) are capable of and want to be involved in decision-making processes around their illness including at the end of life, advance care planning (ACP) with AYAs has become more acceptable (Sisk et al. 2016; Wiener et al. 2013). In a systematic review on pediatric advance care planning, Lotz et al. (2013) reported on the available empirical research on pediatric ACP for severely ill children and adolescents and found only 13 studies; 5 qualitative and 8 quantitative (Lotz et al. 2013). The use of ACP has been shown, through randomized controlled trials of family-centered advance care planning in youth and their families with HIV/AIDS, to be helpful, to decrease anxiety, and to acknowledge the desires of the AYA, regardless of immediate prognosis (Lyon et al. 2009, 2013). A developmentally appropriate guide has been developed for AYA with additional guidance for clinicians on how to start these difficult conversations with patients and families (Wiener et al. 2012; Zadeh et al. 2015). Clinician readiness in the form of skills and beliefs about the importance of quality communication and the clinical culture around the value of open provider-patient communication may inform whether such conversations can proceed (Brook et al. 2008; Feraco et al. 2016).

Recently, experts in pediatric oncology in the United States established 15 evidence-based consensus standards for the psychosocial care of children with cancer and their families; standard 13 specifically states, "Youth with cancer and their families should be introduced to palliative care concepts to reduce suffering throughout the disease process regardless of disease status. When necessary youth and families should receive developmentally appropriate end of life care [which includes bereavement care after the child's death]" (Wiener et al. 2015; Weaver et al. 2015, 2016).

When available, pediatric psychosomatic medicine psychiatrists as well as the pediatric palliative care teams may be involved in helping physicians provide clear information about what to expect at the end of life, working with physicians on how to convey bad news sensitively, and identifying when to include the patient in the discussion when appropriate. Uncertainty and legal and ethical tensions often complicate end-of-life decision-making and can take time to be resolved. Psychiatrists and ethicists may recognize the appropriateness of a competent adolescent to decline aggressive treatment, for example, but some state laws may forbid it (Mack et al. 2005).

Case 15.12

*A 15-year-old girl with cystic fibrosis (*CF*), post lung transplant in acute rejection, presents with dyspnea diagnosed as air hunger by her pulmonary and palliative care teams. Progressive dosing of opiates has not improved her symptoms. Her primary nurse raises the possibility of a psychiatry consult as the patient expresses intense fear and worry that these episodes will not improve.*

Psychiatric consultants have expertise in diagnosing and treating anxiety in the context of medical symptoms. Medical teams may consult for support of anxiety around intense physical symptoms without recognizing that the etiology of primary symptoms may be due to a psychiatric syndrome. Diagnostic clarification and differential diagnosis are the bedrocks of psychosomatic practice and are essential in palliative care and end- of-life patients.

Case 15.13

On mental status exam, the patient is noted to be heavily sedated with complaints of frequent dyspnea. She describes two to three episodes of dyspnea per day. These episodes last 2–10 min and are accompanied by tachycardia, sweating, tremulousness, and thoughts about death. Further history reveals these episodes are brought on by thoughts of her death and possible suffocation. The psychiatrist clarifies that she is experiencing panic attacks and inquires about her medical prognosis.

Panic and other anxiety disorders are often confounding diagnoses for medical clinicians when patients have multiple underlying physical conditions that mimic or exacerbate these symptoms. Linking the symptoms to thoughts and feelings clarifies the diagnosis and broadens opportunities for psychotherapeutic intervention. Diagnostic criteria are helpful in identifying psychotropic options, and knowledge of medical prognosis is important in selecting the most appropriate treatment.

Case 15.14

Given the prospect of months left to live, the psychiatrist starts a selective serotonin reuptake inhibitor. The patient has mild to moderate hepatic failure as part of her CF, *so low-dose citalopram 5 mg once daily is started and titrated to 10 mg once daily over 2 weeks. The psychiatrist also starts concurrent hepatic-adjusted dosing of clonazepam 0.25 mg twice daily, which reduces panic attacks to 2–3 times per week of mild to moderate intensity. The medical team does a gradual taper of opiates without increased dyspnea.*

The psychiatric consultant must gauge risks and benefits along with appropriate timelines for treatment. Given the hepatic impairment of patients with CF, appropriate dose adjustments reduce harm and side effects. Moreover, the consultant must be mindful of using SSRIs such as citalopram and escitalopram, which have the least drug-drug interactions with common CF medication regimens. Planning regarding potential need for agents such as antimicrobials and antibiotics such as linezolid, a weak monoamine oxidase inhibitor, warrants consideration of utilizing serotonergic anxiolytics without long half-lives that would delay treatment of sepsis or make a patient prone to serotonin syndrome (e.g., avoiding fluoxetine). Lastly, appropriate psychotropic treatment can minimize polypharmacy or inappropriate dosing of sedating agents that reduce quality of life.

Case 15.15

There is progressive improvement with follow-up meetings for psychoeducation about panic attacks, relaxation and diaphragmatic breathing and psychotherapy for existential exploration of death and dying. The patient also engages in legacy leaving and advance care planning using "Voicing My CHOiCES™"(Wiener et al.

2012). *At 4 weeks there is further reduction of panic attacks to 1–2 times weekly; each episode lasts for less than 20–30 seconds and is of mild intensity. Citalopram is increased to 15 mg daily with good control of panic. Clonazepam is reduced as needed, mostly around chest physical therapy or during the nighttime.*

This case illustrates the important roles of diagnostic clarification and appropriate psychopharmacologic management to treat the underlying condition and avoid iatrogenic harm. It also highlights the importance of psychotherapy and meaning-making in improving anxiety and panic in patients facing life-limiting illness.

Youth with advanced illness may present with significant multifactorial symptoms that may be related to primary physical symptoms such as dyspnea or pain, as well as fears about their illness and death. These physical and emotional symptoms interfere with their quality of life and must be addressed directly. Discussion and treatment of these concerns may also allow patients and families to thoughtfully consider ACP. Psychiatric consultation can help clarify the contribution of psychiatric issues to distress and provide both pharmacologic and non-pharmacologic interventions.

Impact of Parental Mental Health on End-Of-Life Care

Pediatric palliative care training emphasizes skilled communication with patients and family members to achieve goal concordant care and quality of life for the most seriously ill children. However, PPC clinicians do not have training in the assessment and treatment of adult mental illness and may face challenges when parental mental health issues interfere with parental coping and medical decision-making. Child psychiatrists may therefore have a role in helping to assess these situations and offer targeted parent guidance and family intervention.

Case 15.16

A 5-year-old boy with relapsed stage 4 neuroblastoma and progressive bulky disease in his abdomen is on a phase I trial, which does not stop the progression. He is admitted with a bowel obstruction and increased abdominal girth and pain. His mother is distressed and at bedside, along with maternal grandmother who lives with them. Parents are separated but have shared custody, and the child's father has been only intermittently involved with his medical care. The oncology team approaches the parents about advance care planning, given the poor prognosis and likelihood of perforation and acute decompensation.

Parental separation and different levels of involvement in a child's medical care may complicate decision-making at end of life. It is important to assess both the legal custody arrangement and the emotional and physical engagement of each parent. Even if there are shared legal custody and official decision-making, the parents may have differing levels of understanding about the illness or different levels of prior engagement in everyday medical care and decisions. They may also have different relationships with members of the medical team. Extended family members (e.g., maternal grandmother) may have participated in the care of the child and are invested in the outcome, but do not automatically have legal decision-making authority. The pediatric psychosomatic medicine service could have a role in assessing the family if decision-making becomes conflicted or complicated. Without any expectation of needing to also provide ongoing treatment – including medication prescriptions – to the adults (who generally would not be registered as patients in a pediatric hospital), any of the team psychiatrists, psychologists, or social workers could fulfill this family assessment role.

Case 15.17

The child's mother and grandmother agree that they would like to redirect care to supportive measures only. The child's father feels that more can be done to address the boy's condition, wants a surgical consultation, and does not agree to a Do Not Resuscitate order. He becomes agitated on the unit and yells and threatens to sue the team. Security escorts him to a consultation room, where he calms down and meets with the oncologist, palliative care team, and psychiatry consultant. He is tearful and overwhelmed. Before engaging in further medical decision-making he meets alone with the psychiatrist for additional assessment.

Parental behavior under the stress of a child's life-threatening illness may be mediated by several factors. Containing unsafe behavior must occur first and may require the assistance of security personnel. A compassionate, non-threatening stance from staff, demonstrating a willingness to hear perspectives, can ease tension and provide a platform for calm discussions. Along with medical providers, the psychiatry consultant should clarify the parent's understanding of the child's condition and prognosis and seek to understand their priorities for care.

Case 15.18

The psychiatry consultant provides empathy for the father's suffering, seeing his child so ill, and gently inquires about his relationship with his son and his own personal stressors. On further evaluation, the father reveals a history of anxiety and alcohol abuse and reports that he is in the early stages of recovery. He expresses remorse about not being more available to his son and wants an opportunity to be a better father.

It may be valuable to step back, build rapport, and gather additional personal history from the parent to understand their current mental state and internal experience. A history of mental health and substance abuse issues may affect parental coping with their child's end of life and medical decision-making. Parents may need to be assessed for risk of self-harm, suicidality, and aggression to others, as well as risk of substance abuse relapse. Empathic holding in the face of their child's illness may involve engagement of community resources in addition to support in the hospital.

Case 15.19

Additional meetings with oncology, with further explanation of his son's disease, allow the father to better understand the seriousness of his child's illness. The psychiatrist engages the father's Alcoholics Anonymous sponsor for support and the father's primary care physician in prescribing trazodone for sleep. Over the next week, the father is able to be present at his son's bedside and collaborate with the child's mother to make thoughtful decisions about the child's end-of-life care.

Pediatric/Palliative Care Clinician Distress

Case 15.20

After the child's death on the floor, the multidisciplinary staff gathers for a debriefing session as they usually do after inpatient deaths. One of the child's primary nurses expresses her distress about the child's death, especially as she observed the father's grief about not being present for his son during his earlier life. As a relatively new oncology nurse, she struggled with how unfair it seemed for this little boy and his family; she looked to her more experienced colleagues to learn how they handle their own feelings and continue to care for other children on the floor.

Children and families with comorbid medical and psychiatric issues may present unique personal challenges to primary care and palliative team clinicians. Regular exposure to childhood suffering and death may contribute to compassion fatigue (Rourke 2007), and high expressed emotion or distorted thinking in the child or caregiver may provoke additional strong reactions in clinicians and further erode their coping and resilience. In caring for a seriously ill child, pediatric teams may find it challenging to establish boundaries between their professional and personal responses. Clinicians of any discipline may become overly involved with patients by extending themselves to meet intense demands, sharing personal stories or resources, having trouble setting limits, or connecting through online social networking. These behaviors can pose ethical and confidentiality concerns and create varying patient and family expectations, which can lead to misunderstandings or resentment about why some staff are more flexible than others. On the other hand, clinicians may be overwhelmed or repelled by a patient's psychiatric issues. They may attempt to avoid caring for the patient or blame and criticize the parents.

By providing an outside perspective, psychiatric consultation can provide reflective strategies to enhance clinicians' awareness about their reactions to patients and reestablish professional boundaries. Careful case discussion or regular debriefings can help clinicians distinguish their own feelings and impulses from what is in the best interest of the patient. Psychiatric consultants may also identify overwhelming staff distress and vicarious traumatization and make a referral to outside mental health providers for clinicians needing ongoing support.

Conclusion

Pediatric consultation-liaison psychiatry can play a significant role in helping children and their families during advanced illness and can create opportunities for collaboration with pediatric palliative care clinicians. In bringing expertise about a child's cognitive, emotional, and physical development in the context of serious medical illness, the psychiatry consultant can play an important role in helping families and other clinicians understand how these impact a particular child at the end of life. In cases of significant psychiatric and medical comorbidity, child psychiatrists can improve the recognition and treatment of mental health conditions and improve quality of life and outcomes for dying youth and their surviving families.

References

1984. American Academy of Pediatrics Infant Bioethics Task Force and Consultants: Guidelines for infant bioethics committees. *Pediatrics, 74*, 306–310.

Anghelescu, D. L., Hamilton, H., Faughnan, L. G., Johnson, L. M., & Baker, J. N. (2012). Pediatric palliative sedation therapy with propofol: Recommendations based on experience in children with terminal cancer. *Journal of Palliative Medicine, 15*, 1082–1090.

Bartell, A. S., & Kissane, D. W. (2005). Issues in pediatric palliative care: Understanding families. *Journal of Palliative Care, 21*, 165–172.

Brinkman, T. M., Zhang, N., Recklitis, C. J., Kimberg, C., Zeltzer, L. K., Muriel, A. C., Stovall, M., Srivastava, D. K., Sklar, C. A., Robison, L. L., & Krull, K. R. (2014, January 15). Suicide ideation and associated mortality in adult survivors of childhood cancer. Cancer, 120(2), 271–277. https://doi.org/10.1002/cncr.28385. Epub 2013 Oct 7.

Brook, L., et al. (2008). A plan for living and a plan for dying: Advanced care planning for children. *Archives of Disease in Childhood, 93*(suppl), A61–A66.

Buxton, D. (2015). Child and adolescent psychiatry and palliative care. *Journal of the American Academy of Child and Adolescent Psychiatry, 54*, 791–792.

Feraco, A. M., Brand, S. R., Mack, J. W., Kesselheim, J. C., Block, S. D., & Wolfe, J. (2016). Communication skills training in pediatric oncology: Moving beyond role modeling. *Pediatric Blood & Cancer, 63*, 966–972.

Feudtner, C., Womer, J., Augustin, R., Remke, S., Wolfe, J., Friebert, S., & Weissman, D. (2013). Pediatric palliative care programs in children's hospitals: A cross-sectional national survey. *Pediatrics, 132*, 1063–1070.

DE Graeff, A. & Dean, M. 2007. Palliative sedation therapy in the last weeks of life: A literature review and recommendations for standards. Journal of Palliative Medicine, 10, 67–85.

Groves, A., Traube, C., & Silver, G. (2016). Detection and Management of Delirium in the neonatal unit: A case series. *Pediatrics, 137*, e20153369.

Hays, R. M., Valentine, J., Haynes, G., Geyer, J. R., Villareale, N., Mckinstry, B., Varni, J. W., & Churchill, S. S. (2006). The Seattle pediatric palliative care project: Effects on family satisfaction and health-related quality of life. *Journal of Palliative Medicine, 9*, 716–728.

Himelstein, B. P., Hilden, J. M., Boldt, A. M., & Weissman, D. (2004). Pediatric palliative care. *The New England Journal of Medicine, 350*, 1752–1762.

2016. *International Statistics (Summary of IARC Report)* [Online]. http://www.acco.org/blog/iccd-2017-info-graphics/. American Childhood Cancer Organization. Accessed 24 July 2017.

Jonsen, A. R., Siegler, M. & Winslade, W. J. 2015. *Clinical ethics, 8th edition: A practical approach to ethical decisions in clinical medicine*, 8E, McGraw-Hill Education.

Joyce, C., Witcher, R., Herrup, E., Kaur, S., Mendez-Rico, E., Silver, G., Greenwald, B. M., & Traube, C. (2015). Evaluation of the safety of quetiapine in treating delirium in critically ill children: A retrospective review. *Journal of Child and Adolescent Psychopharmacology, 25*, 666–670.

Kochanek K. D., Murphy, S. L., Xu, J. Q., & Tejada-Vera, B.. (2016). *Final data for 2014*. National vital statistics reports. National Center for Health Statistics [Online], 65.

Lotz, J. D., Jox, R. J., Borasio, G. D., & Fuhrer, M. (2013). Pediatric advance care planning: A systematic review. *Pediatrics, 131*, e873–e880.

Lyon, M. E., Garvie, P. A., Mccarter, R., Briggs, L., He, J., & D'Angelo, L. J. (2009). Who will speak for me? Improving end-of-life decision-making for adolescents with HIV and their families. *Pediatrics, 123*, e199–e206.

Lyon, M. E., Jacobs, S., Briggs, L., Cheng, Y. I., & Wang, J. (2013). Family-centered advance care planning for teens with cancer. *JAMA Pediatrics, 167*, 460–467.

Mack, J. W., Hilden, J. M., Watterson, J., Moore, C., Turner, B., Grier, H. E., Weeks, J. C., & Wolfe, J. (2005). Parent and physician perspectives on quality of care at the end of life in children with cancer. *Journal of Clinical Oncology, 23*, 9155–9161.

Mccullough, L. B., & Ashton, C. M. (1994). A methodology for teaching ethics in the clinical setting: A clinical handbook for medical ethics. *Theoretical Medicine, 15*, 39–52.

Muriel, A. C., Wolfe, J., & Block, S. D. (2016). Pediatric palliative care and child psychiatry: A model for enhancing practice and collaboration. *Journal of Palliative Medicine, 19*, 1032–1038.

2017. *Pediatric Palliative Care* [Online]. www.capc.org/topics/pediatric-palliative-care/. Center to Advance Palliative Care. Accessed 24 July 2017.

Richmond, C. (2005). Dame Cicely Saunders. *BMJ: British Medical Journal, 331*, 238.

Rourke, M. T. (2007). Compassion fatigue in pediatric palliative care providers. *Pediatric Clinics of North America, 54*, 631–644.

Silver, G., Kearney, J., Traube, C., & Hertzig, M. (2015). Delirium screening anchored in child development: The Cornell assessment for pediatric delirium. *Palliative & Supportive Care, 13*, 1005–1011.

Sisk, B. A., Bluebond-Langner, M., Wiener, L., Mack, J., & Wolfe, J. (2016). Prognostic disclosures to children: A historical perspective. *Pediatrics, 138*, e20161278.

Temel, J. S., Greer, J. A., Muzikansky, A., Gallagher, E. R., Admane, S., Jackson, V. A., Dahlin, C. M., Blinderman, C. D., Jacobsen, J., Pirl, W. F., Billings, J. A., & Lynch, T. J. (2010). Early palliative care for patients with metastatic non-small-cell lung cancer. *The New England Journal of Medicine, 363*, 733–742.

Traube, C., Silver, G., Gerber, L. M., Kaur, S., Mauer, E. A., Kerson, A., Joyce, C., & Greenwald, B. M. (2017). Delirium and mortality in critically ill children: Epidemiology and outcomes of pediatric delirium. *Critical Care Medicine, 45*, 891–898.

Weaver, M. S., Heinze, K. E., Kelly, K. P., Wiener, L., Casey, R. L., Bell, C. J., Wolfe, J., Garee, A. M., Watson, A., & Hinds, P. S. (2015). Palliative care as a standard of care in pediatric oncology. *Pediatric Blood & Cancer, 62*(Suppl 5), S829–S833.

Weaver, M. S., Heinze, K. E., Bell, C. J., Wiener, L., Garee, A. M., Kelly, K. P., Casey, R. L., Watson, A., Hinds, P. S., & Pediatric Palliative Care Special Interest Group at Children's National Health System. (2016). Establishing psychosocial palliative care standards for children and adolescents with cancer and their families: An integrative review. *Palliative Medicine, 30*, 212–223.

Wiener, L., Zadeh, S., Battles, H., Baird, K., Ballard, E., Osherow, J., & Pao, M. (2012). Allowing adolescents and young adults to plan their end-of-life care. *Pediatrics, 130*, 897–905.

Wiener, L., Zadeh, S., Wexler, L. H., & Pao, M. (2013). When silence is not golden: Engaging adolescents and young adults in discussions around end-of-life care choices. *Pediatric Blood & Cancer, 60*, 715–718.

Wiener, L., Kazak, A. E., Noll, R. B., Patenaude, A. F., & Kupst, M. J. (2015). Standards for the psychosocial care of children with cancer and their families: An introduction to the special issue. *Pediatric Blood & Cancer, 62*(Suppl 5), S419–S424.

Wolfe, J., Hammel, J. F., Edwards, K. E., Duncan, J., Comeau, M., Breyer, J., Aldridge, S. A., Grier, H. E., Berde, C., Dussel, V., & Weeks, J. C. (2008). Easing of suffering in children with cancer at the end of life: Is care changing? *Journal of Clinical Oncology, 26*, 1717–1723.

Zadeh, S., Pao, M., & Wiener, L. (2015). Opening end-of-life discussions: How to introduce voicing my CHOiCES, an advance care planning guide for adolescents and young adults. *Palliative & Supportive Care, 13*, 591–599.

Part IV
Healthcare Systems and Global Perspectives

Chapter 16
Administrative and Financing Models

Claire De Souza

Whether consulting to a medical/surgical program, starting a consultation-liaison (CL) psychiatry program, or revamping an established one, the consultation-liaison (CL) psychiatrist will inevitably face administrative challenges that require attention. By the end of the chapter, readers will be able to appreciate the knowledge, skills, and attitudes required of a pediatric CL psychiatry clinician; develop a model of care within the context of a medical/surgical program or a pediatric center; and seek collaborative relationships with medical/surgical programs, psychosocial disciplines, and colleagues in the field.

Case Scenario

As a qualified child and adolescent psychiatrist, you have been newly hired to provide consultation to a medical program. You consider the steps that you should follow.

You review the literature to improve your knowledge of the psychiatric and psychosocial needs of the specific medical population. To determine needs and resources, you meet with administrative, medical, and psychosocial staff from the medical program. You develop a model of care, involving direct and indirect patient care, to meet the psychiatric needs of the medical population. As your experience with the program develops, you contribute to education and collaborate on research. You establish connections with colleagues in pediatric and adult CL psychiatry programs.

The original version of this chapter was revised. A correction to this chapter is available at https://doi.org/10.1007/978-3-319-89488-1_23

C. De Souza (✉)
Department of Psychiatry, Hospital for Sick Children, Toronto, ON, Canada
e-mail: claire.desouza@sickkids.ca

A. P. S. Guerrero et al. (eds.), *Pediatric Consultation-Liaison Psychiatry*,
https://doi.org/10.1007/978-3-319-89488-1_16

Appreciating Key Competencies of a CL Psychiatry Clinician

Adopting an engaging, approachable, interested, and flexible stance is key to establishing effective consulting relationships with medical/surgical programs (Ahsanuddin and Adams 1982). CL psychiatry clinicians should:

- Be familiar with recognizing and treating mental health comorbidities of medical illness and/or treatment.
- Understand the determinants of health and advocate when appropriate (Frank et al. 2015).
- Integrate information from a variety of sources to aid in assessment and management.
- Be available and accessible to offer prompt response as needed to provide a tailored impression, including psychiatric diagnosis, understandable biopsychosocial formulation, and practical strategies (Goldman et al. 1983; Leentjens et al. 2010).
- Be skilled in adapting psychotherapy and medication management to the medically ill.
- Have expertise in managing delirium, somatic symptom and related disorders, psychiatric illness secondary to medical/surgical illness, and end of life care (DeMaso et al. 2009).
- Be familiar with medicolegal issues, including risk assessments and risk management.
- Be adept at collaborating within an interdisciplinary context, appreciate various roles and responsibilities, and effectively manage conflict in patient care.
- Efficiently use resources while maintaining patient and staff safety.
- Facilitate the learning of others, including those in the CL psychiatry and medical/surgical programs.
- Maintain an eclectic management style and adapt knowledge and skill to various clinical encounters.
- Become visible as an integral part of the team.

Embedding CL Psychiatry within a Medical/Surgical Program

Embedding CL psychiatry clinicians within medical and surgical programs can help to shape how mental health is managed within a medical/surgical program (Desan et al. 2011). Embedding of staff builds relationships with medical/surgical programs and thereby facilitates the development of a CL psychiatry program. Mental health education, particularly in areas where the CL psychiatrist has expertise, enhances medical/surgical programs' capacity to find cases, to appropriately refer to mental health, and to effectively use resources (Kishi et al. 2004). In turn, these educational activities can address mental health stigma. Case finding can occur through attending rounds. Furthermore, specialized patient care models can be developed along with collaborative education and research.

Points to consider when embedding CL psychiatry clinicians include ensuring adequate staffing, minding wait times, determining coverage, balancing the service demands of the hospital against those of the medical/surgical program, mitigating against silos, and considering the population's mental health comorbidity, service utilization, and CL psychiatry clinician's academic interests.

The embedded CL psychiatry clinician may begin the process by meeting with medical directors, managers, and psychosocial team members to review the mental health needs and opportunities for clinical care, education, and collaboration. The embedded CL psychiatry clinician may then participate in medical/surgical team meetings and rounds, provide direct and indirect clinical care depending on availability and larger team processes, and facilitate education of the team through patient rounds or in-services and of families through education days. Integrated clinics with medical/surgical programs may also be created, wherein CL psychiatry clinicians see patients with medical/surgical colleagues in clinic. The model necessitates creation of a process for urgent care coverage, whether by the CL psychiatry clinician, the CL psychiatry program, or the whole department of psychiatry.

Connecting with CL Psychiatry Colleagues

Online discussion forums connect pediatric CL psychiatry colleagues across institutions and enable discussion about clinical, administrative, research, and educational issues as related to CL psychiatry and collaborative work. Pediatric organizations and child psychiatry networks may also provide other opportunities for collaboration. Collaborating on pathways and guidelines enables standardization and optimization of care for patients seen by CL psychiatry: for example, children with somatization and children with delirium.

Opportunities for collaboration, support, and mentorship are important to recruit and sustain the workforce. Gatherings of CL psychiatry colleagues at conference special interest groups, committees, or symposia can facilitate national and international collaborations to advance pediatric CL psychiatry (De Souza 2010; De Souza et al. 2011; De Souza 2012; De Souza et al 2012; De Souza et al. 2013a; De Souza et al. 2013b; De Souza 2014; De Souza et al. 2014; De Souza et al. 2015; De Souza et al. 2016). Such forums can facilitate the sharing of expertise in clinical care, research, administration, and teaching; provide support and mentorship; and create opportunities for collaboration. Collaborating with adult CL psychiatry programs can aid education, clinical care, and research.

Case Scenario

Other medical and surgical programs hear of your work and also request psychiatry consultation for their patients. You consider the additional steps that you should follow.

You meet with the various programs to determine reasons for referral and resources. You outline a process for referral as well as the type of services offered. You ascertain hospital resources to optimize collaboration.

Referral Sources

Inpatient and outpatient medical and surgical programs may refer to a CL psychiatry program. In some countries and settings, community primary care physicians may also seek consultation. Tracking the referral sources and reasons for referral and comparing this data to that found in the literature can identify opportunities for collaboration and education and can help with establishing and refining referral criteria.

Based on the literature, up to 14% of pediatric admissions in certain settings are referred to psychiatry. The patients referred tend to be complex, with severe problems and ambiguous presentations (Shugart 1991; Knapp and Harris 1998a). Based on a survey of pediatric CL psychiatry programs (Shaw et al. 2006; Shaw et al. 2016), common reasons for referral include suicide risk assessments, delirium, disruptive behavior, treatment refusal, nonadherence, depression, anxiety, psychosis, adjustment issues, and somatic symptoms. Of note, the stated and actual reasons for referral may differ due to challenges related to risk, ethical aspects, and/or countertransference. There may be problems identifying mental health problems by type and urgency. Urgency may be related to factors other than safety risk and may include desire to access services prior to discharge and impending discharge.

A CL psychiatry outpatient service may require the patient to be concurrently followed by a hospital medical/surgical program or to have been hospitalized in the last year. In addition, a CL psychiatry outpatient service can address patients who have a medical condition/treatment affecting their mental health, a mental health condition affecting their other medical condition or treatment adherence, and/or patients with significant somatic symptoms. Patients may require preparation for hospitalization and procedures. Referral criteria are affected by the availability of CL psychiatry resources (Table. 16.1).

Type of Service

According to a survey of pediatric CL psychiatry programs, services offered include diagnostic clarification, therapy, medication, behavioral modification, preparation for procedures, liaison, and education (Shaw et al. 2006; Shaw et al. 2010; Shaw et al. 2016). In addition to direct patient care, liaison work may include attending rounds or meetings within medical/surgical programs for case finding and education to highlight the mental health comorbidities of a medical/surgical population (Bierenbaum et al. 2013). These forums can also address concerns about stigma of mental illness and of psychiatry in general and/or the medical/surgical team's tendency to overlook mental health problems in the presence of an acute medical/surgical problem, especially when symptoms do not interfere with medical/surgical treatment (Shugart 1991).

Interdisciplinary case conferences can be helpful in bringing different team members together to arrive at a shared understanding of a case, to process team

Table 16.1 Reasons for referral to CL psychiatry

Level of urgency	Reason for referral
Urgent	Suicide attempt/self-harm
	Delirium
	Psychosis
	Mania
	Aggression
	Intellectual disability/autism spectrum disorder with self-injurious and/or disruptive behavior
	Treatment refusal
	Assistance with capacity assessment
Semi-urgent	Depression (without safety concerns)
	Poor coping/adjustment to catastrophic injury, illness, and/or disability
	Anxiety
	Somatization
	Sleep problems
	Eating/Feeding problems
	Chronic nonadherence
	Parent-child relationship problem
	Complex family dynamics (without risk of abuse/neglect of child)

members' countertransference and to develop an integrated care plan, especially in cases that are complex and where multiple teams are involved (DeMaso and Meyer 1996; Williams and DeMaso 2000). The CL psychiatry clinician may suggest a team meeting and outline the purpose, process, content, and participants to support family engagement. The CL psychiatry clinician can assist with formulation of the case and address issues of team countertransference. In cases where there is conflict, it may be helpful to involve risk management, ethics, administrative leadership, and/or the patient advocate. At the meeting, the CL psychiatry clinician may take the role of chairing or facilitating the process. Families may be brought in after the teams have reached some consensus; the meeting may then provide an opportunity to discuss the impression and plan and to address families' questions and concerns.

Therapy is often eclectic, reflecting the CL psychiatry clinician's ability to adapt treatment to the patient's needs (including comfort and privacy), to the acuity and setting, and to the inevitable multiple interruptions by interdisciplinary team members on a medical/surgical unit. Therapy may help to address nonadherence or treatment refusal, preparation for procedures, somatization, sick role development, and mental health conditions in the context of medical illness. Theoretical frameworks may derive from cognitive behavioral therapy for anxiety, depression, and/or somatic symptoms; dialectical behavioral therapy for suicidal thinking; brief interpersonal therapy, acceptance and commitment therapy, supportive-expressive therapy, strength-based therapy, or narrative approaches for adapting to illness; and mindfulness, imagery, relaxation, hypnosis, and desensitization for procedural anxiety. Therapy can be directed at the individual or family or offered in groups. Medical/surgical teams can be counseled on therapeutic strategies, such as relaxation exercises and other behavioral approaches, that may be helpful in supporting care. Rehabilitation efforts can be supported by physical and occupational therapists. Case management can be directed at the more complex CL psychiatry patients who cross multiple sectors. Medication recommendations need to consider drug interactions and organ functioning as well as family and team preference. Consultation with the hospital/medical team pharmacist is beneficial.

Enhancing Collaboration

Understanding what the disciplines and programs offer and how they are accessed and organized is important to ensuring effective collaboration and efficient use of resources (Richardson et al. 2014). Based on a survey of US pediatric CL psychiatry programs (Shaw et al. 2006), a lack of coordination and/or integration with other psychosocial services was noted as a problem. It is important to determine the allied health support available to a medical or surgical program. This support may include social workers, case managers, discharge planners, psychologists, neuropsychologists, advanced practice nurses, child life specialists, child and youth counselors, art therapists, music therapists, chaplaincy and therapeutic clowns. In addition, various programs may offer psychosocial support through palliative care programs, pain programs, and adolescent medicine. Additional hospital programs that may aid management include ethics and risk management. Collaborating with organizations such as community mental health agencies, primary care, rehabilitation centers, and school boards can aid transition to and care in different settings (Martini et al. 2012; Kelly et al. 2002). Case conferences, knowledge exchange, and warm handovers can help to demystify the patient population and culture of the various sectors and can bridge the service gap in caring for this population. Through these forums, care pathways and partnerships can be developed.

Case Scenario

You have been promoted to medical director of an established CL psychiatry program. You consider the most appropriate first steps in this new role.

You ascertain the context and gather input from the CL psychiatry program and from medical/surgical programs with respect to communication, collaboration, care coordination, and consistency. You outline the mandate, vision and mission, reasons for referral, and interdisciplinary service delivery model. You develop a database, quality improvement initiatives, and scorecard to reflect outcomes. You support a model for interdisciplinary education and training. You support a research mandate.

Context

It is important to contextualize the CL psychiatry program within the department's and hospital's strategic directions. Aligning the CL psychiatry program with hospital initiatives, for instance, by addressing quality metrics involving patient safety or cost, can be helpful in building a case for growth or sustainability of the program. Quality, effectiveness, and responsiveness of a CL psychiatry program in meeting the hospital's needs reflect on the department of psychiatry as a whole because of the program's central position and visibility (Campo et al. 2000). As such, attention to the workings of a CL psychiatry program ensures the reputation of the department of psychiatry. Defining the relationships between the CL psychiatry program and the inpatient psychiatry unit, emergency psychiatry services, and ambulatory psychiatry programs is important in establishing patient flow within the department. Additionally, reviewing the literature for administrative aspects and benchmarking against similar programs enable an evidence-informed approach to building the CL psychiatry program.

Mandate

Establishing a mandate, which may include a vision and mission statement, can be important to orienting the program within the department and hospital. The purpose of a CL psychiatry program is to provide support for patients with mental and other medical illness and those with somatic symptoms. Specifically, the mandate may define care for the critically ill, chronically complex, perpetually ill, and occasionally ill populations. Inherent in this mandate is the need for an interprofessional model of care that delivers efficient care that is effective from the perspectives of CL psychiatry, medical/surgical teams, and families. In addition to direct patient care, support and education for medical/surgical teams are important. Furthermore, there may be a need to build capacity, collaborative networks, and care pathways within the hospital's and community's health system. These care pathways may follow collaborative or integrative care guidelines, clinical care pathways, or bundled care algorithms to improve care access and coordination. A case may be made for mental health screening in medical/surgical programs. Patients may then be triaged, based on positive screening results, to receive CL psychiatry care. Based on the availability of resources, the mandate may also include research, advocacy, and training. There must be built-in accountability to the department, hospital, university, and other funding sources and stakeholders.

Workflow Processes

Where electronic health records are available, a computerized order set to request CL psychiatry involvement enables data tracking. Furthermore, consult requests can be triaged more effectively by mandating certain fields: level of urgency, reason for referral, and if the family is aware of the referral. Clinical staff may then triage by level of urgency: emergent, urgent, semi-urgent, or non-urgent. Response time may be determined by the program and/or by the hospital and may differ depending on patient location and/or referral source: emergency room, medical/surgical inpatient unit, or medical/surgical outpatient clinic. It is beneficial to set timeframes for booking patients based on urgency and available resources. To enable data gathering on symptom severity and functioning, standard questionnaires may be sent in advance of patients being seen. To ensure process consistency and transparency, the CL psychiatry program may benefit from standardizing assessments, documentation, types and duration of treatment, and case closures (Fig. 16.1). Hospital process improvement teams can help support process mapping.

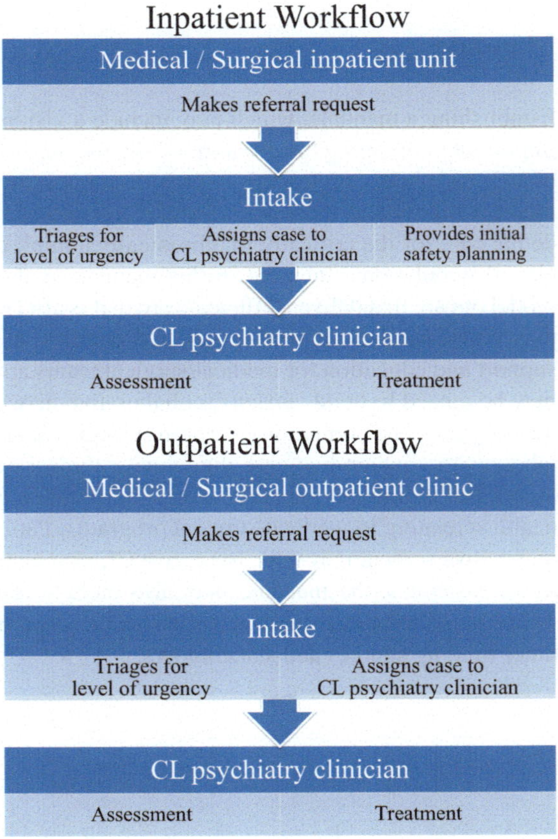

Fig. 16.1 CL psychiatry patient workflow

In addition, there is a need to improve patient navigation from intake through assessment, treatment and transition to the community and a need to attend to response times, wait times, care access, transparency, and accountability. Expectations need to be set for clinical work, research, education, and administration; and the schedule needs to support protected time for each of these components.

CL psychiatry administrative meetings enable discussion of patient safety and workflow concerns and enable process standardization. CL psychiatry patient rounds facilitate patient care through case review, interprofessional collaboration, and education. A handover document can be updated during rounds and used to communicate with the on-call service (Table 16.2). The duration and frequency of CL psychiatry patient rounds will depend on the service's workload and team size; the service's need for collaboration, coordination, education, and supervision; and financial resources to support indirect patient care.

Service Delivery

A CL psychiatry program supports medical and surgical programs by being available to respond to urgent concerns on medical/surgical inpatient units. Depending on the psychiatry department's organization and size, services may also be extended to emergency and outpatient settings. Offering outpatient consultation and

Table 16.2 CL psychiatry handover template

Level of urgency/ complexity	Patient information Name Age Gender Record # Inpatient unit Date admitted: Date referred:	Patient summary Medical diagnoses: Psychiatric diagnoses: Situation: Background: Asessment: Recommendations:	Psychiatric Medications	Roles of CL psychiatry team members involved + Other psychosocial staff involved	Plan for on call
Urgent					
Non-urgent					
On hold					
Signed off					
At rehabilitation centre					
Recent discharges					
Acute outpatients					

follow-up of patients followed in medical and surgical programs can address issues that may be different from what may arise in inpatient settings and can promote continuity of care, support for high-risk patients, and prevention of unnecessary hospitalization. Depending on available resources, a CL psychiatry program may also offer availability – either in-person or via telephone – to respond to urgent concerns in the medical/surgical outpatient clinics. Telehealth or videoconferencing can enable care for patients who live out of town and can support healthcare professionals in other hospitals or community clinics. At times, the family may not be interested in, available for, or agreeable to a referral; in this case, there must be communication with the referral source.

Medical/surgical programs generally appreciate a CL psychiatry service's continued and collaborative care and consultation to the team, program, or division/department when needed. Consultation may be based on a protocol and may proactively anticipate a patient population's needs. Programs may be built around illness groups such as delirium and treatment nonadherence and may focus on improving health outcomes and decreasing healthcare costs. Furthermore, the CL psychiatry program may take on an advocacy role and create hospital-wide processes to ensure patient safety and optimize patient and family experience.

A CL psychiatry clinician rotation enables urgent and intensive responses. An on/off service model like that of other consulting services minimizes disruption to outpatient work and enables protected time when a clinician is off-service. It supports a generalist model of care wherein the clinician is expected to see all referrals unless there are referrals unique to a certain available clinician's area of expertise. The model permits a CL psychiatry clinician to work in a variety of clinical settings and helps to balance team members' workload. Interprofessional staff may become involved based on the referral's urgency, complexity, and/or time intensity. This model needs to ensure effective handover of cases and, particularly for complex cases, continuity of care. The on-service duration may be 1 or 2 weeks, for example. The longer the duration, the more likely the impact on continuity of care for CL psychiatry outpatients.

Combining an on/off service model for general CL psychiatry inpatients while also embedding CL psychiatry clinicians into medical/surgical programs ensures prompt response to all medical/surgical programs; preserves continuity of care for complex patients; and builds areas of expertise with medical/surgical populations. Urgent or time-intensive inpatient cases may be assigned to the on-service CL psychiatry clinician, while specialized or complex inpatient cases may be assigned to the embedded CL psychiatry clinician if available.

Medical-psychiatry units and day hospitals offer intensive treatment, serve as an alternate to medical/surgical inpatient units, and offer an interdisciplinary team approach focused on the holistic needs of this population. They may focus on psychiatric illnesses causing nonadherence and thereby impacting medical treatment or psychiatric illnesses requiring medical evaluation or intervention (e.g., somatic symptoms, eating disorders). Co-management by pediatrics and psychiatry enables progression toward functional goals and symptom reduction.

Critical to the success of these models is ensuring that all CL psychiatry clinicians have basic comfort and skill in seeing all populations; that there is always coverage; that there is a streamlined and equitable approach to case assignment; and that there is good handover and collaboration, with opportunities for team learning and support.

Regardless of which model is chosen, attention to scheduling and workload is required. Assisted by the hospital's corporate development, communications, and/or business strategy department, a SWOT (Strengths, Weaknesses, Opportunities, Threats) analysis can aid in selecting from various possible models.

Interdisciplinary Staffing

A CL psychiatry program that includes interdisciplinary team members is ideal and enables expansion of services beyond what can be provided by psychiatrists alone (Table 16.3).

Mutual respect for and understanding of distinct and overlapping roles enables team members to work to the full scope of their training and to appropriately cover team tasks. The CL psychiatry program's organization appropriately considers the number and types of interdisciplinary staff members (Shaw et al. 2016).

The interprofessional model of care should be based on a set of operating principles: patient care for a defined group of patients and catchment area and efficient and ethical use of time and resources. This model may include delineating the team's tasks and scope of practice for the interdisciplinary staff. In addition, pathways, guidelines, and standardized approaches can further outline roles and tasks.

Table 16.3 CL psychiatry interdisciplinary roles

Discipline	Role
Psychiatrist	Provides assessment, diagnosis, formulation, therapy, medication, monitoring
Psychologist	Provides assessment, diagnosis, formulation, therapy, monitoring, program evaluation and psychometric testing
Advanced Practice Nurse	Provides assessment, care coordination, safety planning, coaching, monitoring, protocol development
Nurse	Provides triaging of cases, safety planning
Social Worker	Provides individual, family and group therapy
Case Manager	Provides care coordination, transition planning care plans, advocacy for complex patients between the hospital and community
Behavioural Therapist	Provides assessment and management of behavior
Physiotherapist	Provides a functional assessment, graded exercise programs, pool therapy, guidelines for equipment
Occupational Therapist	Provides a functional assessment, addresses activities of daily living

Database

A database is important for capturing CL psychiatry patient complexity, determining a CL psychiatry program's productivity, facilitating quality improvement and research, and supporting business plans to optimize staffing (Ellen et al. 2006).

Helpful data to collect are shown in Table 16.4.

Quality Improvement, Scorecard

Quality improvement initiatives aim to improve patient care processes and may address handover systems, patient workflows, and patient safety metrics (Huyse et al. 1992). Program outcomes data, gleaned from qualitative and quantitative evaluations, may inform further service delivery refinements and may potentially develop a case for funding to support increased staffing (Harden et al. 2005). Outcomes to be measured and tracked include patient outcomes related to quality of life, satisfaction (Kitts et al. 2013; De Albuquerque Citero et al. 2008), and improvement in symptoms and functioning (Trauer 2004); service delivery outcomes, including volumes and types of care, timeliness of care (response time, wait time) (Lyne et al. 2009; O'Keefe et al. 2007), medical/surgical team satisfaction (Solomons et al. 2011), referral patterns, and cost-effectiveness; and staff

Table 16.4 CL psychiatry datapoints

Database	
Patient descriptor	Name
	Medical record number
	Date of birth
	Language
	Region (city/municipality)
	Location – inpatient (date of admission, unit)/ outpatient
	Medicolegal status
	Patient previously seen by CL psychiatry
	Psychosocial risk factors
Referral details	Date, Time
	Urgency
	Service
	Reason for referral
CL psychiatry consultation	Urgency
	Diagnoses
	Recommendations
CL psychiatry treatment	Duration, frequency, type
CL psychiatry members involved	By discipline
Disposition	Home/transfer, Referral/ongoing care
Outcomes	Satisfaction, symptoms, functioning, quality of life

safety, including staff injuries from patients' aggressive behavior. Documented decreases in lengths of stay, emergency department visits, and readmission rates can demonstrate improved healthcare utilization and can help to secure funding.

Education and Training

Education should include training of various disciplines. Although it may be challenging to meet the learning needs of trainees and staff from different disciplines and levels, collaboration with various disciplines can facilitate mutual education. A CL psychiatry rotation should include training objectives, expectations, graded responsibilities, case log requirements, a didactic curriculum, supervision, a schedule and timetable, and an evaluation process (Heinrich et al. 2014; Leentjens et al. 2011). Beyond the formal curriculum, any unintentional "hidden curriculum" should be acknowledged and addressed.

The CL psychiatry clinician must also work to optimize recruitment, often through trainee and junior faculty mentorship.

Interprofessional education and coaching with medical and surgical programs can enhance knowledge, skill, and comfort in recognizing and managing comorbid mental health issues. Depending on the mandate of the CL psychiatry program, education may be aimed at enhancing mental health literacy in the hospital and raising awareness of comorbid mental illnesses, mental health resources, care pathways, and the need for integrated interprofessional care. Education is particularly important to address the international shortage of CL psychiatrists.

In addition, collaborating with adult CL psychiatry programs on educational initiatives can address developmental and transitional age issues and can enhance the development of CL psychiatry curricula, educational tools, and training objectives.

Supervision of trainees by discipline, level, and school as well as number and types of educational sessions should be tracked as an outcome of the CL psychiatry program.

Research

Research could focus on pediatric patients with complex comorbid mental and other medical conditions, validation of an integrated model of care, and evaluation of innovative tools and interventions (Knapp and Harris 1998b). Educational research may focus on the efficacy of the CL psychiatry program's training or other educational efforts.

Challenges to engaging in CL psychiatry research include securing sufficient funding and time, obtaining statistical support and mentorship cultivating research relationships, and determining appropriate measures to use. Overcoming these challenges may be achieved through identifying research gaps, building research relationships with medical/surgical programs, conducting outcomes-based research, utilizing a database, "following the money" or funding opportunities starting with small grants, building a grant profile, obtaining mentorship locally or through networks, and supervising research students. Research productivity can be tracked as a program outcome. Collaborative opportunities with colleagues in the field can be identified from lists of grants and funding agencies and from mentorship (De Souza et al. 2015).

Case Scenario
Your CL psychiatry program is quite busy. You feel that more staff are required to meet the need.

You begin by reflecting on the challenges and possible solutions. You review the literature and consult with colleagues in the field on administrative aspects, staffing, quality improvement, cost, and impact. You develop a business case proposal, obtain approval from leadership, and secure funding. You develop a service delivery rollout plan, including a communication plan. You address change management.

Reflecting on and Overcoming Challenges

The literature cites difficulties with coordination of CL psychiatry services and variability in funding, service structure, and service delivery (Shaw and DeMaso 2006). Surveys of CL psychiatry programs have reflected increased clinical demands and limited or decreased staffing impacting important liaison work (Shaw et al. 2006; Shaw et al. 2016). These challenges can be daunting for those new to the field and stressful for those who are already established. Staff working in the area can feel a sense of isolation. There can be limited opportunities for dialogue about CL psychiatry experiences in clinical care, administration, education, and training.

Challenges include managing roles, tasks, expectations, and heavy workloads in the context of a broad scope of practice; inadequate staffing; limited time, funding, and evidence base; the need to secure and satisfy various stakeholders; the need to nurture and optimize interdisciplinary collaborations; different languages and cultures among the medical/surgical teams; and mental health stigma that must be addressed through advocacy (De Souza et al. 2011; De Souza et al. 2012; De Souza et al 2013b; De Souza et al. 2014; De Souza et al. 2015).

Solutions developed by pediatric CL psychiatry programs include defining the CL psychiatry population and mandate and positioning CL psychiatry as an essential service. From a logistical point of view, it is important to connect with key stakeholders through a needs assessment; to outline patient flow processes from initial referral (via centralized intake, electronic order for CL psychiatry, CL psychiatry pager) to triage, assessment, treatment, follow-up and referral; to develop service delivery models (including co-location with pediatrics), guidelines, and best practices; to determine adequate staffing and to define roles; to ensure pediatrics' advocacy for CL psychiatry services; to serve on hospital committees; to develop templates for documentation; to determine coverage and day call systems; and to secure dedicated space (De Souza et al. 2011; De Souza et al. 2012; De Souza et al 2013b; De Souza et al. 2014; De Souza et al. 2015).

To grow the CL psychiatry program, workload – inclusive of important liaison activities – needs to be accurately captured, a database needs to demonstrate the program's impact, and a business plan must be developed. Quality improvement projects not only improve the program but also demonstrate impact. Any proposal for CL psychiatry program growth must appreciate limits on time and not duplicate what has already been developed. It is important to share useful tools, including a toolkit for how to "justify" the CL psychiatry service, amongst colleagues (De Souza et al. 2011; De Souza et al. 2012; De Souza et al 2013b; De Souza et al. 2014; De Souza et al. 2015).

Developing a Business Case

Overview

Making a business case for increased funding involves detailing the current program, what is required ("the ask"), the rationale for such, the current clinical and administrative staffing, and the clinical demand as indicated by data (Holmes et al. 2011; Kunkel et al. 2010). It is essential to link positive outcomes (such as early stabilization and discharge, decreased length of stay, decreased costs, and better treatment adherence) with specific CL psychiatry program elements, including specialized delivery of complex care for patients (in inpatient and/or outpatient settings) with comorbid mental and other medical illnesses, rapid response availability, medical and surgical team support, consultation, education, and safety planning (Bujoreanu et al. 2015). It is also important to outline short- and long-term consequences or risks of not expanding the CL psychiatry program. It is helpful to benchmark the new or established CL psychiatry program against comparable organizations and to reference the literature.

Rationale

To support the need for mental health support of medical/surgical programs and CL psychiatry program growth, the business case proposal can note the growth of the medical and surgical programs, the rates of psychiatric illness in the medically ill population (Bardach et al. 2014; Doupnik et al. 2016), and the impact of untreated psychiatric illness on medical and surgical outcomes. The business case proposal can highlight limited system capacity, medical/surgical teams' variable knowledge and comfort regarding mental health problems, and potentially affected referral rates, referral routes, and triaging processes. Under these circumstances, cases may be referred "late" or not at all by medical/surgical programs and may therefore be at higher risk for nonadherence and adverse outcomes. Where appropriate, the business case proposal can also highlight the limited availability of inpatient child psychiatry beds and community supports; in this context, the hospital's capacity may be reduced by delays and other challenges in transferring medical/surgical inpatients to psychiatry units or discharging them with community follow-up. Where appropriate, the business case proposal can highlight the often poor coordination of psychosocial services related to a lack of clarity of roles and level of psychosocial care required, both within the hospital (emergency department, medical/surgical inpatient units, psychiatry inpatient unit, day hospital, affiliated outpatient clinics) and within the community (other hospitals, children's mental health agencies). The business case proposal may also note that high clinical volumes and limited resources on the CL psychiatry team affect academic productivity and increase the risk for clinician burnout. Finally, the business case proposal should note that the stigma of co-occurring mental and other medical conditions can affect care access within both the general healthcare and mental healthcare systems. Indeed, patients with medical problems may be excluded from general psychiatry clinics.

Data

Clinical volumes, case complexity, response times, wait times, and catchment area should be described. Case examples may be helpful to showcase the need. Children with comorbid mental and other medical illnesses reflect complex/severe presentations and can be time- and resource-intensive, requiring expertise of a CL psychiatry program. With limited resources, a case may be built for ensuring that a CL psychiatry program not be required to also serve patients with general mental health conditions in the absence of an acute medical condition.

Initiatives

Initiatives to improve efficiency and effectiveness through pathways and standardized protocols should be highlighted. Describing the educational productivity can demonstrate the program's reach through capacity-building practice change. Similarly, describing research productivity can highlight the creation of new knowledge. As noted earlier, referencing key contextual factors such as impact on patient safety or finances can build the case.

Costs

Business plans may need to include costs for facilities and technology, including data management and telehealth. Although remuneration from health plans often covers direct patient care, CL psychiatry work requires funding to support indirect patient care, education, and research and funding for interdisciplinary and administrative staff.

Funding

Depending on the country, funding of CL psychiatry programs may be through a combination of some or all of the following: the hospital, the university, research grants, the government, insurance plans, and philanthropy (Shaw et al. 2006; Shaw et al. 2016). Funding may be channeled through the department of psychiatry or through a medical/surgical program or department. The funding source dictates the accountability framework and shapes the program.

As an example, the Medical Psychiatry Alliance (MPA), established in Ontario, Canada, in 2014, is funded over 5 years through a generous private donor, the Ontario government (Ministry of Health and Long-Term Care), and four organizations: The Hospital for Sick Children, the University of Toronto, the Centre for Addiction and Mental Health, and Trillium Health Partners, as well as their associated networks. The aim of the MPA is to transform care for people with physical and mental health conditions through the development of integrated models of care, education, and research (https://www.medpsychalliance.ca/).

Final Reflections

A comprehensive approach to CL psychiatry program development can aid in collaboration within the hospital and among colleagues in the field. Evidence-informed protocols can optimize a number of referrals and increase opportunities for collaborative approaches to complex patient populations. Role clarity is paramount to defining a service delivery model. Utilization of existing psychosocial resources decreases duplication of work and reduces confusion. Community partners are paramount in the continuum of care for CL psychiatry patients, and case management enables coordination with community partners.

It is important to communicate the program's contextualized mandate, as it is developed and as it evolves, and to provide information about referral criteria, service delivery model, staffing, and evidence-informed interprofessional models of care and care pathways. It is also helpful to highlight research, quality improvement, and education efforts. Communication can be maintained via a website. The hospital communications department can also assist.

Model sustainability must be supported through data collection, analysis, and evaluation. Having a developed program and database can help inform service delivery, develop business case proposals, and secure funding.

Interdisciplinary models of care are informed by partnerships: medical/mental health as well as hospital/community (Gordon et al. 2007; Kelly et al. 2002; Martini et al. 2012). The Canadian Institute for Health Information noted that improved coordination between primary care, hospitals, and community agencies may decrease the need for hospitalizations and emergency room visits (Canadian Institute for Health Information 2015). Also, collaboration in patient care promotes interprofessional education. Education, both within the hospital and within the community and school systems, can serve to enhance system capacity for managing patients with medical/mental health needs (Kutcher 2011; Mental Health Commission of Canada 2012).

References

Ahsanuddin, K. M., & Adams, J. E. (1982). Setting up a pediatric consultation-liaison service. *Psychiatric Clinics of North America, 5*(2), 259–270.

Bardach, N. S., Coker, T. R., Zima, B. T., Murphy, J. M., Knapp, P., Richardson, L. P., Edwall, G., & Mangione-Smith, R. (2014). Common and costly hospitalizations for pediatric mental health disorders. *Pediatrics, 133*(4), 602–609.

Bierenbaum, M. L., Katsikas, S., Furr, A., & Carter, B. D. (2013). Factors associated with non-reimbursable activity on an inpatient pediatric consultation–liaison service. *Journal of Clinical Psychology in Medical Settings, 20*, 464–472.

Bujoreanu, S., White, M. T., Gerber, B., & Ibeziako, P. (2015). Effect of timing of psychiatry consultation on length of pediatric hospitalization and hospital charges. *Hospital Pediatrics, 5*(5), 269–275.

Campo, J. V., Kingsley, R. S., Bridge, J., & Mrazek, D. (2000). Child and adolescent psychiatry in general Children's hospitals: A survey of chairs of psychiatry. *Psychosomatics, 41*(2), 128–133.

Canadian Institute for Health Information. (2015). *Care for children and youth with mental disorders*. Ottawa: CIHI.

De Albuquerque Citero, V., De Araujo Andreoli, P. B., Nogueira-Martins, L. A., & Andreoli, S. B. (2008). New potential clinical indicators of consultation-liaison psychiatry's effectiveness in Brazilian general hospitals. *Psychosomatics, 49*, 29–38.

De Souza, C. (2010). Special interest group: Consultation-liaison psychiatry. In scientific proceedings of the 30th annual meeting of the Canadian Academy of the Child and Adolescent Psychiatry. Toronto, ON, Canada.

De Souza, C. (2012). Special interest study group: Pediatric consultation-liaison psychiatry. In scientific proceedings of the 32nd annual meeting of the Canadian Academy of Child and Adolescent Psychiatry. Montreal, QC, Canada.

De Souza, C. (2014) Special interest study group: Pediatric consultation-liaison psychiatry. In scientific proceedings of the 34th annual meeting of the Canadian Academy of Child and Adolescent Psychiatry. Toronto, ON, Canada.

De Souza, C., Pirlot, T., Giles, L., & Pao, M. (2011). Special Interest Study Group: Pediatric consultation-liaison psychiatry. In scientific proceedings of the Joint American and Canadian Academy of Child and Adolescent Psychiatry Annual Meeting. Toronto, ON Canada.

De Souza, C., Pirlot, T. Giles, L., & Pao, M. (2012). Special Interest Study Group: Pediatric consultation-liaison psychiatry. In scientific proceedings of the 59th annual meeting of the American Academy of Child and Adolescent Psychiatry. San Francisco, CA, USA.

De Souza, C., Pirlot, T., Russell, R., Gandy, H. & Saran, K. (2013). Special interest study group: Pediatric consultation-liaison psychiatry. In scientific proceedings of the 33rd annual meeting of the Canadian Academy of Child and Adolescent Psychiatry. Vancouver, BC, Canada.

De Souza, C., Pirlot, T., Giles, L., Silver, G., & Pao, M. (2013b). Special interest study group: Pediatric consultation-liaison psychiatry. In scientific proceedings of the 60th annual meeting of the American Academy of Child and Adolescent Psychiatry. Orlando, FL ,USA.

De Souza, C., Pirlot, T., Giles, L., Silver, G., & Rackley, S. (2014). Special interest study group: Pediatric consultation-liaison psychiatry. In scientific proceedings of the 61st annual meeting of the American Academy of Child and Adolescent Psychiatry. San Diego, CA, USA.

De Souza, C., Rackley, S., Giles L, Pirlot, T., & Silver, G. (2015). Special interest study group: Pediatric consultation-liaison psychiatry. In scientific proceedings of the 62nd annual meeting of the American Academy of Child and Adolescent Psychiatry. San Antonio, TX, USA.

De Souza, C., Russell, R., Cohen, J., & Anang, P. (2016). Special interest study group: Pediatric consultation-liaison psychiatry. In scientific proceedings of the 22nd annual meeting of the International Association for Child and Adolescent Psychiatry and Allied Professions World Congress. Calgary, AB, Canada.

DeMaso, D. R., & Meyer, E. C. (1996). A psychiatric consultant's survival guide to the pediatric intensive care unit. *JAACAP, 34*(10), 1411–1413.

DeMaso, D. R., Martini, D., Cahen, L., et al. (2009). Practice parameter for the psychiatric assessment and management of physically ill children and adolescents. *JAACAP, 48*(2), 212–233
Desan, P. H., Zimbrean, P. C., Weinstein, A. J., Bozzo, J. E., & Sledge, W. H. (2011). Proactive psychiatric consultation services reduce length of stay for admissions to an inpatient medical team. *Psychosomatics, 52*, 513–520.
Dosa, N., Boeing, N., Ms, N., & Kanter, R. (2001). Excess risk of severe acute illness in children with chronic health conditions. *Pediatrics, 107*(3), 499–504.
Doupnik, S. K., Lawlor, J., Zima, B. T., Coker, T. R., Bardach, N. S., Hall, M., & Berry, J. G. (2016). Mental health conditions and medical and surgical hospital utilization. *Pediatrics, 138*(6), e20162416–e20162416.
Ellen, S., Lacey, C., Kouzma, N., Sauvey, N., & Carroll, R. (2006). Data collection in consultation-liaison psychiatry: An evaluation of Casemix. *Australasian Psychiatry, 14*(1).
Frank, J. R., Snell, L., & Sherbino, J. (Eds.). (2015). *CanMEDS 2015 physician competency framework*. Ottawa: Royal College of Physicians and Surgeons of Canada.
Goldman, L., Lee, T., & Rudd, P. (1983). Ten commandments for effective consultations. *Archives of Internal Medicine, 143*(9), 1753–1755.
Gordon, J., Colby, H., Bartelt, T., Jablonski, D., Krauthoefer, M., & Havens, P. (2007). A tertiary care-primary care partnership model for medically complex and fragile children and youth with special health care needs. *Archives of Pediatrics & Adolescent Medicine, 161*(10), 937–944.
Harden, et al. (2005). Redevelopment of a CL service at a tertiary pediatric hospital. *Australasian Psychiatry, 13*(2), 169–172.
Heinrich, T. W., Schwartz, A. C., Zimbrean, P. C., Lolak, S., Wright, M. T., Brooks, K. B., Ernst, C. L., & Gitlin, D. F. (2014). Recommendations for training psychiatry residents in psychosomatic medicine. *Psychosomatics, 55*, 438–449.
Holmes, A., Handrinos, D., Theologus, E., & Salzberg, M. (2011). Service use in consultation-liaison psychiatry: Guidelines for baseline staffing. *Australasian Psychiatry, 19*(3), 254.
Huyse, F. J., Lyons, J. S., Zwaan, T., Strain, J. J., Rijssenbeek, A. J. M. M., Herzog, T., & Malzu, U. F. (1992). Audit in C-L psychiatry. *International Review of Psychiatry, 4*, 5–14.
Kelly, A. M., Kratz, B., Bielski, M., & Rhinehart, P. M. (2002). Implementing transitions for youth with complex chronic conditions using the medical home model. *Pediatrics, 110*(6), 1322–1327.
Kishi, Y., Meller, W. H., Kathol, R. G., & Swigart, S. E. (2004). Factors affecting the relationship between the timing of psychiatric consultation and general hospital length of stay. *Psychosomatics, 45*, 470–476.
Kitts, R. L., Gallagher, K., Ibeziako, P., Bujoreanu, S., Garcia, G., & DeMaso, D. R. (2013). Parent and young adult satisfaction with psychiatry consultation services in a children's hospital. *Psychosomatics, 54*(6), 575–584.
Knapp, K., & Harris, E. (1998a). Consultation-liaison in child psychiatry: A review of the past 10 years. Part 1: Clinical findings. *JAACAP, 37*(1), 17–25.
Knapp, P. K., & Harris, E. (1998b). Consultation-liaison in child psychiatry: A review of the past 10 years. Part II: Research on treatment approaches and outcomes. *JAACAP, 37*(2), 139–146.
Kunkel, E. J. S., del Busto, E., Kathol, R., Stern, T. A., Wise, T. N., Stoddard, F. R., Straus, J., Saravay, S. M., Muskin, P. R., Dresner, N., Harrington, C. J., Weiner, J., Barnhill, J., Becker, M., Joseph, R. C., Oyesanmi, O., Fann, J. R., Colon, E., Epstein, S., & Weinrieb, R. (2010). Physician staffing for the practice of psychosomatic medicine in general hospitals: A pilot study. *Psychosomatics, 51*, 520–527.
Kutcher, S. (2011). Facing the challenge of care for child and youth mental health in Canada: A critical commentary, five suggestions for change and a call to action. *Healthcare Quarterly, 14*, 14–21.
Leentjens, A. F. G., Boenink, A. D., & van der Feltz-Cornelis, C. M. (2010). Can we increase adherence to treatment recommendations of the consultation psychiatrist working in a general hospital? A systemic review. *Journal of Psychosomatic Research, 68*, 303–309.
Leentjens, A. F. G., Rundell, J. R., Diefenbacher, A., Kathol, R., & Guthrie, E. (2011). Psychosomatic medicine and consultation-liaison psychiatry: scope of practice, processes, and

competencies for psychiatrists or psychosomatic medicine specialists. *Psychosomatics, 52*(1), 19–25.

Lorenz, J. (2000). Survival of the extremely preterm infant in North America in the 1990s. *Clinics in Perinatology, 27*(2), 255–262.

Lyne, J., Hill, M., Burke, P., & Ryan, M. (2009). Audit of an inpatient liaison psychiatry consultation service. *International Journal of Health Care Quality Assurance, 22*(3), 278–288.

Martini, R., Hilt, R., Marx, L., Chenven, M., Naylor, M., Sarvet, B., et al. (2012). *Best Principles for Integration of Child Psychiatry into the Pediatric Health Home*. AACAP.

Matlow, A., Wright, J., Zimmerman, B., Thomson, K., & Valente, M. (2006). How can the principles of complexity science be applied to improve the coordination of care for complex pediatric patients? *Quality & Safety in Health Care, 15*(2), 85–88.

Mental Health Commission of Canada. (2012). *Changing directions changing lives: The mental health strategy for Canada*. Calgary: Mental Health Commission of Canada.

Merikangas, K. R., Calkins, M. E., Burstein, M., He, J. P., Chiavacci, R., Lateef, T., Ruparel, K., Gur, R. C., Lehner, T., Hakonarson, H., & Gur, R. E. (2015 Apr). Comorbidity of physical and mental disorders in the neurodevelopmental genomics cohort study. *Pediatrics, 135*(4), e927–e938.

O'Keefe, N., Ramaiah, U. S., Nomani, E., Fitzpatrick, M., & Ranjith, G. (2007). Benchmarking a liaison psychiatry service: A prospective 6 month study of quality indicators. *Psychiatric Bulletin, 31*, 345–347.

Richardson, D., Calder, L., Dean, H., Glover Takahashi, S., Lebel, P., Maniate, J., Martin, D., Nasmith, L., Newton, C., & Steinert, Y. (2014). *The CanMEDS 2015 collaborator expert working group report*. The Royal College of Physicians and Surgeons of Canada: Ottawa.

Shaw, R. J., & DeMaso, D. R. (2006). *Clinical manual of pediatric psychosomatic medicine – Mental health consultation with physically ill children and adolescents*. Washington, DC: American Psychiatric Publishing.

Shaw, R. J., Wamboldt, M., Bursch, B., & Stuber, M. (2006). Practice patterns in pediatric consultation–liaison psychiatry: A National Survey. *Psychosomatics, 47*, 43–49.

Shaw, R. J., Pao, M., Holland, J. E., & DeMaso, D. R. (2016). Practice patterns revisited in pediatric psychosomatic medicine. *Psychosomatics, 57*(6), 576–585.

Shugart, M. A. (1991). Child psychiatry consultations to pediatric inpatients: A literature review. *General Hospital Psychiatry, 13*, 325–336.

Solomons, L. C., Thachil, A., Burgess, C., Hopper, A., Glen-Day, V., Ranjith, G., & Hodgkiss, A. (2011). Quality of psychiatric care in the general hospital: Referrer perceptions of an inpatient liaison psychiatry service. *General Hospital Psychiatry, 33*, 260–266.

Srivastava, R., Stone, B., & Murphy, N. (2005). Hospitalist care of the medically complex child. *Pediatric Clinics of North America, 52*, 1165–1187.

Stern, A., & Markel, H. (2002). *Formative years: Children's health in the United States, 1880–2000*. Ann Arbor: University of Michigan Press.

Trauer, T. (2004). Use of a routine outcome measure in a consultation-liaison mental health service. *Australasian Psychiatry, 12*(2), 139.

Williams, J., & DeMaso, D. R. (2000). Pediatric team meetings: The mental health Consultant's role. *Clinical Child Psychology and Psychiatry, 5*(1), 105–113.

Additional Readings

Kutcher, S., & McLuckie, A. for the Child and Youth Advisory Committee, Mental Health Commission of Canada. (2010). *Evergreen: A child and youth mental health framework for Canada*. Calgary: Mental Health Commission of Canada.

Shaw, R. J., & DeMaso, D. R. (2010). *Textbook of pediatric psychosomatic medicine*. Washington, DC: American Psychiatric Publishing.

Chapter 17
Patient Experience, Safety, and Quality

Tyler Pirlot and Eden McCaffrey

Introduction: The Value of the Psychosomatic Model

With awareness of the significant morbidity and mortality associated with medical error, and of how poorly healthcare has compared with other service industries in terms of customers' experience, there has been a growth, over the past two decades, in initiatives to improve patient safety, quality of care/quality of service, and patient experience. In this context, we believe that pediatric psychosomatic medicine plays an indispensable role in simultaneously promoting these three important and closely related aspects of healthcare, not just for somatic symptom disorders, which classically are associated with psychosomatic medicine, but for all clinical situations.

Consider the following case vignette:

Vignette 17.1

At 3:30 P.M. on a Friday, a pediatrician from an inpatient unit of a children's hospital contacts the on-call psychiatrist about a well-known patient who had been admitted for 4 weeks. The patient, a 14-year-old female, had been extensively worked up, with consultation and investigations from other health areas, without any positive findings and without progress. Initially presenting with gastrointestinal concerns, the patient has had morphing somatic symptoms and has become wheelchair bound. During the preceding 4 weeks while in hospital, the psychiatry team attempted to manage the case via *a purely consultative role, to no avail, as multiple services, agencies, and professionals have been called in at various times with no*

T. Pirlot (✉)
Alberta Health Services, Edmonton, AB, Canada

University of Calgary, Calgary, AB, Canada
e-mail: tyler.pirlot@ahs.ca

E. McCaffrey
Alberta Health Services, Edmonton, AB, Canada
e-mail: eden.mccaffrey@ahs.ca

A. P. S. Guerrero et al. (eds.), *Pediatric Consultation-Liaison Psychiatry*,
https://doi.org/10.1007/978-3-319-89488-1_17

cohesive plan in place. Further complicating the case, the other health professionals, who suspected that the patient's parents were perpetuating the symptoms, called Children's Protective Services. The parents are dumbfounded that the doctors cannot explain why their daughter is in a wheelchair and are now threatening lawsuits in view of the patient's lack of progress and their perception that the doctors have "found nothing!" The pediatrician, citing the "expense" and "waste of a bed" on a medical unit, is now demanding that the consulting psychiatrist take over the care of the patient and move the patient to a psychiatric unit, and the conversation between the two professionals devolves into threats and screaming.

What led to this high conflict situation between the family and the healthcare system?
What led to this high conflict situation between systems and healthcare providers?
What led to this poor outcome for the patient?
Why was this admission viewed as unsuccessful and/or an inefficient use of healthcare resources?
Why would a consulting psychiatrist refuse admission to a mental health unit?
Why did the parents think that they found "nothing," when in fact everyone knew that the patient had mental distress?
Why the urgency on the part of the pediatrician after the patient had been in hospital for 4 weeks?

The global shift in disease patterns toward chronic diseases and the substantial public health impact of mental disorders together imply that there can be no health without mental health (Prince et al. 2007). During the twentieth century, there has been an emerging epidemiological transition, whereby chronic noncommunicable illnesses, rather than acute infectious diseases, are the most significant causes of mortality globally (Bauer et al. 2011). Further, chronic illness accounts for almost 80% of health expenditures (Bodenheimer et al. 2002). It has been during this same period that the proliferation of the biopsychosocial (BPS) model across clinical and theoretical research has shown biopsychosocial mechanisms to be preluding, causal to, coexisting with, or consequences of many medical conditions. With this, medicine is globally becoming, and will further evolve into, an integrated science. Fassino (2010) argues that human illness and health may be better understood if all medical disciplines are considered as a whole, working in collaboration. Just as we all have health, we humans all have mental health; the mind is one part of the body and works together with the various systems to function. This perspective is supported by increasing evidence that care of a person's mental health is essential for effective care of the body (Huffman et al. 2014). As such, global healthcare resources are being challenged to address the connections between mental health and other medical disorders. It is in addressing these challenges that the field of psychosomatic medicine, home to the theoretical tradition of the BPS model, is especially well-suited to lead (Prince et al. 2007).

There is increasing awareness of the disease-oriented healthcare approach's limitations, which have paved the way for patients to become "consumers" of healthcare and which have created an opportunity for patients to work in partnership with their healthcare providers (Leventhal et al. 2008). This patient-centered and partnered humanistic approach to healthcare strives to understand how patients experience their care as a means of better supporting their healing. Despite this approach, stigma and discrimination in mental health are global concerns. A study looking at stigma in pediatric psychiatry found that three quarters of children struggling with mental health are not diagnosed, and of those diagnosed, only about a quarter of those children receive treatment (Pescosolido et al. 2008). Furthermore, a recent exploration of healthcare utilization patterns reveals a very serious system-based stigma, whereby pediatric patients with identified psychiatric disorders suffer systemic consequences when utilizing health services for other medical disorders (Ghuttora and Cawthorpe 2013). Stigma pertaining to mental health permeates our society globally across personal, professional, and even institutional operations, which has negative ramifications on patient experience and safety. The above case illustrates how stigma toward patients with psychiatric conditions can adversely impact the healthcare team's engagement with the patient and family, the overall quality and safety of healthcare, and ultimately the patient and family's experience of care.

Consider that in the general medical setting, as many as 30% of patients have a psychiatric disorder (Bronheim et al. 1998) and that medically unexplained symptoms, often referred to or known as somatic symptoms, occur in up to 30–40% of medical patients (Kroenke 2002). It is in caring for these patients where psychosomatic medicine is well positioned to advance global healthcare by tackling critical needs related to resources and stigma. The primary goal of psychosomatic medicine is to correct the disease-oriented approach in healthcare by incorporating advanced strategies into clinical practice. Psychosomatic medicine addresses globally emerging healthcare needs through: (1) the holistic approach to patient management that acknowledges and incorporates the psychosocial factors and (2) the clinical reasoning mode that reflects a multifactorial frame of reference (Fava et al. 2016). Bauer et al. (2011) emphasize that psychosomatic medicine extends beyond psychiatric management to include knowledge of the individual, cultural, and contextual factors that interact with a wide array of behavioral contributors to health. This humanistic approach is rooted in the BPS model and improves healthcare quality and outcomes.

Quality healthcare is comprised of three important areas: (1) patient experience, (2) clinical effectiveness, and (3) patient safety (Doyle et al. 2013). The current status quo of segregated care systems, which perpetuates stigma and discrimination, renders poor outcomes with regard to patient experience, safety, and quality. While an entire textbook could be devoted to this topic, this chapter will look at this topic in more detail and highlight the need to embody and actualize the principles and theory of psychosomatic medicine into clinical practice. To date, this translation into practice is still lacking, but if we move forward in this direction, the psychosomatic approach can improve quality of care across all health systems globally.

Reflecting upon the opening illustrative vignette (17.1), this chapter aims to answer the questions posed by systematically reviewing the concepts of patient experience, patient safety, and patient quality and subsequently proposing a more effective, efficient, and ethical psychosomatic approach to these cases that will reduce and even eliminate the current and ongoing dysfunctional dynamics.

Defining the Patient in Pediatric Psychosomatic Medicine

Prior to looking at patient experience, safety, and quality, it is imperative to define the patient in pediatric psychosomatic medicine. Rask et al. (2010) noted a relative scarcity of literature characterizing the services and clients seen in pediatric psychosomatic medicine. This scarcity is understandable because, contrary to other areas of medicine where the patient is the individual presenting with a medical condition, in pediatric psychosomatic medicine, the "identified patient" is expansive and requires consideration of the unique situation. In efforts to integrate a developmentally informed BPS formulation of the *identified patient* in pediatric psychosomatic medicine, one must consider that the individual child receiving healthcare services inherently presents with an array of both biological and social aspects, including the family and healthcare providers that comprise the child's larger social environment and the biological and psychological factors associated with the child's development. In defining that a "patient" is the recipient of healthcare services delivered through a BPS approach, the patient in pediatric psychosomatic encompasses:

1. The individual child/adolescent.
2. The family.
3. The primary healthcare providers.

Each of these three presents with factors worthy of consideration. Without understanding the unique aspects specific to this patient population, problems with regard to ethics (i.e., engagement, effectiveness, and experience) and efficiency (i.e., role confusion) occur.

Acknowledging that psychosomatic medicine explores the relationship between comorbid psychiatric and other medical conditions (Shaw and DeMaso 2007), the complexity of "the patient" continues to unfold. Unlike a cardiologist, specializing in the cardiovascular system, psychosomatic medicine encounters patients experiencing difficulties across all systems of the body and embraces the interaction of the psyche and the soma. In sharp contrast to the medical model view of the patient in their medical "silo," psychosomatic medicine moves away from the "chicken or the egg" paradox, which only serves to increase stigma, and explores the relationship between systems (Shaw and DeMaso 2007). The psychosomatic approach to illness classifications is integrative (see Fig. 17.1) and considers the multitude of BPS factors affecting vulnerability to, course of, and outcome of any type of illness a patient may have. The chart below offers examples of the interplay between BSP factors that ought to be considered in identifying the pediatric psychosomatic patient (see Fig. 17.2). Additionally, the context of the illness and the context of the experiences need to be considered in pediatric psychosomatic medicine patients. For example, while Crohn's disease may not be acute, the unpredictable and relapsing nature may arguably cause the patient long-standing and great distress (see Fig. 17.3).

Global Issues for Health Systems	Psychosomatic Solutions
Disease oriented approach	**BPS approach**
Chronic and Costly	**Integrated and Humanistic**
Acute and Urgent	**Process and Partnership-focused**
Discriminatory	**Collaborative**
Stigmatizing	**Holistic, mind and body integrated**

Fig. 17.1 Psychosomatic solutions for current global health issues

By considering the illness-specific factors to a diagnosis, the psychosomatic approach to patients reduces risk for over-pathologizing and iatrogenic harm inherent in the current disease-oriented approach (Fava et al. 2012). Rather than dangerously assuming that, if other medical conditions cannot explain the presentation, there must be a psychiatric illness, psychosomatic medicine patients are viewed not only by their symptoms and illness classification but by the potential interplay between the psyche and the soma. As such, in considering the patient in psychosomatic medicine, one must be mindful of the various unique patient factors and consider a broader view of illness-specific factors. It is within this definition and understanding of the pediatric psychosomatic patient where we see improved patient experience, patient safety, and quality of care.

With the initial case vignette in mind (17.1), we propose that the outcome could have been much different had the primary medical team and psychiatry teams applied the psychosomatic model from the beginning of the admission and considered the described patient factors, with early involvement of psychiatric liaison (not just consultation); regular collaborative rounding to discuss, fine-tune, and share (with the patient and family) a working biopsychosocial formulation and a mutual commitment (without trying to "turf" from one specialty to the other) to improving the patient's well-being and functioning; and psychiatrically informed intervention for dysfunctional team dynamics (e.g., threats and screaming) that are not clearly conducive to thoughtful and safe patient care.

Patient Experience in Pediatric Psychosomatic Medicine

Vignette 17.2

One month following a sports injury incurred during a rugby match, a 13-year-old male is admitted to the hospital for unexplained chest pain and weakness. During a lengthy inpatient stay, the child has an extensive medical work-up. Following consultations from neurology, complex pain management, and physical medicine and rehabilitation, the inpatient pediatrician discharges the patient and tells him and

The Patient	Key Unique Aspects of this Patient Population
Individual child/ adolescent	• Pediatric patients often do not request mental health assistance and areoften not aware that psychiatric involvementis being requested by their primary health provider. • Stigma perpetuated by archaic medical models and societal myths are problematic and when psychiatry becomes involved, the individual may feel like they are a "bad patient", that they are disbelieved, and/or that the problems are 'all in their head'(Griffin & Christie, 2008). • Developmental stages affect a child's understanding of illness. It is developmentally abnormal to incorporate health and illness into a child'sidentity and illness-based management is at odds with normal development (Holmbeck, 2002). • Children, compared with adults, tend to be more naïve and trusting of "authority figures" and are more concrete and literal in their thinking and expression (Caplan et al., 2013). • For a child, admission to the hospital can be a traumatic experience and can isolate them from their typical environments, inclusive of friends and family and school (Ortiz, 1997). • A wide variety of reactions and symptoms can occur during and following hospitalization (Graham, 1991). • The child's age; personality; temperament; and language, cognitive and emotional development all need to be considered in assessment and treatment formulations. • Illness-specific factors must be considered within the pediatric developmental context. For example, static, chronic illness may leave a child feeling over-controlled, while a chronically relapsing illness can worsen magical thinking (i.e., that the illness has 'disappeared'in between episodes) • Somatic symptoms may cause the child iatrogenic harm through unnecessary testing and/or treatment. If BPS factors are not thoroughly considered, there is potential negative impact on patient experience, safety and quality of care.
Family	• The family often presents seeking medical explanations for symptoms. Due to stigma, they hold preconceived notions, perceptions and beliefs related to psychiatric services and are in turn surprised by and/or resistant to the introduction of psychiatric services. • Families are often unaware of psychiatric resources and may feel angry, blamed, and invalidated when psychiatry and/or psychosomatic medicine is introduced (Hardwick, 2005). • The family provides both genetic and environmental contributions. • Parents are interlocutors of children (especially young children) in both sickness and health (Ortiz, 1997; Bingley et al., 1980). • Family involvement renders better outcomes in pediatrics (Heru, 2006). • Family involvement in illness management evolves in tandem with the child's increasing cognitive sophistication which may also bring forth issues related to privacy, trust, control and acceptance (Holmbeck, 2002). • "Medical Parenting" (i.e., through guilt, control, and restriction) is associated with higher levels of problem behaviors for the child (Logan et al., 2002).
Primary Health Care Providers	• Psychosomatic medicine services include consultation and liaison with other healthcare providers, who in turn may be the intended beneficiaries of this psychiatric involvement (Bronheim et al., 1998). • Primary health care providers may not have informed their patient that they would be consulting with psychiatry. • When patients have atypical symptom presentations or somatic symptoms accompanying a known illness, primary health care providers may feel at a loss, and consult psychiatry out of the "righting reflex" (the need to fix every problem encountered in clinical practice)

Fig. 17.2 Patient aspects to consider in pediatric psychosomatic medicine

the family that the medical investigations found "nothing," and therefore the discharge diagnoses is "conversion disorder." The discharge plan is for the family to see their community primary care provider if necessary and refers them for mental health services. Following discharge, the child and his family, frustrated with their care, discontinue services with all healthcare providers. The boy's symptoms persist and his impairment prevents him from engaging in social and academic activities. Very sadly, the child completes suicide 8 months later.

	ACUTE PRESENTATION	NON-ACUTE PRESENTATION
INTERMITTENT COURSE	Usually presents with acute symptoms and is diagnosed in an acute context; however, course is unpredictable and potentially episodic *(i.e. Acute Lymphoblastic Leukemia)*	May not present with acute symptoms or be diagnosed in an acute context; however, the illness can be unpredictable and intermittent even with optimal management and adherence *(i.e., Crohn's Disease)*
CHRONIC COURSE	Medical symptoms are persistent but unexplained, with a sense of acuity. *(i.e., Somatic Symptom Disorder)*	May not present with acute symptoms or be diagnosed in an acute context; and symptom presentation and management are chronic and generally predictable. *(i.e., Non-Insulin Dependent Diabetes)*

Fig. 17.3 Illness-specific factors across subspecialty clinics

Although recognition of the mind-body interaction dates from antiquity, it has only been in modern times that a vocabulary to conceptualize its manifestations has arisen. With these developments came the notion of *psychosomatic disorders*, which is how all psychiatric disorders were initially conceptualized in the *Diagnostic and Statistical Manual of Mental Disorders* (DSM) (Oken 2007). Patients experiencing serious symptoms dread the possibility of having a devastating diagnosis and hope that the problem is trivial or at least treatable. The individual's reaction depends on many factors (i.e., temperament, coping abilities, underlying assumptions and beliefs). Patients may either face head-on ("fight") or avoid/deny ("flight") the potential diagnosis. This reaction applies to both somatic symptom disorders and other medical conditions; however, patients with the former may experience not only dread but also fear that undecipherable symptoms may be attributed to being "all in one's head" because of the pervasive stigma surrounding mental illness (Atkins and Hodges 2010).

These poorly disguised judgments that often accompany the communication of the psychosomatic opinion reveal our societies' continued conceptual separation of mind and body and the ongoing stigmatization of mental health. Psychological and biological factors are involved in all aspects of human function, healthy or disordered; therefore, all health and disease states are psychosomatic. Under current practices, however, affect and emotions are not considered in relation to medical illness, and this shortcoming has very serious negative ramifications on the patient experience. Vignette 17.2 highlights this point all too well, with negative impact on all three identifiable "patients."

Individual Patient Experience

When a patient's report of symptom severity and characteristics does not match the healthcare provider expectations, the provider may doubt the validity of the reports and may feel challenged to arrive at a specific diagnosis. When no diagnosis is apparent, the medical care provider may hope that involving psychiatry will reassure the patient and the family that the problem is not medically serious and facilitate access to continued psychiatric care. Often, however, neither of these goals is accomplished. Patients report that the process of moving from medical illness identification to psychosomatic medicine brings forth new and serious problems, including stigmatization, undermining of personal identity, and worsening of symptoms (Atkins and Hodges 2010).

Compared with adults, children are developmentally more concrete, less verbally expressive, and more likely to speak in terms of symptoms associated with illnesses that they have identified with than in terms of abstract feelings. For example, the patient described in Vignette 17.2 may be more likely to report chronic chest pain as opposed to palpitations triggered by performance anxiety and panic. As such, the patient typically receives a detailed medical work-up and often experiences distress, fear, and vulnerability related to this illness identification. At times, they may even be isolated from others during hospital admissions and tests.

Children are very trusting of those in positions of power, and when the illness that they are identifying with is invalidated, there is a strong message that they are disbelieved. It is easy for patients to feel dismissed by care providers and worried that their concerns are not being taken seriously. This embarrassing and isolating experience is often expressed as anger and a sense of entitlement (Campo and Fritz 2001). These experiences make it extremely difficult to reassure the concerned child, who in turn becomes very mistrusting of the healthcare professionals. Pediatric psychosomatic medicine patients often describe their experience as being both frightening and humiliating.

Family Experience

Childhood illness confronts the whole family with threats and uncertainties that undermine parents' inherent role in caring for their child's biological needs and providing support, guidance, and safety. Uncertainty can lead to fear and worry in the parents, who are expected to model effective coping and hope. As parents try to navigate this uncertainty, they often feel unfairly judged and scrutinized. These feelings may confound their own judgment as parents (Campo and Fritz 2001).

Parents' experience can be improved by anticipating and considering parental expectations. When parents present their child to health professionals, they expect their child to be assessed, diagnosed, and treated, and they expect an experience similar to taking a car to a mechanic (Hardwick 2005). Some parents do not expect to be asked psychosocial questions and may feel dismissed or blamed if these questions are asked. Parents often come with self-judgments and with feelings of defeat and self-blame. For example, in a genetic illness like cystic fibrosis, parents already experience guilt over the possibility of their own contribution; they may then feel that any new symptoms are "another thing," possibly associated with social stigma, that they may have to confront and feel responsible for.

Following the inevitable grieving over the loss of their "normal" child, parents may alter their identity to encompass the sick role and the need to act as part of the care team, assisting in treatment and advocating for their child. Parents may be deeply entrenched into this role as their lifestyle has been altered. Further, parents may balance their losses related to caregiving (i.e., with regard to career advancement, social, economic), with relatively few gains (i.e., extra support, family unity) Globally, society holds the discriminatory premise that symptoms are only genuine and worthy of parents' care if "physically" caused and that mental health problems represent moral weakness. As such, parents may be reluctant to accept psychological components to the formulation and may be reluctant to reach out for social support. They may feel confused, isolated, frustrated, and humiliated (Andrews and Istvanffy 2011).

Healthcare Providers' Experience

Almost half of all primary care visits are for several common "physical" symptoms, which, when studied over a 1-year period, are only explained by other medical illness 10% of the time (Katon and Walker 1998). Symptoms are currency for attention and interaction with healthcare providers, who often feel pressured, in their rushed schedule, to act on these symptoms and to offer more investigations. They may feel anxious about wrongfully or belatedly diagnosing a patient and may feel unable to express formulations that incorporate the psychosocial experience. Unfortunately, this approach – rather than thoughtfully incorporating psychosocial aspects into the formulation – entrenches the medicalization of the patient and the patient's family's medical view (Hardwick 2005) and leads the provider to feel "damned if I do and damned if I don't" and more challenged in caring for patients in psychosomatic medicine.

Another important part of the healthcare providers' experience is related to the intensity of working with children and adolescents. Pediatric work requires maintaining good boundaries while facilitating working relationships. The intense feelings provoked by medically ill children's regression and their families' anxiety may lead to either over-involvement or emotional distancing (Ortiz 1997). These reactions, along with transference and countertransference, may then lead to internal conflicts and confusion among healthcare providers, as illustrated in Vignette 17.1. Without insight into these dynamics, healthcare providers may be compromised in their ability to provide safe, quality patient care. This is inline with what is stated by McCaffrey and colleagues (2017) that "the gaps between perceived, actual and ideal performance in healthcare are real" (p.123).

Reflecting on Vignette 17.2, we believe that the patient and family would have been more likely to follow up with recommended care if they had a better experience during the hospitalization. Applying the psychosomatic model described in the previous section, the team could have empathized more effectively with the patient and the family, comprehensively managed and "owned" the patient as an emotionally insightful and well-functioning team, and insured continuity of the psychosomatic model in outpatient follow-up (e.g., via an integrated primary care/behavioral health team further described in Chap. 18). As this vignette illustrates, poor patient experience can lead not only to low satisfaction ratings or unreturned survey forms but also to potentially preventable tragic outcomes. Indeed, the combination of feeling invalidated, hopeless, and isolated and the lack of appropriate follow-up care were likely important risk factors for suicide and/or serious psychiatric disturbance in this patient. Ineffective engagement often associated with feelings of shame and stigma, likely, further increased the suicide risk (Berg et al. 2017).

Patient Safety in Pediatric Psychosomatic Medicine

Vignette 17.3

Over a 2-year span, an outpatient primary care provider refers a 13-year-old female with chronic and complex pain for consultation with musculoskeletal specialists, a neurologist, pain management services, and eventually a psychiatrist. Ultimately, she is diagnosed with somatic symptom disorder and generalized anxiety, for which psychosocial interventions are recommended. The family opts not to engage in these interventions and instead continues their own research into other potential medical etiologies. They even leave the country for ongoing assessments. Upon returning from abroad, the patient/family requests that the primary care provider start the child on an opioid pain medication. The primary care provider agrees, despite knowing there is no evidence to support opioid use and that this is against the psychiatrist's advice. Over time, the child develops tolerance, and the medication is increased. One year later, the child, very unfortunately, dies via *an accidental overdose.*

Patient safety is an issue for all counties that deliver healthcare services. Healthcare systems are products of the society and culture wherein they evolve, and to the degree that the culture stigmatizes psychiatric illness and psychosocial adversities, stigma will adversely impact not only patient experience but also patient safety and well-being. Traditionally, patient safety has focused on mitigating adverse events associated with physiological harm. In mental health, these events obviously include self-harm, suicide, and violence toward staff and other patients. Following the psychosomatic model, and recalling the missed opportunities for earlier intervention in Vignette 17.3, we propose that there is a genuine need to redefine patient safety in the context of the BPS approach. We support a preliminary framework for evaluating patient safety and patient harm in pediatric psychosomatic medicine: this framework includes not only traditionally defined and retrospectively

	Definitions and examples	Metrics
Adverse Events	Attempted or completed suicide Violent events)	• Suicide rate • Frequency of security activations
Ineffective Treatment	No improvement in function over what would have been achieved without intervention.	• % of cases where guidelines exist but are not being followed • % of cases on waiting lists outside of target times
Ineffective Engagement	Patient terminating contact with service providers prior to receiving necessary and or recommended intervention.	• Drop-out rate

Fig. 17.4 Patient safety framework with defined classifications of harm and metrics to monitor. (Adapted from Wolpert et al. 2015)

monitored adverse events but also metrics to proactively monitor effectiveness of engagement and treatment (Wolpert et al. 2015) (Fig. 17.4).

It has been said that having a psychological label is an early warning sign of trouble ahead for the patient (Atkins and Hodges 2010). In Canada, only 4.8% of the health budget is allocated to and spent on mental health services (Ghuttora and Cawthorpe 2013). Prospective population studies substantiate the role of support and resources in relation to mortality, psychiatric, and other comorbidity and adjustment to and recovery from chronic illness (Fava et al. 2012). While most global systems mean well, inadequate investment into mental healthcare directly and indirectly causes physical, mental, and emotional harm. Compared with other patients, patients in psychosomatic medicine are at higher risk of harm because of discrimination bias and the inadequacy of resources available to them, their families, and their healthcare providers.

Because of the value of the psychosomatic model in appropriately identifying quality and safety metrics and in identifying important BPS factors in vulnerable patients (e.g., with psychiatric comorbidities), we propose that consultation-liaison psychiatrists should be regular members of healthcare teams tasked with insuring the safety and quality of care for patients – not just with somatic symptom disorders (as illustrated in the vignettes thus far) but other medical conditions as well.

Individual and Family Perspective

Patients with psychological disturbances generally use medical care more frequently, stay in the hospital longer, and are more likely to be readmitted (Bronheim et al. 1998). However, studies show that children with psychiatric disorders (in comparison with those without) are also at risk of receiving inequitably less care for other medical disorders, rendering them at higher risk for adverse events, ineffective engagement (illustrated by Vignette 17.2), and ineffective treatment (illustrated by Vignette 17.3) (Ghuttora and Cawthorpe 2013). Furthermore, with non-psychosomatically informed treatment, children with psychiatric conditions may be at risk for iatrogenic harm caused by unnecessary or improper investigations and treatments.

Vignette 17.4
The mother of an 11-year-old female with type 1 diabetes frequently presented to the primary care provider for various symptoms and impairments unrelated to the diabetes. Over a 4-year period, the child underwent a multitude of investigations, mostly prompted by the mother's insistence as well as the primary care provider's desire to provide reassurance. Years later, the child was diagnosed with a type of cancer thought to be caused by iatrogenic radiation exposure.

For patients who become entrenched in the sick role, further medicalization carries risk for side effects, trauma, and even death. Professionals, unsure of what to do for patients/families when the symptoms are unexplained, find themselves writing more prescriptions in efforts to treat the symptoms that in fact are the currency to remain in the sick role. Furthermore, the contemporary obsession with diagnosis under the medical model is partly fueled by fear of litigation, especially with families having easier access to knowledge through the Internet (Campo and Fritz 2001).

Ironically, the risks of unnecessary investigation and/or treatment include further medicalization from side. An unnecessary medical investigation purely to reduce anxiety does not justify the risk associated with adverse events (i.e., radiation exposure).

Healthcare Provider Perspective and Role

Patient safety and healthcare provider safety interact in unique and complex ways. The contemporary obsession with diagnosis under the medical model is partly fueled by fear of litigation as well as the stigma pertaining to mental health that exists globally at professional and institutional levels. With families having easier access to knowledge through the Internet, an overly medically focused view and threats of litigation are becoming more commonplace (Campo and Fritz 2001).

Research indicates that providers have a considerable impact on the rate of patient safety incidents (Wolpert et al. 2015). Mascherek and Schwappach (2016) found several common errors – including communication errors, interface of care errors, structural errors, diagnostic errors, and treatment errors – that increase safety risk in global healthcare systems.

Vignette 17.5
A 16-year-old female was admitted to an inpatient unit at the children's hospital after presenting with unusual and unexplained symptoms. Following a lengthy

medical work-up, the medical teams felt strongly that there was no other medical etiology and that the patient needed to be transferred to a psychiatric unit. The medical team insisted that their safety was being compromised, as the patient was at times very aggressive and unmanageable on a medical unit. However, the psychiatric team insisted with equal vigor that their safety would be compromised if the patient were transferred, given the need for intravenous lines and other medical equipment that they felt would be dangerous to keep on a psychiatric unit. The managers of both units did not want to "set a precedent" in regularly accepting such patients and grew concerned that their "safety scores," routinely measured by hospital administration, would be adversely impacted. For over a month, various professionals argued their positions and even threatened litigation.

The child was subsequently found to have anti-NMDA receptor encephalitis. Challenged by this diagnosis, the healthcare providers committed to working collaboratively in managing the patient on a medical unit with psychiatric consultation and liaison. The patient improved with appropriate treatment and was subsequently discharged. There were no injuries related to patient aggression, and the family expressed – through an inspiring thank you note and a generous gift – their significant gratitude to the hospital.

Additionally, the medical and psychiatric teams committed to creating a task force focused on the optimal management of patients with acute medical and acute psychiatric needs and to conducting collaborative liaison rounds once weekly. They noted that, on both units, several quality and safety measures – as diverse as patient satisfaction, use of restraint and/or seclusion, and staff engagement – all seemed to improve over the next several months.

This vignette illustrates – in addition to the challenge in deciding which medical investigations are necessary for behavioral symptoms (addressed further in Chap 9) – the essential value of the psychosomatic model in creating an environment conducive to safe and high-quality patient care. Unlike the previous vignettes, which ended with a dysfunctional healthcare team and a suboptimal patient outcome, this vignette ended with a team that was unified around treating a condition needing both psychiatric and other medical management of acute symptoms and able to effectively problem-solve around complex safety issues.

Patient Care Quality in Pediatric Psychosomatic Medicine

The greater the gap between the healthcare provider's objectives and the patient's expectations, the larger the potential for negative impact on the patient experience in terms of satisfaction, treatment compliance, treatment outcomes, safety, and overall quality. As quality in healthcare is comprised of three distinct components (experience, safety, and clinical effectiveness) (Doyle et al. 2013), we propose that these be regarded as the three necessary pillars to support patient care quality (Fig. 17.5).

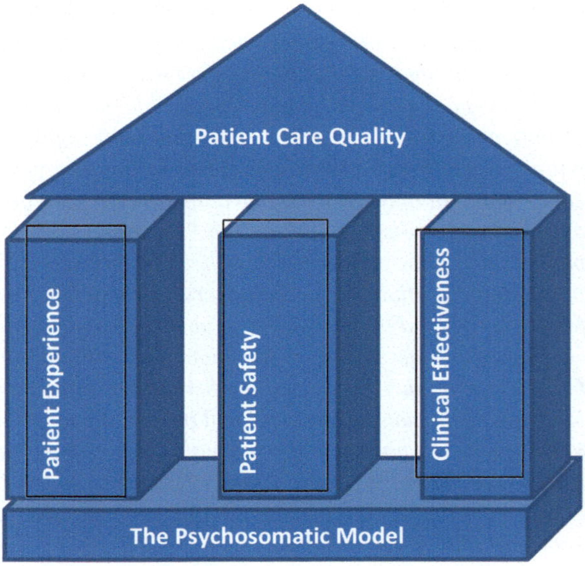

Fig. 17.5 The three pillars and foundation to support patient care quality in pediatric psychosomatic medicine

Research has identified a correlation between somatic symptoms and impaired health, indicated by increased use of care, unnecessary diagnostic procedures and non-indicated treatments, high patient dissatisfaction, and poor prognosis and a correlation between the quality of healthcare and the doctor-patient relationship (Wu et al. 2015). These findings are consistent around the world and demonstrate that patients in psychosomatic medicine experience an overall lower quality of care and quality of life (Zhang et al. 2014). It is not surprising that in psychosomatic medicine, the doctor-patient relationship, upon which a successful outcome hinges, is often under considerable strain because of the patient's anxiety that can also be experienced by the family and the healthcare professionals. Given what is known about the importance of the patient-doctor relationship (Wu et al. 2015), patient experience measures ought to be considered, rather than dismissed as being too subjective, as another important component of accurately measuring patient safety and clinical effectiveness (Doyle et al. 2013). Ultimately, the three should be considered as a group and included in all levels of clinical work, including measurement of and improvement of effectiveness.

As illustrated in the opening scenario of this chapter, healthcare systems that operate in silos, that exclusively rely on a biomedical model, that ineffectively engage patients, and that perpetuate societal stigma render unsafe, low-quality, and unethical care for patients (Fig. 17.6).

The connections between the three pillars are evident in pediatric psychosomatic medicine: instability in any one pillar has the potential to collapse patient care quality. The pillars are grounded in the psychosomatic model, which unfortunately is under siege from global stigma and the false dichotomy between "mind" and "body" and "psychological" and "physical." We propose that much somatization and excessive medicalization is iatrogenic and unwittingly encouraged by aspects of contemporary medical care and the culture in which healthcare professionals practice. We

Patient	Experience	Safety impacts	Outcomes
Individual Patient	Frightened Humiliated Isolated Invalidated Accused	Hyper-Identification with illness Suicidality Iatrogenic harm Adverse events Disengagement	
Family	Blamed Confused Isolated Frustrated Dismissed	Disengagement Overly medicalization Iatrogenic Harm Adverse Events	Poor Suboptimal
Healthcare Provider	Confused Unsettled Self-Doubting Dissatisfied Rushed	Ineffective/potentially harmful treatment Adverse events Ineffective engagement System and communication breakdowns Litigation	

Fig. 17.6 Quality in pediatric psychosomatic medicine as informed by the three pillars

believe that there is a significant potential for the psychosomatic approach, practiced by consultation-liaison psychiatrists, to concretely improve patient experience, safety, and quality in a variety of settings and contexts.

Pediatric Psychosomatic Approach to Improve the Quality of Global Healthcare

With longer lifespans, rising healthcare costs, and growing prominence of chronic illness, a psychosomatic approach is timely and essential for global healthcare. The psychosomatic approach is genuinely informed by and practiced within the BPS model; emphasizes cross-disciplinary collaboration and integration of mental health into primary care; accounts for individual and contextual influences on health to reduce stigma-related barriers; and aims to improve experience, safety, and quality across all health systems.

In advancing the psychosomatic model, we offer the following three guiding principles:

Guiding Principle 1: **To address the contextual influences on health, psychosomatic medicine must eliminate the mind-body dichotomy to address stigma and improve patient experience.**

Giffin and Christie (2008) argue that the term "psychosomatic" has drawbacks in implying that some conditions are psychosomatic while others are not. We advocate that all illnesses, with inherent biological, psychological, and social aspects, be considered psychosomatic, without the false dichotomy that perpetuates global stigma.

Prince et al. (2007) highlight three priorities necessary for adopting a psychosomatic perspective: increasing the evidence base supporting the interactivity between mental health and overall health, improving the understanding of the bidirectional mechanisms that link mental health and overall health, and uncovering the ways that psychosocial interventions improve health. While supporting these priorities as information-building, future-oriented goals, we believe that it is critical to apply the psychosomatic approach in current day-to-day practice. Following the BPS model, one can observe clinical phenomena in terms of (1) circular causality, wherein feedback underpins specific behavioral patterns over time, and (2) structural causality, wherein cause-effect relationships involve precipitant causes, maintaining forces, and event combinations (Fassino 2010). By modeling a unified system approach, healthcare systems can eliminate the stigma that separates psychological health from overall health.

This psychosomatic approach calls for healthcare professionals to routinely explore psychological aspects of illness in a way that reduces patients' negative experiences and feelings of stigma. In understanding that there are psychological aspects to all illnesses, patients do not need to use symptoms as currency to engage in a patient-doctor relationship.

Guiding Principle 2: To address individual influences on health and to improve safety, psychosomatic medicine must consider the patient's biology and psychology.

The pediatric psychosomatic approach, grounded in the BPS model, is developmentally appropriate, considers the family as a part of the pediatric patient, and thereby promotes a strong patient-doctor relationship that reduces risks to patient safety and care quality. Relationship ethics emphasizes that healthcare professionals and patients *together* ensure prudent and deliberative decision-making that improves patient safety (in Fava et al. 2012). When BPS influences are not considered, patient safety is unintentionally compromised (Wolpert et al. 2015).

Based on the concept of the complete person, pediatric psychosomatic medicine facilitates coping and adjustment and optimizes developmental trajectory. A sole focus on psychopathology leads to safety concerns for the patient, family, and healthcare professionals (Fava et al. 2012). A genuine BPS approach links individual aspects of illness to biological, psychological, and social factors unique to the patient and offers an individually tailored approach that is truly humanistic and client-centered (Fassino 2010). Evidence shows that this practice improves patient and provider experience, is positively associated with safety and effectiveness and reduced adverse events (Doyle et al. 2013). The transactional nature of patient and provider safety suggests that efforts to improve one must consider the other.

Guiding Principle 3: To address changing healthcare needs and to improve quality of patient care, psychosomatic medicine must be practiced collaboratively among healthcare providers.

Guiding principle 1 focuses on working as one system to remove stigma and improve patient experience, and guiding principle 2 focuses on facilitating the patient-doctor relationship by appreciating factors unique to the patient. Guiding principle 3 builds on both principles and focuses on working collaboratively among healthcare providers to further improve quality.

Collaborative practice is an evidence-based way to increase quality, to address emerging and changing global healthcare needs, to improve population health, and to reduce healthcare costs (Huffman et al. 2014). We take the position that collaborative care improves patient and population experience, safety, and quality outcomes.

Furthermore, care integration insures equitability in psychological healthcare (i.e., Wilkes and Cawthorpe 2008) and removes segregated care systems that perpetuate stigma, discrimination, and medicalization (i.e., Ghuttora and Cawthorpe 2013). There is a severe shortage of psychiatrists worldwide, with less than 1 psychiatrist per 100,000 people for nearly half of the world's population (Bauer et al. 2011). Collaborative practice involving psychosomatic medicine is a promising model to address global needs for stigma reduction and healthcare accessibility and affordability.

Clinical Pathways in Pediatric Psychosomatic Medicine

Based on what has been covered thus far, and with the goals of improving experience, safety, and quality, we propose the clinical pathways depicted in Fig. 17.7.

This psychosomatic approach develops collaborative skills, models professional behaviors, and addresses limitations in specialty services by utilizing them for consultation, support, and education. Informed by the BPS model these pathways are clinically integrated, grounded in evidence, and able to offer a deliberative process. This approach advocates that healthcase systems move away from service fragmentation, which encourages and perpetuates stigma and discrimination. Accordingly, these pathways utilize a partnership paradigm of collaborative care across disciplines and across the patient-doctor relationship.

To implement, on a global level, the psychosomatic approach, current and future healthcare professionals need to be educated in this perspective. As global healthcare needs are changing, a new direction in policy and practice is needed, and psychosomatic medicine is ideally suited to lead in this change.

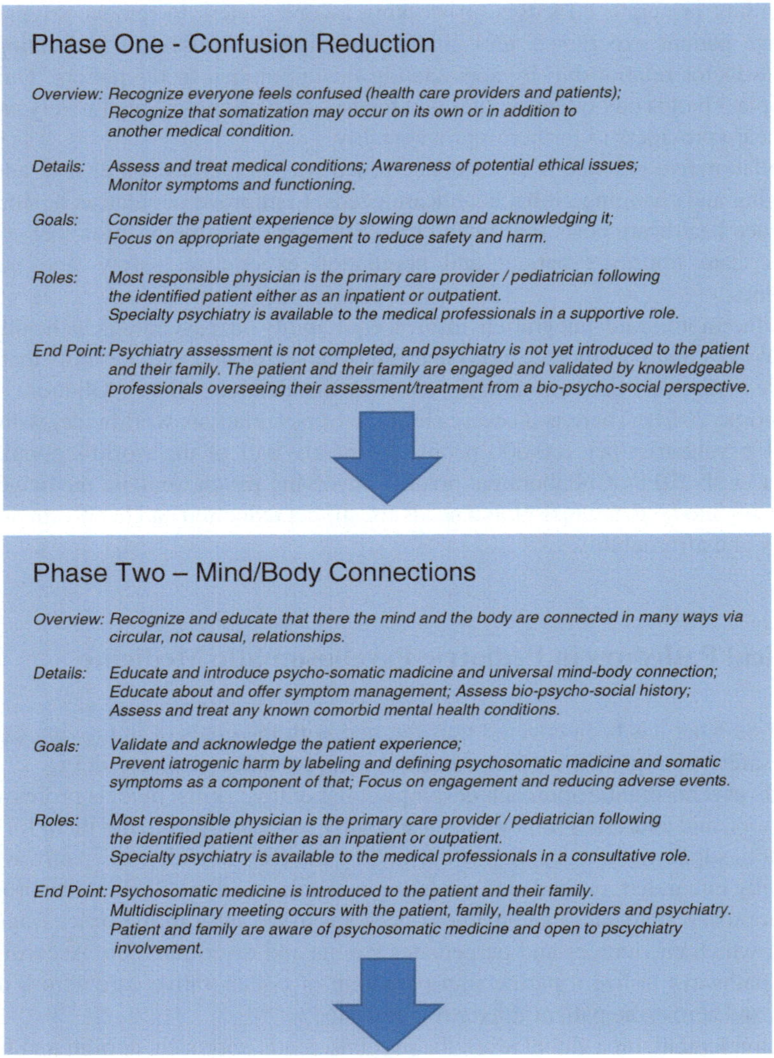

Fig. 17.7 A four-phase model for clinical pathways in pediatric psychosomatic medicine

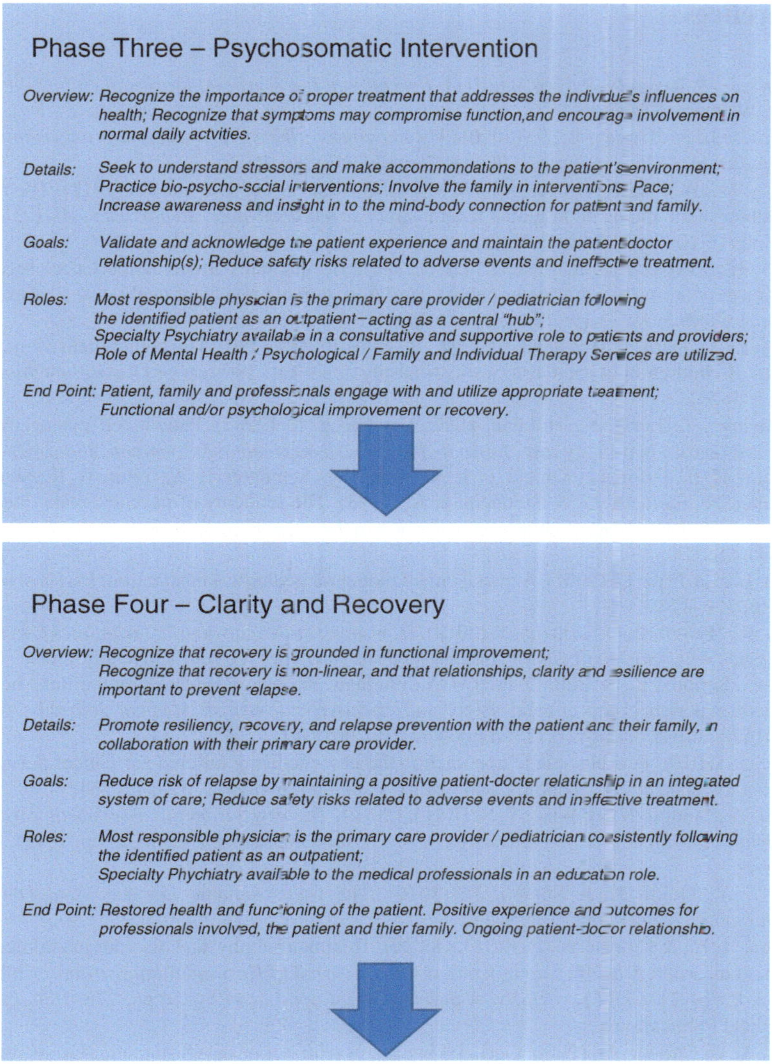

Fig. 17.7 (continued)

References

Andrews, J., & Istvanffy, P. (Eds.). (2011). *Exceptional life journeys: Stories of childhood disorder*. Waltham: Elsevier.

Atkins, C. G., & Hodges, B. D. (2010). *My imaginary illness: A journey into uncertainty and prejudice in medical diagnosis*. Ithaca: Cornell University Press.

Bauer, A. M., Bonilla, P., Grover, M. W., Meyer, F., Riselle, C., & White, L. (2011). The role of psychosomatic medicine in global health care. *Current Psychiatry Reports, 13*, 10–17. https://doi.org/10.1007/s11920-010-0162-2.

Berg, S. H., Rørtveit, K., & Aase, K. (2017, Jan 23). Suicidal patients' experiences regarding their safety during psychiatric in-patient care: A systematic review of qualitative studies. *BMC Health Services Research, 17*(1), 73.

Bingley, L., Leonard, J., Hensman, S., Lask, B., & Wolff, O. (1980). The comprehensive management of children on a paediatric ward: A family approach. *Archives of Disease in Childhood, 55*, 555–561.

Bodenheimer, T., Lorig, K., Holman, H., & Grumbach, K. (2002). Patient self-management of chronic disease in primary care. *Journal of the American Medical Association, 288*, 2469–2475.

Bronheim, H. E., Fulop, G., Kunkel, E. J., Muskin, P. R., Schindler, B. A., Yates, W. R., Shaw, R., Steiner, H., Stern, T. A., & Stoudemire, A. (1998). The academy of psychosomatic medicine practice guidelines for psychiatric consultation in the general medical setting. *Psychosomatics, 39*(4), S8–S30.

Campo, J. V., & Fritz, G. (2001). A management model for pediatric somatization. *Psychosomatics, 42*(6), 467–476.

Caplan, R., Bursch, B., & Leipzig, A. (2012). *How many more questions?: Techniques for clinical interview of young medically ill children*. Oxford/New York: Oxford University Press.

Doyle, C., Lennox, L., & Bell, D. (2013). A systematic review of evidence on the links between patient experience and clinical safety and effectiveness. *British Medical Journal Open, 3*, e001570. https://doi.org/10.1136/bmjopen-2012-001570.

Fassino, S. (2010). Psychosomatic approach is the new medicine tailored for patient personality with a focus on ethics, economy, and quality. *Panminerva Medica, 52*, 249–264.

Fava, G. A., Sonino, N., & Wise, T. N. (Eds.). (2012). *The psychosomatic assessment. Strategies to improve clinical practice, Advances in psychosomatic medicine* (Vol. 32, pp. 1–18). Basel: Karger.

Fava, G. A., Guidi, J., & Sonino, N. (2016). The psychosomatic practice. *Acta Dermato-Venereologica, 96*(Suppl 217), 9–13.

Ghuttora, H. K., & Cawthorpe, D. (2013, Oct 29). Treatment of physical disorder in children with mental disorder: A health care utilization study. *Journal of Hospital Administration., 3*(2), 24.

Graham, P. (1991). *Child psychiatry: A developmental approach* (2nd ed.pp. 276–280). Oxford: Medical Publications.

Griffin, A., & Christie, D. (2008, Oct). Taking the psycho out of psychosomatic: Using systemic approaches in a paediatric setting for the treatment of adolescents with unexplained physical symptoms. *Clinical Child Psychology and Psychiatry, 13*(4), 531–542.

Hardwick, P. J. (2005, Oct). Engaging families who hold strong medical beliefs in a psychosomatic approach. *Clinical Child Psychology and Psychiatry, 10*(4), 601–616.

Heru, A. M. (2006). Family psychiatry: From research to practice. *The American Journal of Psychiatry, 163*, 962–968.

Holmbeck, G. N. (2002, Jul 1). A developmental perspective on adolescent health and illness: An introduction to the special issues. *Journal of Pediatric Psychology, 27*(5), 409–416.

Huffman, J. C., Niazi, S. K., Rundell, J. R., Sharpe, M., & Katon, W. J. (2014). Essential articles on collaborative care models for the treatment of psychiatric disorders in medical settings: A publication by the academy of psychosomatic medicine research and evidence-based practice committee. *Psychosomatics, 55*, 109–122.

Katon, W., & Walker, E. (1998). Medically unexplained symptoms in primary care. *The Journal of Clinical Psychiatry, 59*(suppl 20), 15021.

Kroenke, K. (2002). Psychological medicine. *British Medical Journal, 324*, 1536–1537.

Leventhal, H., Weinman, J., Leventhal, E. A., & Phillips, L. A. (2008). Health psychology: The search for pathways between behavior and health. *Annual Review of Psychology, 59*, 477–505.

Logan, D. E. (2002). Parent factors and adolescent sickle cell disease: Associations with patterns of health service use. *Journal of Pediatric Psychology, 27*(5), 475–484.

Mascherek, A. C., & Schwappach, D. L. B. (2016). Patient safety priorities in mental healthcare in Switzerland: A modified Delphi study. *British Medical Journal Open, 6*, e011494. https://doi.org/10.1136/bmjopen-2016-011494

McCaffrey, E. S. N., Chang, S., Farrelly, G., Rahman, A., Cawthorpe, D. (2017). Mental health literacy in primary care: Canadian Research and Education for the Advancement of Child Health (CanREACH). *Evidence Based Medicine, 22*(4):123–131.

Oken, D. (2007). Evolution of psychosomatic diagnosis in DSM. *Psychosomatic Medicine, 69* 830–831.

Ortiz, P. (1997). General principles in child liaison consultation service: A literature review. *EuropeanChild and Adolescent Psychiatry, 6*, 1–6.

Pescosolido, B. A., Jensen, P. S., Martin, J. K., et al. (2008). Public knowledge and assessment of child mental health problems: Findings from the national stigma study-children. *Journal of the American Academy of Child and Adolescent Psychiatry, 47*(3), 339–349.

Prince, M., Patel, V., Saxena, S., et al. (2007). No health without mental health. *Lancet, 370*, 859–877.

Rask, C. U., Borg, C., Søndergaard, C., Schulz-Pedersen, S., Thomsen, P. H., & Fink, P. (2010, Apr 30). A medical record review for functional somatic symptoms in children. *Journal of Psychosomatic Research, 68*(4), 345–352.

Shaw, R. J., & DeMaso, D. R. (2007). *Clinical manual of pediatric psychosomatic medicine: Mental health consultation with physically ill children and adolescents*. Washington, DC: American Psychiatric Publishing.

Wilkes, C., & Cawthorpe, D. (2008). The need for more children's mental health services. *Canadian Medical Association Journal, 178*(11), 1465–1466. https://doi.org/10.1503/cmaj.1080017

Wolpert, M., Deighton, J., Fleming, I., & Lachman, P. (2015, Jan 1). Considering harm and safety in youth mental health: A call for attention and action. *Administration and Policy in Mental Health and Mental Health Services Research, 42*(1), 6–9.

Wu, H., Zhao, X., Fritzsche, K., Leonhart, R., Schaefert, R., Sun, X., & Larisch, A. (2015). Quality of doctor-patient relationship in patients with high somatic symptom severity in China. *Complementary Therapies in Medicine, 23*(1), 23–31. http://dx.doi.org.ahs.idm.oclc.org/10.1016/j.ctim.2014.12.006.

Zhang, Y., Fritzsche, K., Leonhart, R., et al. (2014). Dysfunctional illness perception and illness behavior associated with high somatic symptom severity and low quality of life in general hospital outpatients in China. *Journal of Psychosomatic Research, 77*(3), 187–195. http://dx.doi.org.ahs.idm.oclc.org/10.1016/j.jpsychores.2014.06.005.

Chapter 18
Primary Care Integration

Alexis Aplasca and Daniel Alicata

The principles of high-quality healthcare include strategies for prevention, acute care management, and chronic disease management, all of which have been embraced by pediatrics. With the advent of vaccines, anticipatory guidance, and structured well-child visits, children are living longer and healthier lives. Unfortunately, these types of screenings for health and developmental risks have not been applied broadly and systematically to mental health issues. Furthermore, individuals with mental disorders experience disproportionally higher rates of disability and mortality. For example, individuals with major depression and schizophrenia have a 40–60% greater chance of dying prematurely than the general population due to lack of attention of physical health needs and access to preventive healthcare. Conversely, mental health disorders often affect (e.g., through treatment nonadherence) the course of other chronic illnesses (such as diabetes or asthma), thus highlighting the needs for an integrated approach to healthcare. Prevention and early intervention efforts for both psychiatric and other medical conditions are key to promoting the optimal development of children.

The various components of primary healthcare for children are provided by a spectrum of practitioners including community health workers, nurses, nurse aides, medical assistants, physician assistants, general practitioners, and pediatricians. The setting in which this care is provided also varies from within the home to hospitals. Unfortunately, there is a chronic shortage of well-trained healthcare workers, especially in low-income countries. "Task shifting," or delegation of a task to the "lowest" category provider who can adequately complete it, is one strategy that has been used to address this shortage (Lehmann and Sanders 2007). In many

A. Aplasca (✉)
Magellan Health, Inc, Glen Allen, VA, USA
e-mail: aplascaa@magellanhealth.com

D. Alicata
Department of Psychiatry, University of Hawaii, JABSOM, Honolulu, HI, USA
e-mail: alicatad@dop.hawaii.edu

A. P. S. Guerrero et al. (eds.), *Pediatric Consultation-Liaison Psychiatry*,
https://doi.org/10.1007/978-3-319-89488-1_18

Table 18.1 Caplan's types of prevention

Type of prevention	Definition	Focus	Example
Primary	Aims at reducing the incidence of new cases of mental disorder in the population	Focuses on modifying the environment and strengthening individual capacities	A community health worker provides weekly group sessions at a local school to provide education on preventing bullying
Secondary	Aims at reducing the duration and severity of mental illnesses	Focuses on early detection and treatment	The medical assistant at the primary care clinic conducts depression screening at annual exams. The physician is notified when patients are screened positive to address concerns during that visit without delay
Tertiary	Aims at reducing the rate of relapse and acute exacerbation of mental illness	Focuses on ensuring that individuals who have recovered from mental illness are able to return to full participation in the community	The psychiatrist ensures regular follow-up for a patient with schizophrenia after hospitalization to monitor medication and therapy adherence and promotes return to work

Adapted from Caplan and Grunebaum (1967)

low-income and low-middle-income countries, much of the preventive care is provided by community health workers utilizing a population health approach. Mental healthcare intervention programs are also adopting the use of community health workers.

Integration of mental health into primary care practices can occur along a continuum. This can be conceptualized using Caplan's idea of primary, secondary, and tertiary prevention (Table 18.1). Taking this approach also makes task shifting feasible.

The Substance Abuse and Mental Health Services Administration describes a four-quadrant clinical integration model (Fig. 18.1), which considers the varying behavioral and other healthcare needs of patient populations and suggests care models which might best meet these characteristics. These models include facilitation, co-location, and integration (SAMHSA-HRSA Center for Integrated Health Solutions 2013). The following case examples highlight pertinent factors to consider when choosing among integration models and practical systems of care implementation.

Facilitate, Co-locate, or Integrate: Three Examples of Service Delivery Structures

Please refer to Table 18.2 for model definitions.

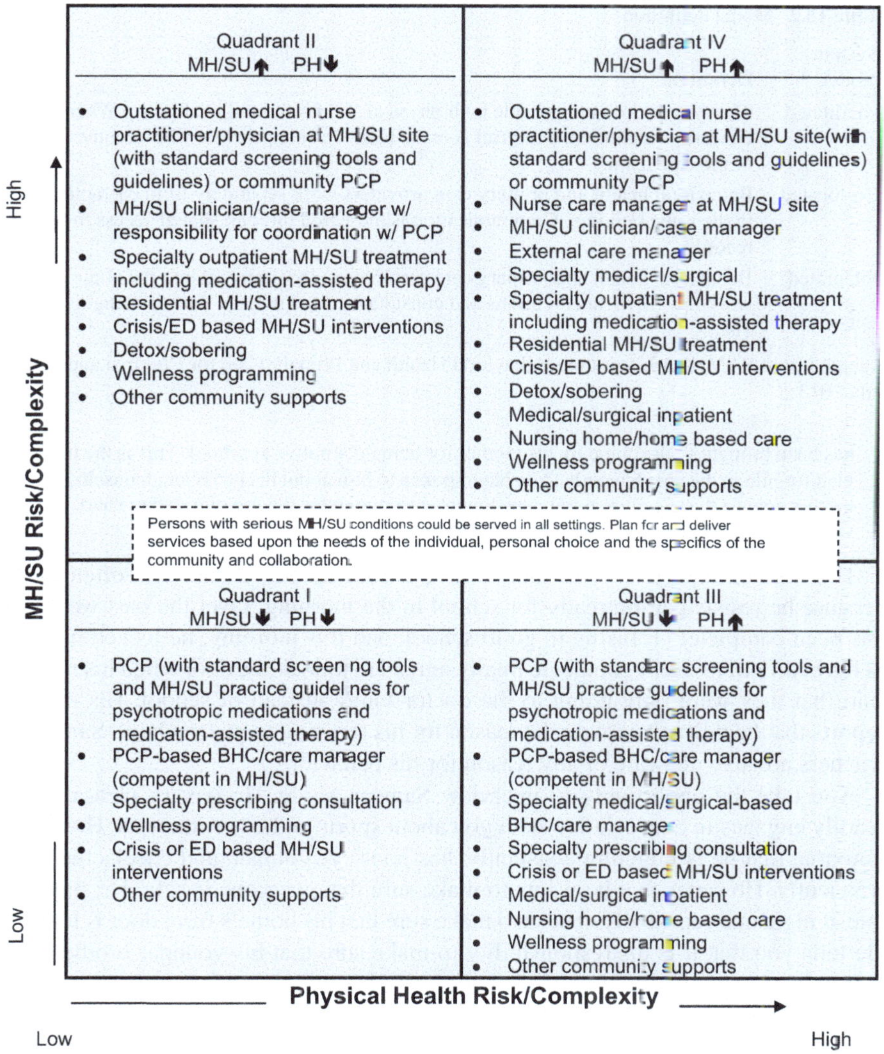

Fig. 18.1 SAMHSA four quadrants (Citation: Mauer, Barbara J.. "Behavioral Health/Primary Care Integration and the Person Centered Healthcare Home". April 2009. The National Council for Behavioral Health Care [accessed 1/12/2018, reproduced with permission])

Case 18.1: Facilitated Delivery

You are a general practitioner in a large community health clinic, which employs nurses and medical assistants as part of the healthcare team. You see approximately 40 patients per day, half of which are children and adolescents. Your clinic has done well to educate its patients about vaccines and the prevention of many infectious diseases. The biggest challenge facing your clinic is the increasing number of behavioral health concerns in young children. Today, you are seeing Samson, a healthy, 7-year-old male, with normal development, who

Table 18.2 Model definitions

System model	Definition
Facilitated	The system does not provide both physical and behavioral healthcare. When a concern is identified, a referral is made to an outside provider who becomes a part of the care team.
Co-located	Behavioral health and primary care providers work separately from each other but in the same building. Communication is increased through shared access to health records.
Integrated	Behavioral health and primary care services are incorporated into the clinic workflow. Brief interventions and consultations are utilized during a single patient visit.

Adapted from SAMHSA Integrating Behavioral Health and Primary Care for Children and Youth, July 2013

has been brought to the clinic by his mother for being disruptive at school. This is the third visit for him in the past 6 months. You have spoken to him about his behavior, counseled his mother against the use of corporal punishment, recommended the use of a sticker chart, and written a letter to the school requesting additional support.

His mother reports to you that, over the past month, Samson is often tardy because he resists getting ready for school in the morning. Over the past week, he has been completely refusing to go to school, and this morning, he locked himself in his bedroom to avoid going. He finally agreed to unlock the door when his mother said that they were only going to the doctor today instead of school. His mother reports that he will not explain the reason for his refusing to go to school. Samson's teachers are also unaware of any reason for his behavior.

You take the opportunity to interview Samson alone. He is very pleasant and readily engages in conversation with you about sports and other interests. However, you note that he is fidgeting constantly, has poor eye contact, and checks the door frequently. He states that he wants to make sure that everyone is safe. He stays up late at night and repeatedly checks to make sure that his home's front door is locked. He tells you that it is his responsibility to make sure that his younger brothers are safe.

His mother tells you that the family home was burglarized last month, but no one was injured. The intruder stole a few items and left a threatening note, instructing the family not to notify the police. They decided against involving the police, since the stolen items were easily replaceable. You suspect that this traumatic event may be the cause of the child's behavioral issues, but his mother does not understand the relationship between the burglary and school avoidance. However, she agrees with your recommendation to have Samson see a mental health specialist to address these issues further. When making the referral, you find that the earliest available appointment is in 4 months. By that time, the school year will have ended.

The Traditional Model of Mental Healthcare and its Pitfalls

This case describes the traditional facilitated model of healthcare, in which the primary care provider (PCP) identifies and manages a behavioral health concern until a point at which specialty services are needed. This is the predominant model for most behavioral health and other healthcare in the United States. Unfortunately, as mentioned in the case, the numbers of behavioral and emotional health concerns presenting to primary care clinics are growing exponentially. Epidemiological data reveals a worldwide prevalence of approximately 20% for child and adolescent mental health disorders, and in high-income countries like the United States, it has been reported that 70% of children and adolescents in need of treatment do not receive any mental health care (U.S. Department of Health and Human Services 1999). There are not enough specialty-trained mental health providers, and as a result, professionals with suboptimal training in mental healthcare are struggling to meet these needs. This phenomenon is known as the mental health service gap. Like in primary care, a variety of professionals provide mental healthcare. Child and adolescent psychiatrists are rare outside developed countries. Most countries in the African, Eastern Mediterranean, South East Asian, and Western Pacific regions have only one to four child and adolescent psychiatrists per million children (WHO Department of Mental Health and Substance Abuse 2005).

Lack of access to specialists is only one of many barriers for individuals seeking mental healthcare. Lack of awareness of mental health conditions in children and stigma also play large roles. Additionally, much of mental health care is crisis driven, in which individuals with emergent issues such as acute suicidality, homicidality, psychosis, and agitation receive more timely access to care. The case highlights a common problem encountered in the traditional facilitated model, extended waiting periods to receive specialty care. This delay poses a significant risk for worsening of symptoms, further social and academic impairment in the child, loss of workdays for caregivers, and development of emergent situations.

This case also highlights the large volume of patients seen in primary care clinics each day in most current practice models. Few PCPs find the time allotted for routine office visits sufficient to adequately address mental health issues. Together with the mental health service gap, these factors have led to an urgent call for innovation to address the persistent unmet mental health needs of children.

Case 18.2: Co-located Delivery

The mental health clinic to which you referred Samson notified you that there was a cancellation and he can be seen at an earlier appointment. You arrange to have Samson return to see you 1 month after his initial mental health appointment to see what recommendations were made. You are disappointed to learn that Samson missed his mental health appointment because his mother could not arrange transportation there, which is located 25 miles from your clinic. Since his last visit with you, Samson's mother met with the school, and they have provided him with an on-site counselor. His mom started with him a consistent bedtime routine, and she insured that he checks only once whether the home's front door is locked. With this intervention, he has been less fearful at night. Samson continues to tell you that it is his job to keep everyone in the house safe from intruders, and he adds that his mom has given him super powers to be brave and that he now has a special shield to protect people. While the situation may have improved somewhat, you continue to be concerned about Samson's perseveration on safety and would still like him to be evaluated by a mental health specialist. This time, however, you plan to address the potential barriers to accessing care.

You learn that only 30% of the patients whom you referred to mental health specialists over the past year were able to access this care. You advocate for integrating mental health services into your clinic. Resources are limited, so your clinic manager asks that you to provide a proposal outlining the costs, benefits, and resources needed to provide these services. You have investigated different models of care and are certain that if you and the patients had easier access to specialists, you could more optimally coordinate care and reinforce treatment plans. You propose a co-location model of service delivery. You contact the mental health clinic to where you referred Samson and most of your other patients needing services. You arrange a meeting with their staff to brainstorm ideas about a collaboration, and you emphasize the high no-show rate as a major barrier to accessing care.

You discuss piloting a shared space, and you offer a reserved office for a mental health provider to see patients in your clinic once a week. You are confident that your patients are more likely to show for their appointments with a mental healthcare provider at your clinic because transportation is less likely to be a barrier, as they already present themselves to that location for their primary care visits. They are also familiar with the clinic's administrative procedures and staff. Additionally, you believe that, because of the perceived stigma associated with going to a psychiatric clinic, patients may prefer obtaining mental healthcare services at the same location where they receive their other medical care. Within this partnership, you offer to provide quick medical consultation as needed for the patients who do not regularly see any doctor other than the mental healthcare provider. The potential benefits are clear, and together, you develop the co-location delivery model for your clinic.

Addressing Access to Care

This case highlights the stark reality that less than half of the families of children referred to mental healthcare providers follow through on those referrals (Kelleher et al. 2006). While lack of timely access to care is a system problem, factors inherent to patients and families, such as perceived stigma associated with cultural views of mental health conditions and their treatment, can also impede care even when services are readily available. Thus, it is important to take into account multiple factors when deciding the type of service delivery model to be implemented, including the array of available services in the community, the capacity of those services to meet the need, patient preference in where they receive care, the competency and skill of the mental healthcare providers, organizational support, and financial reimbursement for the model (SAMHSA-HRSA Center for Integrated Health Solutions

2013). In regard to the care providers, a plan should be included to build the competencies of those working in integrated models. A 2009 policy statement on mental health in primary care developed by the American Academy of Pediatrics described the opportunities to build the capacity for mental healthcare service provision in the primary care setting. A key characteristic of the family-centered medical home, which is conducive to this effort, is the longitudinal and trusting relationship with children and their families integral to the comprehensive care of children (Committe on Psychosocial Aspects of Child and Family Health and Task Force on Mental Health 2009).

There are several advantages to co-located delivery models. Co-located mental health and primary care services have been found to decrease the use of general healthcare services by children with unidentified and untreated mental health problems. Health outcomes are improved, and costs are reduced (William et al. 2006). Additional benefits with this service delivery model include:

- Improved communication between treatment providers through shared medical records and informal consultation, allowing frequent interchange
- Less stigma for families seeking mental healthcare
- Increased exchange of knowledge and skill between mental health and primary care providers (Rosman et al. 2005)
- Earlier identification and referral to mental health by a primary care provider

Case 18.3: Co-located Delivery Continued

Samson has been seeing a mental health specialist in your clinic now for the past 4 months. His mother reports that he has been going to school without difficulty for the past 1 month, but she continues to have concerns about his behavior at home. He seems to cry easily, and his mother asks if it is possible to have depression at such a young age. You meet with Samson alone, and he tells you that his mother is expecting another child, and, although he is excited to be a big brother, he is mad about having to share his room and give away some of his belongings to make room for his new sibling. His mother notes that she has been cleaning their home in anticipation of the new baby, and every time she donates Samson's old toys, he starts crying, even though they are broken, and he has not played with them in several years. You provide some counseling and reassurance about Samson's adjustment to a new sibling, and you focus on his significant improvements over the past few months.

Since your clinic started the co-located delivery model, the no-show rate for your patients' mental healthcare appointments has decreased from 70% to 20%. Both the primary care and mental health providers have noted that patients benefit from increased communication and more efficient use of time. However, due to the increase in mental health referrals, the wait time for an appointment is starting to increase. Like Samson's mother, many families have expressed concerns about common behavioral health issues, such as ADHD, depression, anxiety, suicidal thoughts, and self-injury in their children. The mental health providers have suggested that the PCPs use screening tools and first-line treatment strategies to minimize the delay in care. There is some hesitation among the busy and time-pressured PCPs in incorporating screening tools, but a compromise is reached to screen children 12 years and older with a depression screening tool: the Patient Health Questionnaire-2 (PHQ-2), which is a 2-item screening tool that, if positive, expands to a nine-question scale (PHQ-9) to determine the potential severity of depression. This tool was chosen because of its ease of use, availability in multiple languages, and validation in the primary care setting. The PCPs also liked that the total time to use the PHQ-2 is 30 seconds if negative and less than 3 min if using the PHQ-9. Moving toward true integration will continue to take time and will require evaluation of the successes and pitfalls, but this progress has already proven to be beneficial for Samson.

Case 18.4: Complex Health Needs and Integrated Care

Alia is a 10-year-old female living with her family in Panama. She has a history of autism spectrum disorder and mild intellectual developmental disorder. She was identified with a developmental disorder by age 3 and was able to receive early intervention services for speech, motor, and sensory development. These services have significantly improved her overall functioning. She has received accommodations and services through the school system to help support her success. However, her mom has recently become more concerned because Alia will be transferring to a different school next year. Alia has significant difficulty with transition, and, when anxious, she exhibits atypical self-soothing behaviors such as skin picking and pulling out her own hair. A community health worker comes to the home once a week to work with the family in helping Alia to develop skills to become more independent in her daily activities. Additionally, Alia has asthma, for which she uses a rescue inhaler, for which she has required treatment with steroids twice in the past for severe exacerbations, and for which she has seen an asthma specialist once in the past. She has a history of seizures, which have been well controlled on a daily antiepileptic medication and for which she has also seen a neurologist once in the past. As her PCP, you manage all her medical and behavioral health issues, as access to specialty providers is limited. You anticipate that the transition to a new school and the onset of adolescence will pose new challenges for Alia. Although currently there are no acute problems, your practice has adopted the Chronic Care Model for children and adolescents who have high levels of behavioral and other healthcare needs and who require ongoing treatment and monitoring. As the manager of Alia's medical home, you facilitate a treatment team meeting that includes the family, her medical and behavioral specialists, and community health workers and that aims to enhance strengths and to anticipate problems. The team identifies that, because of anticipated school-related issues in the early part of the academic year, she will need more frequent sessions (approximately 2–3 times per week) with the community health worker. Overall, although difficult to coordinate, this approach has been very rewarding, and, as a PCP, you have been able to see its long-lasting benefits for your patients. A local advocacy organization has asked you to volunteer time to supervise community health workers so that they can support other children with complex needs both in homes and schools. Currently, the community health workers in your area are involved in home visitations to promote maternal-infant health efforts; to assist children with complex healthcare needs and their families with daily activities, including home healthcare and personal assistance needs; and to provide health education materials from the Ministry of Health. Many of the community health workers have a limited literacy level and education, and part of your supervisory role is to determine how to best delegate tasks and provide support to minimize rapid turnover of personnel. The resources are limited in your community, and so you decide to focus on the essential elements and foundational building blocks for helping children and families meet their potential.

Comprehensive Care for Complex Needs

Internationally, children with high needs and their families commonly face lifelong challenges in accessing basic resources. This lack of access to resources is an even more serious concern when managing children with co-occurring medical and mental health conditions. There are several chronic health conditions associated with higher rates of behavioral and mental health issues. Adequate treatment of the mental health conditions can significantly impact the course of physical well-being. For example, children with more severe asthma have higher rates of comorbid depression, anxiety, and learning disabilities (University of Virginia Health System 2007). Individuals with sickle cell disease who have comorbid mental health disorders experience higher admission rates and longer hospital stays for sickle cell-related pain (Myrvik et al. 2013). Because of unmanaged health conditions, individuals with serious mental health conditions die earlier than the general population (Colton and Manderscheid 2006). Although many people recover from their mental health problems, they may chronically experience symptoms and/or some level of impaired functioning (Committe on Psychosocial Aspects of Child and Family Health and Task Force on Mental Health 2009).

SAMHSA's four-quadrant model recommends the Chronic Care Model in caring for individuals with high levels of mental and other healthcare needs. This model has been found to be effective in the management of children with complex needs. The essential elements of this model include:

- Emphasis on the patient and family's central role in managing the patient's health and priorities
- Support of the patient and family in self-management
- Delivery system design that promotes team-based, proactive care
- Decision support, which integrates evidence-based practices into daily treatment and which includes health screenings for early detection of problems
- Clinical information systems for performance and clinical outcome monitoring
- Community linkages to promote wellness by utilizing comprehensive services from schools, local organizations, and care programs
- Health systems that create a culture, practice, and mechanisms that promote high-quality care (Wagner et al. 2001)

Mental health conditions, such as mood disorders, can be chronic, with intermittent periods of acute exacerbation and remission. The Chronic Care Model incorporates strategies to prevent relapsing episodes or minimize their severity. For lifelong mental health conditions such as schizophrenia, it is necessary to provide tertiary prevention strategies to avoid the development of secondary medical comorbidity. During periods of exacerbation, other health needs are often overlooked. If co-occurring medical conditions already exist, the stability of those conditions can be placed at risk with poor self-care associated with increasing severity of psychiatric symptoms. With the Chronic Care Model, a fully integrated care team can optimally manage complex cases by incorporating psychosocial supports and by addressing the relevant social determinants of health.

Using Telepsychiatry to Facilitate Care Integration

Developing integrated care programs incorporating telepsychiatry can address the critical goals of increasing both the capacity and access to behavioral healthcare, especially in rural and underserved communities (Fortney et al. 2015).

With continually developing technological advances, many telepsychiatry programs are now using secured (in the United States, Health Insurance Portability and Accountability Act or HIPAA-compliant) cloud-based videoconferencing systems, which have the potential to dramatically increase access to child and adolescent psychiatric care even in otherwise low-resource settings. Users simply download an application or link to a website to join a session. Primary care providers and specialists can connect with each other through various devices, such as desktop computers, laptops, tablets, and smartphones. Administrative, clinical, and technical guidelines for using telepsychiatry to provide behavioral health services for children and adolescents, including integrated care, are described in the Policy and Practice Guidelines for Telemental Health (TMH) for Children and Adolescents (Myers et al. 2017) and in the Clinical Update: Telepsychiatry With Children and Adolescents (AACAP 2017).

Cloud-based videoconferencing technology provides geographically separated integrated care and behavioral health teams with affordable, reliable, flexible, and encrypted collaboration opportunities. As the demand for behavioral health access and capacity rapidly increase, telepsychiatry-facilitated integrated care will be most important for rural primary care patients. Guerrero et al. (2017) describe how the use of telepsychiatry allows the consulting telepsychiatrist to adapt to the rapidly growing and dynamically changing behavioral health needs in an isolated rural community's federally qualified community health center (FQHC). In this highly adaptive and flexible integrated care model, the telepsychiatrist consultant located at a distant site and the FQHC teams utilize cloud-based video teleconferencing (VTC) to maintain convenient, reliable, user-friendly, and, most importantly, secured (HIPAA-compliant) communication between the primary care and behavioral health teams. Telepsychiatry provides the flexibility to define and adapt the consultant's role to the changing needs of the primary care team and can include guidance on behavioral health screenings, ongoing collaboration and discussion with integrated care teams around selected patients, scheduled telepsychiatry consultations on select patients, participation in team conferences, in-service educational presentations focusing on high yield topics, and in-person visits to reinforce team-building, problem-solving, and familiarity with community resources (Guerrero et al. 2017).

Project Extension for Community Healthcare Outcomes (ECHO) is another example of using telepsychiatry in a hub-spoke model to provide integrated care and increase behavioral health capacity (Komaromy et al. 2016). The specialist hub can be centralized at a single location or distributed across multiple sites, and it is not uncommon for international specialists to participate in an ECHO clinic. The behavioral health specialist hub can include psychiatrists, psychologists, primary care providers, social workers, case managers, and pharmacists. The hub staff meet weekly to review and discuss clinical cases presented by a distributed spoke network of integrated care teams in private clinical practices and community health centers. Participant learners can include physicians (e.g., family and internal medicine, pediatrics, and psychiatry) and non-physicians (e.g., nurses, nurse practitioners, physician assistants, community health workers, social workers, pharmacists, and administrators).

Komaromy et al. (2016) described outcome data for an ECHO Integrated Addiction and Psychiatry Program at the University of New Mexico. Since 2008, over 950 cases were discussed; over 9000 hours of continuing medical education credit were awarded; 285 participants attended, with each attending an average of 12.4 clinics; and over 375 New Mexico physicians participated in the buprenorphine waiver training, with certification provided by the American Academy of Addiction Psychiatry and American Osteopathic Association of Addiction Medicine. Another Project ECHO Behavioral Health Program was started in Hawaii in January 2016. Integrated care teams at community health centers representing the Republic of the Marshall Islands (Majuro) and the Federated States of Micronesia (Pohnpei) have been consistent spoke participants. Cloud-based telepsychiatry efficiently and reliably connects a distributed network of participants across Hawaii, the Pacific Islands, and the continental United States.

There is a rapidly growing evidence base for sustained outcomes supporting the use of telepsychiatry and integrated care (Fortney et al. 2013, 2015). The American Psychiatric Association (APA) and the American Academy of Child and Adolescent Psychiatry (AACAP) have developed integrated care education and training initiatives. The APA received a $2.9 million grant from the Center of Medicare and Medicaid Services with the goal of training 3500 psychiatrists to work in collaborative care settings (Duncan 2017). Access to the APA training in integrated care website can be found at https://www.psychiatry.org/psychiatrists/practice/professional-interests/integrated-care. Additionally, Dr. Gregory Fritz, President of the AACAP, made the development of integrated care training initiatives and collaborative care resources for child and adolescent psychiatrists his presidential initiative for the 2015–2017 term (Moran 2017). Access to the Pediatric Integrated Care Resource Center can be found at http://www.integratedcareforkids.org/.

The APA and AACAP have created goals to train and develop a workforce of psychiatrists to participate in integrated care programs. With increasing global and rural community demands for behavioral health capacity and access, it makes sense for psychiatry residency programs to develop integrated care and telepsychiatry training opportunities, whether elective or required, and make them available to psychiatry residents and child and adolescent psychiatry fellows. Recommended integrated care competencies in psychiatry training include communication skills, role flexibility, ability to build trust, collaborative management of complex patients, risk management, and mentorship of non-psychiatrists (Sunderji et al. 2016). Recommended child and adolescent telepsychiatry competencies in training are described by Shore et al. (2011), Sunderji et al. (2015), Hilty et al. (2015), and AACAP (2017). Hilty et al. (2015) described telepsychiatry training competencies that closely align with the Accreditation Council for Graduate Medical Education (ACGME) psychiatry milestone competencies including patient care, system- and practice-based learning, professionalism, communication, knowledge, and technology. Crawford et al. (2017), leaders in the rapidly developing field of telepsychiatry-facilitated provide integrated care, described training competencies that include collaborative care, interprofessional teamwork, communication, patient care, documentation, health advocacy, medicolegally informed and ethical practice, population-based care, and health system leadership.

Successes of Integrated Care

Integrated care is a promising option to address the mental health gap. Since integrated care has not been universally adopted, implementing programs at the local level and then scaling up based on the successes of those programs can be an effective strategy to eventually reach broader populations and settings.

One exemplary model is the Massachusetts Child Psychiatry Access Program (MCPAP), whose goal is to increase access to behavioral health treatment by making child psychiatric services available to primary care providers across the state of Massachusetts. MCPAP is grounded in the medical home model of care for children and aims to enhance pediatric mental health practice by aiding in the implementation of universal screenings in primary care, by increasing immediate access to consultation, by improving utilization of existing resources, and by aiding with coordination of care between systems. Much of the consultation rendered is through immediate phone and limited face-to-face consultation, with the pediatrician providing the recommended behavioral health services. This program was initiated in 2003 and piloted at the University of Massachusetts Medical School in Worcester. With its success and the support of the Massachusetts Chapter of the American Academy of Pediatrics, the program was expanded statewide. Now more than 30 states throughout the United States have developed child psychiatry consultation programs based on the MCPAP model (Massachusetts Child Psychiatry Access Program n.d.).

Additionally, several resources exist to educate both primary care and mental health providers on integration. Integrated care is an emerging field, and as more models are developed, universally applied terminology aids in organizing collaborative efforts to contribute toward a shared vision. The Agency for Healthcare Research and Quality (AHRQ) published the Lexicon for Behavioral Health and Primary Care (Agency for Healthcare Research and Quality 2013) to provide functional definitions and a set of concepts developed by expert consensus. This resource enables effective communication and action among clinicians, care systems, health plans, payers, researchers, policy makers, business modelers, and patients (Agency for Healthcare Research and Quality n.d.). At a national level, organizations such as AHRQ and SAMHSA provide frameworks for integration. However, more regional information and connections are necessary to promote further development at the grass roots level. In California, Integrated Behavioral Health Partners (IBHP) was launched in 2006 to provide guidance and funding for the integration of behavioral health services into primary care settings. IBHP-funded projects have shown statistically significant improvements in the mental and overall health of patients (Integrated Behavioral Health Partners n.d.). IBHP provides an implementation toolkit, which helps to implement long-lasting culture change through an integration readiness assessment; establishment of goals; identification of workforce and roles; and procedures for client engagement, referrals, and financial reimbursement for sustainability. The toolkit also includes process measures for patient and provider satisfaction and effectiveness, which are important components to maintain support and long-term investment.

Internationally, the lack of workforce in child mental health is even more striking, and integrated care can similarly provide an important step forward. In 2013, when Typhoon Haiyan struck the Philippines, an extensive scale-up of the Mental Health Gap Action Programme of the World Health Organization was undertaken in the community and general healthcare settings. The effect of this intervention resulted in four million people having access to mental healthcare in the most affected disaster areas (World Health Organization n.d.).

The persistent mental health gap and these examples of success underscore the continued need to further develop innovative integrated care programs. Utilizing the available tools and resources and coordinating with organizations implementing similar programs can lead to effective, long-lasting changes to better address the global mental health gap and promote optimal well-being.

References

(n.d.). Retrieved March 14, 2017, from Massachusetts Child Psychiatry Access Program: http://www.mcpap.org

(n.d.). Retrieved April 5, 2017, from World Health Organization: http://www.who.int/mental_health/emergencies/mhgap_philippines/en/

Agency for Healthcare Research and Quality. (2013). *Lexicon for behavioral health and primary care integration*. Rockville, MD.

Agency for Healthcare Research and Quality. (n.d.). Retrieved February 1, 2017, from The Academy- Integrating Behavioral Health and Primary Care. http://integrationacademy.ahrq.gov/lexicon

American Academy of Child and Adolescent Psychiatry (AACAP) Committee on Telepsychiatry and AACAP Committee on Quality Issues. (2017). Clinical update: Telepsychiatry with children and adolescents. *Journal of the American Academy of Child and Adolescent Psychiatry, 56*(10), 875–893 Epub 2017 Jul 25.

Caplan, G., & Grunebaum, H. (1967). Perspectives on primary prevention. A review. *Archives of General Psychiatry, 17*(3), 331–346.

Colton, C. W., & Manderscheid, R. W. (2006, April). Congruencies in increased mortality rates, year of potential life lost, and causes of death among public mental health clients in eight states. *Prevention of Chronic Disease, 3*(2), A42.

Committee on Psychosocial Aspects of Child and Family Health and Task Force on Mental Health. (2009, July). The future of pediatrics: Mental health competencies for primary care. *Pediatrics, 124*(1), 410–421.

Crawford, A., Sunderji, N., Serhal, E., Teshima, J.. (2017). Proposed competencies for providing integrated care via telepsychiatry. *Journal of Technology in Behavioral Science*. https://doi.org/10.1007/s41347-017-0014-6. Published online: 08 February 2017.

Duncan, M. (2017, September 15). Collaborative care model effective for addition treatment. *Psychiatry News, 52*, 18. Published online September 14, 2017. Available from http://psychnews.psychiatryonline.org.prx.hml.org/doi/full/10.1176/appi.pn.2017.9b9 Accessed 10/1/2017

Fortney, J. C., Pyne, J. M., Mouden, S. B., Mittal, D., Hudson, T. J., Schroeder, G. W., Williams, D. K., BynumCA, M. R., & Rost, K. M. (2013). Practice-based versus telemedicine-based collaborative care for depression in rural federally qualified health centers: a pragmatic randomized comparative effectiveness trial. *American Journal of Psychiatry, 170*(4), 414–425.

Fortney, J. C., Pyne, J. M., Turner, E. E., Farris, K. M., Normoyle, T. M., Avery, M. D., Hilty, D. M., & Unützer, J. (2015). Telepsychiatry integration of mental health services into rural primary care settings. *International Review of Psychiatry, 27*(6), 525–539.

Guerrero, A. P., Takesue, C. L., Medeiros, J. H., Duran, A. A., Humphry, J. W., Lunsford, R. M., Shaw, D. V., Fukuda, M. H., & Hishinuma, E. S. (2017). Primary care integration of psychiatric and behavioral health services: A primer for providers and case report of local implementation. *Hawai'i Journal of Medicine & Public Health, 76*(6), 147–151 PMID: 28607831.

Hilty, D. M., Crawford, A., Teshima, J., Chan, S., Sunderji, N., Yellowlees, P. M., Kramer, G., O'neill, P., Fore, C., Luo, J., & Li, S. T. (2015). A framework for telepsychiatric training and e-health: Competency-based education, evaluation and implications. *International Review of Psychiatry, 27*(6), 569–592.

Integrated Behavioral Health Partners. (n.d.). Retrieved April 14, 2017, from http://www.ibhpartners.org

Kelleher, K., Campo, J. V., & Gardner, W. P. (2006). Management of pediatric mental health disorders in primary care: Where are we now and where are we going? *Current Opinion in Pediatrics, 18*, 649–653.

Komaromy, M., Duhigg, D., Metcalf, A., Carlson, C., Kalishman, S., Hayes, L., Burke, T., Thornton, K., & Arora, S. (2016). Project ECHO (Extension for Community Healthcare Outcomes): A new model for educating primary care providers about treatment of substance use disorders. *Substance Abuse, 37*(1), 20–24.

Lehmann, U., & Sanders, D. (2007). *Community health workers: What do we know about them? The state of the evidence on programmes, activities, costs and impact on health outcomes using community health workers*. School of Public Health University of the Western Cape. WHO evidence and information for policy.

Moran, M. (2017, September 15). AACAP integrated care initiative aims to change culture of care for Youth. *Psychiatry News,* 52, 18. Published online: September 14, 2017. Available from http://psychnews.psychiatryonline.org.prx.hml.org/doi/full/10.1176/appi.pn.2017.9a1 Accessed 10/1/2017

Myers, K., Nelson, E. L., Rabinowitz, T., Hilty, D., Baker, D., Barnwell, S. S., Boyce, G., Bufka, L. F., Cain, S., Chui, L., Comer, J. S., Cradock, C., Goldstein, F., Johnston, B., Krupinski, E., Lo, K., Luxton, D. D., McSwain, S. D., McWilliams, J., North, S., Ostrowsky, J., Pignatiello, A., Roth, D., Shore, J., Turvey, C., Varrell, J. R., Wright, S., & Bernard, J. (2017). American telemedicine association practice guidelines for telemental health with children and adolescents. *Telemedicine Journal and E-Health, 23*(10), 779–804 PMID: 28930496.

Myrvik, M. P., Burks, L. M., Hoffman, R. G., Dasgupta, M., & Panepinto, J. A. (2013). Mental health disorders influence admission rates for pain in children with sickle cell disease. *Pediatric Blood & Cancer, 60*(7), 1211–1214.

Rosman, E. A., Perry, D. F., & Hepburn, K. S. (2005). *The best beginning: Partnerships between primary health care and mental health and substance abuse services for young children and their families*. Washington, DC: National Technical Assistance Center for Children's Mental Health.

SAMHSA-HRSA Center for Integrated Health Solutions. (2013). *Integrating behavioral health and primary care for children and youth: Concepts and strategies*. Washington, DC: Substance Abuse and Mental Health Services Administration.

Sunderji, N., Waddell, A., Gupta, M., Soklaridis, S., & Steinberg, R. (2016). An expert consensus on core competencies in integrated care for psychiatrists. *General Hospital Psychiatry, 41*, 45–52 PMID: 27302722.

U.S. Department of Health and Human Services. (1999). *Mental health: A report of the surgeon general*. Rockville: Substance Abuse and Mental Health Services Administration, Center for Mental Health Services, National Institutes of Health, National Institute of Mental Health, U.S, Department of Health and Human Services.

University of Virginia Health System. (2007, April 12). Retrieved April 1, 2017, From developmental and behavioral problems can plague children with asthma: http://newsroom.uvahealth.com/about/news-room/archives/developmental-and-behavioral-problems-can-plague-children-with-asthma/

Wagner, E. H., Austin, B. T., Davis, C., Hindmarsh, M., Schaefer, J., & Bonomi, A. (2001). Improving chronic illness care: Translating evidence into action. *Health Affairs, 20*(6), 64–78.

WHO Department of Mental Health and Substance Abuse. (2005). WHO atlas child and adolescent mental health resources. In *Global concerns: Implications for the future*. Geneva: World Health Organization.

William, J., Shore, S. E., & Foy, J. M. (2006). Co-location of mental health professionals in primary care settings: Three North Carolina models. *Clinical Pediatrics, 45*, 537–543.

Chapter 19
Preventive Models for Reducing Major Causes of Morbidity and Mortality in Childhood

Jeanelle J. Sugimoto-Matsuda and Deborah Goebert

Introduction and Overview

Increasingly, pediatric providers are partnering with educational, public health, social service, and child welfare entities in interdisciplinary teams to identify various factors contributing to children's well-being and illness and to participate in advocacy on multiple levels. These factors include biological, psychological, educational, economic, and other social influences (American Academy of Pediatrics 2013). Collaboration between pediatric providers and consultation-liaison (CL) psychiatry, in both the inpatient and outpatient settings, creates opportunities to address and prevent leading causes of morbidity and mortality Toward this goal, it is essential for pediatric practitioners to understand the public health approach and integrate a community dimension into their practice. While most clinicians are accustomed to focusing on the treatment of individual patients and their immediate social support, such a narrow focus can lead to missed opportunities for effective prevention in the context of the patient, family, and larger community. The public health approach encourages providers to not limit their attention to the individual, but also consider the patient's various interpersonal relationships and organizational and community memberships, as well as larger societal influences that impact people's health. The goal of this chapter and associated vignettes is to provide an overview of key public health principles, approaches, and tools that pediatric CL psychiatrists may find useful and relevant for day-to-day application.

J. J. Sugimoto-Matsuda (✉) · D. Goebert
Department of Psychiatry, John A. Burns School of Medicine,
University of Hawai'i at Mānoa, Honolulu, HI, USA
e-mail: sugimotoj@dop.hawaii.edu; goebertd@dop.hawaii.edu

A. P. S. Guerrero et al. (eds.), *Pediatric Consultation-Liaison Psychiatry*,
https://doi.org/10.1007/978-3-319-89488-1_19

Table 19.1 Leading causes of death for youth and young adults in the United States, from birth through age 24 (excerpted from CDC 2015c)

Rank	<1 year old	1–4 years old	5–9 years old	10–14 years old	15–24 years old
1	Congenital abnormalities	Unintentional injury	Unintentional injury	Unintentional injury	Unintentional injury
2	Short gestation	Congenital abnormalities	Malignant neoplasms	Malignant neoplasms	Suicide
3	SIDS	Homicide	Congenital abnormalities	Suicide	Homicide
4	Maternal pregnancy complications	Malignant neoplasms	Homicide	Homicide	Malignant neoplasms
5	Unintentional injury	Heart disease	Heart disease	Congenital abnormalities	Heart disease

Trends in Morbidity and Mortality Among Youth

Globally, the leading causes of death among adolescents are traffic injury, HIV, suicide, lower respiratory infections, and interpersonal violence (World Health Organization [WHO] 2017). Depression, road injuries, HIV, and suicide are major causes of disability-adjusted life years lost in 10- to 19-year-olds and account for nearly 35% of the global burden of disease rooted in adolescence. The most recent data on the leading causes of death in the United States from the Centers for Disease Control and Prevention (2015c) are presented in Table 19.1. Except for in the newborn and infant age group, unintentional injuries are the leading cause of death for youth and young adults up to 24 years of age. Unintentional injuries for these age groups include drowning (leading cause for 1- to 4-year-old age group), motor vehicle crashes (leading cause for the 5- to 24-year-old age groups), suffocation, fire/burns, poisoning, and other land transport (CDC 2015b). With respect to nonfatal injuries, unintentional falls were the leading reason for treatment in an emergency department (ED) for youth up to 14 years old (CDC 2015a). Being struck by or against an object (i.e., blunt force trauma) was the leading cause for those in the 15- to 24-year-old group (CDC 2015a).

It is also important to highlight violence-related causes of fatal and nonfatal injuries for youth. Interpersonal violence (i.e., child abuse/neglect, youth fights/violence/homicide, intimate partner violence, and sexual violence) and suicide are paramount issues for clinicians and public health practitioners alike.

Violence Among Youth

Youth violence is a major public health problem, with the United States having the highest rate of serious youth violence among developed nations (Thornton et al. 2002; US Department of Health & Human Services [DHHS] 2001; World Health

Organization [WHO] 2002). In 2012, 4787 youth between the ages of 10 and 24 years were victims of homicide, and another 599,000 were treated in EDs for physical assault injuries (CDC 2012). In addition, more than 1.1 million juvenile arrests occur annually, with more than 350,000 of those for violent crimes (Federal Bureau of Investigation 2012). Each year, youth homicides and assault-related injuries result in an estimated $16 billion in medical costs and work loss (CDC 2012).

Youth Suicide

Globally, while suicide is the 15th leading cause of death overall, it is the 2nd leading cause of death among youth and young adults ages 15–29 (WHO 2014). Furthermore, suicide rates of adolescents and young adults have generally increased in the last few decades throughout societies across the world. Suicide is becoming one of the fastest-growing causes of death among American youth, with more dying from suicide than motor vehicle traffic-related injuries (DHHS 2012). In addition, approximately 157,000 youth receive medical care for self-inflicted injuries nationwide every year (Kochanek et al. 2011). Epidemiologic studies have confirmed that youth and young adults have higher rates of ED visits for suicide attempts and self-inflicted injuries, compared to adults (Larkin et al. 2008; Ting et al. 2012).

These intentional injuries take a substantial toll on communities, affecting individuals and families from all areas, ethnicities, age groups, and life circumstances. As with unintentional injuries, those who survive intentional violent events or situations may suffer physical, mental, and/or emotional issues throughout the rest of their lives. Violence also impacts our whole society. It decreases academic and occupational productivity and property values, and increases the burden on social service programs.

Case Vignette 19.1: Multiple Suicides in a Community

A 16-year-old girl is admitted to the hospital with severe injuries sustained from being struck by a car on a rural road late at night. She had been out walking because she was unable to sleep. You are consulted because the treating physician is concerned that the patient may be depressed.

During the interview, she does indeed admit to feeling sad for the past several months following her breakup with her boyfriend of 8 months. She admits to difficulties with insomnia, decreased interest in activities she previously enjoyed doing, and social withdrawal. Her grades have declined as she has had increasing difficulty concentrating on her academics. She denies substance use beyond occasional use of marijuana, and her labs were unremarkable. She denies being sexually active. She has never previously suffered from mental health issues.

You assess for suicidality using the IS PATH WARM mnemonic for warning signs and risk factors (Ideation, Substance abuse, Purposelessness, Anxiety, Trapped, Hopelessness, Withdrawal, Anger, Recklessness, Mood changes (American Association of Suicidology [AAS] n.d.*)). You learn that she has had suicidal thoughts* *but does not have a plan. You develop a treatment and safety plan with her and her family. You also note that this is the third adolescent from her community that has been seen with suicidality and wonder what is being done in this community to address this issue.*

You speak with the patient's primary care doctor, who shares that, in recent months, they have been seeing several teens in their office with suicidality. He says this phenomenon also happened a few years ago, and the community banded together to do gatekeeper trainings and awareness activities, but over time, their interest waned. He said that he would soon be meeting with concerned community members and that he would keep you informed. He thought there was some sort of plan that had been developed by the Department of Health and Human Services. You call the department's suicide prevention contact and obtain a copy of the plan and their working group meeting schedule. You decide to attend their meeting to collaborate with other organizations on this important issue.

Because of your diligent efforts, your regular attendance, and your willingness to learn public health approaches (different from what you had learned in medical school, residency, and fellowship training), you eventually emerge as a leader in this area and become more involved in several important initiatives to "hard wire" improved screening for suicidality and accessibility to urgent mental healthcare in the community.

The Public Health Approach

Public health approaches and models are valuable tools for health providers. There are three aspects of public health that differentiate it from partner disciplines such as clinical medicine. First, in contrast with the medical model, which centers intervention and treatment around the individual patient, public health approaches view health issues from a community and population perspective. Second, public health programs and interventions tend to emphasize the promotion of wellness and primary prevention, as opposed to disease treatment and management. Finally, public health emphasizes the translation and application of research to the community. Some practitioners describe their work as "where the rubber meets the road" or "the 'so what' of research." Public health strives to provide the maximum benefit for the largest number of people (CDC n.d.).

There are three core functions of public health:

1. Assessment, the surveillance of health issues, which includes monitoring trends, analyzing causes, and identifying needs.
2. Policy development through community engagement, promotion of evidence in decision-making, and strategic planning/approaches.
3. Assurance, monitoring, and evaluation of the implementation of interventions and ensuring high-quality services through legislative mandates, statutory

responsibilities, health services, and financing (Johns Hopkins University 2008; Schneider 2006).

Ten specific "essential services (ES)" are defined under the three overarching functions of public health (CDC 2014). These ten services provide a foundation at the community, state, and national levels, and are also used as a framework for reviews and evaluation according to national performance and educational accreditation standards.

- Assessment
  - ES1 – Monitor health to identify and solve community health problems.
  - ES2 – Diagnose and investigate health problems and health hazards in the community.
- Policy Development
  - ES3 – Inform, educate, and empower people about health issues.
  - ES4 – Mobilize community partnerships to identify and solve health problems.
  - ES5 – Develop policies and plans that support individual and community health efforts.
- Assurance
  - ES6 – Enforce laws and regulations that protect health and ensure safety.
  - ES7 – Link people to needed personal health services, and assure the provision of healthcare when otherwise unavailable.
  - ES8 – Assure a competent public and personal healthcare workforce.
  - ES9 – Evaluate effectiveness, accessibility, and quality of personal and population-based health services.
- Crosscutting Service
  - ES10 – Research for new insights and innovative solutions to health problems.

Within the discipline, there are several major specializations that work in concert to address public health issues, including epidemiology, social and behavioral sciences, and health policy and management. *Epidemiology* is the study of the distributions and determinants of health-related events in human populations. A basic tenet of epidemiology is that health conditions are not randomly distributed in the population. Determining the prevalence and risk factors associated with these events, as well as measuring the magnitude of such occurrences, is a key driver in epidemiology. This information then serves as the basis of public health action. An essential part of this determination involves the utilization of epidemiologic and biostatistical methods to evaluate the effectiveness of disease control measures. Epidemiologic tools and strategies have direct relevance for physicians and other clinical providers in areas such as monitoring of disease and treatment trends, both within an identified patient pool as well as in the larger community.

Social and behavioral health sciences (SBHS) address public health issues by motivating changes in people's behaviors, by reducing unhealthy behaviors, and by emphasizing healthy ones. This field also investigates the ways in which people and communities interface with each other and their environments, and how these interactions impact health outcomes. The major tools of SBHS include health communication, needs/assets assessments, intervention planning and implementation, and process and outcome evaluation of interventions. There is also a growing emphasis on the use of community-based participatory research methods for intervention assessment, design, implementation, and evaluation. SBHS tools and strategies have direct relevance for physicians and other clinical providers in areas such as program/intervention implementation and evaluation, which includes quality assurance/improvement initiatives.

Public health practitioners who serve in senior-level leadership positions in health services are often engaged in the work of *health policy and management (HPM)*. The challenge of delivering high-quality, cost-effective healthcare and developing public policies that maintain or improve health is becoming increasingly complex as the trend toward globalization permeates all living systems. HPM research generally aims to advance the organization, financing, and delivery of health services, systems, and policies. HPM tools and strategies have direct relevance for physicians and other clinical providers in areas such as healthcare financing and systems, patient/health advocacy, and program/organizational management.

In public health practice, the above specializations are applied to health issues and work in concert to carry out the public health functions and essential services. For example, both clinicians and public health practitioners alike have identified underage drinking as a concerning health issue (National Institute on Alcohol Abuse and Alcoholism 2017). In this example, epidemiologists may gather, analyze, and interpret data to ascertain the extent of the underage drinking problem within a community or population. They may also conduct an analysis to identify subgroups that are particularly susceptible to early alcohol initiation or to propose potential risk/protective factors that may increase/decrease the risk for underage drinking. Social and behavioral health scientists may partner with epidemiologists to interpret the data collected and translate it to public health practice. They may help to integrate data and prevention best practices into training programs that target those who interface with youth. They may also design, implement, and evaluate drinking prevention programs that target the youth themselves. HPM practitioners may help to establish policies and best practices for organizations that work to prevent underage drinking. They may also design, implement, and evaluate public policies that expand funding for underage drinking prevention or increase penalties for individuals or businesses that provide alcohol to minors.

Fig. 19.1 The three levels of prevention in public health

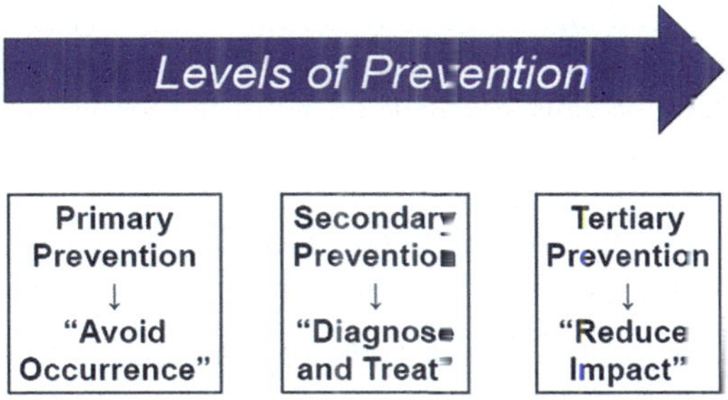

Levels of Prevention

As previously discussed, wellness and prevention of disease in communities and populations are paramount goals for public health. It is important to note that public health practitioners define three levels within the broader term "prevention" (see Fig. 19.1). *Primary prevention* refers to the most "upstream" type of prevention – that is, preventing the occurrence of an illness or conditions before onset. Primary prevention activities promote health and protect against exposure to risk factors that lead to health problems (Owen et al. 1999). Primary prevention involves addressing individual lifestyle behaviors, family and social networks, and the larger community and environment. For example, in suicide prevention, programs teach youth about positive coping skills and ensure connections to positive adult role models.

Secondary prevention refers to early detection and/or intervention of an illness or condition, as well as strategies to stop or slow the progression of disease. Secondary prevention includes programs such as early screening and treatment and appropriate follow-up. Secondary prevention activities may target those who are more susceptible to health problems because of factors such as family history, age, lifestyle, health condition, or environmental factors (Owen et al. 1999). For example, suicide prevention involves efforts to institutionalize routine screening for risk factors such as depression, anxiety, and suicidal thoughts.

Tertiary prevention refers to the management and rehabilitation of those who have been affected by an illness or condition. Interventions are aimed at those with diagnosed health conditions and reduce complications, improve quality of life, and extend years of productivity (Owen et al. 1999). For example, in suicide prevention behavioral therapy, medication treatment, and crisis plans prevent future suicide attempts.

When conceptualizing the three levels of prevention, it is useful to consider the ideas of working "upstream" (with primary prevention efforts) or "downstream" (with tertiary prevention efforts). When one works upstream, it is common to discover that not all contributors to a health issue are related to an individual's biology. Providers must consider broader contributors that impact the health of people in a community, as well as factors that account for differences in the health status and outcomes of different groups. Social determinants of health refer to the conditions of daily life that impact health, as well as factors such as access to power, money, and resources (Solar and Irwin 2010). The health of a community depends not only on the genetics and behaviors of its individual residents but also the social, political, economic, and environmental conditions that exist. Health disparities occur when there are different conditions across different groups.

Vignette 19.2: Youth Violence and Family and Organizational Responses

A 13-year-old boy presents to the ED with an ocular injury. The boy's father states that the injury occurred during soccer practice. You are consulted because the treating physician is concerned that the boy's presentation is inconsistent with the father's story. The physician also noted that the father would not allow his son to respond to questions, and the boy seemed ashamed of presenting with this type of injury.

You gain the father's permission to speak to the patient alone. During your interview with the boy, he admits struggling in school for the past year. He eventually reveals that he disclosed to his parents that he is gay. While his mother has been generally supportive, his relationship with his father has become fragmented. Although not expressing outright anger, his father avoids discussing the issue, and the patient believes that his father is disappointed in him. The boy also reveals having increasing difficulties in school due to several other students suspecting that he is gay. For the past 6 months, he has endured verbal taunting and harassment over social media. He sought help from his school counselor, who was not able to offer assistance other than to advise him to avoid the individuals harassing him. This bullying culminated in a physical alteration on campus today and resulted in the patient's ocular injury. Although he admits to feeling depressed since the bullying and harassment started, he denies having suicidal thoughts or using substances.

After ensuring that the boy's injury was attended to, you speak privately with the boy's father. He admitted that he had convinced his son to tell the providers that the injury was due to a sports injury. While it is evident that the father continues to struggle with the fact that his son is gay, he seems to genuinely care for his son. You encourage the father to speak openly with his son and wife on how to come together as a family, even possibly seeking family counseling if appropriate. You also make him aware of the Family Acceptance Project (https://familyproject.sfsu.edu/), which provides online resources on ways families can support their lesbian, gay, bisexual, transgender, and questioning/queer (LGBTQ) children.

You contact a colleague who has an ongoing relationship with the boy's school. Without discussing the patient's details, you express concerns over the school's ability and readiness to support bullied students, as well as LGBTQ youth. You learn that a group of parents concerned about different situations related to bullying and harassment have already contacted the school. You then contact a local bullying prevention resource group and help to facilitate a meeting with this group of parents and the school personnel.

At the meeting, the bullying prevention resource group provides you, the school staff, and the concerned parents with resources and suggestions for best practices. During the discussion, the school staff articulate some of their resistances to changing their current practices, but they ultimately acknowledge that, in view of the data presented to them, "something needs to change." The school agrees to arrange trainings for its staff in both bullying and suicide prevention. Furthermore, the principal commits to monitoring the data on incidents at the school and will investigate how similar information is being tracked across the state. The parents are appreciative of the school's response and efforts to be more preventative.

Social Determinants of Health

This case vignette provides an example on how the various levels of social ecology can contribute to a youth's health condition, as well as how the various levels of prevention and response provide solutions. There are nine general categories of social determinants (adapted from Brennan-Ramirez et al. 2008):

1. Stress: While brief episodes of stress may be manageable chronic stress can have significant negative impacts on health. For example, it can lead to anxiety, insecurity, social isolation, a sense of lack of control, and low self-esteem.
2. Early life: This category includes childhood factors such as early education, eating habits, and lifestyle. It also includes prenatal contributors such as nutrition, maternal stress, smoking, and drug use.
3. Social exclusion: This category can result from a variety of circumstances, including poverty, deprivation, and discrimination. Social exclusion may hinder access to necessities and services, as well as participation in activities.
4. Work: Having a job is better than not, and a healthy workplace contributes to good health. In addition, having a sense of control over one's job or workplace is also a positive factor. In general, work not only provides income to secure necessities, but it also supports important aspects of life such as healthy relationships.
5. Employment: Additional factors around employment such as job stability and job satisfaction also contribute to health. Instability or stress around employment can lead to financial and psychological stress.
6. Social support: Social interaction and healthy relationships help to bolster health. Relationships provide emotional and physical support, allow people to build social networks, and have an overall sense of feeling valued.
7. Addiction: Substance use disorders are unfortunately present in our communities. Some use substances as means of escape or coping, but this behavior often exacerbates problems. On a broader level, addiction can also lead to social breakdown and unemployment.

8. Food: Food is a basic necessity. Related considerations include the need to maintain a healthy diet and consume a proper amount. This category considers both ends of the spectrum, from malnutrition to overeating which contributes to obesity and other chronic diseases.
9. Transportation: Access to transportation has a variety of health benefits. These include exercise (e.g., cycling, walking), increased social interaction, and access to goods and services.

The Social Ecological Model

Ecological approaches are one of the cornerstones of public health planning and practice. Such approaches conceptualize health broadly, including physical, mental, and social well-being (WHO 1947). Ecological approaches also consider the multiple factors that contribute to the health of an individual and population and how those different levels of influence interact with one another (Israel et al. 2003; National Institutes of Health [NIH] 2011; Sallis et al. 2008; Wallerstein and Duran 2003). In addition to individual-level attitudes and behaviors, there are many relational, structural, environmental, and policy factors that influence a person's health outcomes, including social determinants of health. A multilevel, public health approach is recommended to effectively address complex community-wide topics such as those that contribute to the leading causes of morbidity and mortality among youth.

The Social Ecological Model (SEM), seen in Fig. 19.2, is a valuable tool that helps to frame and organize the multitude of factors that influence a health topic or

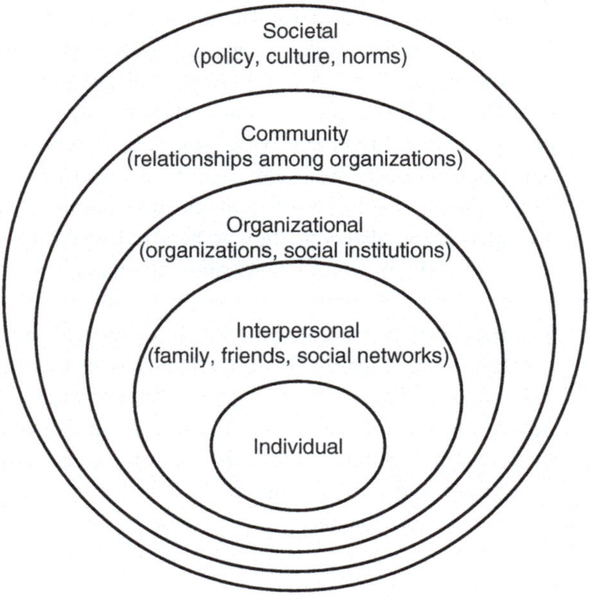

Fig. 19.2 The social ecological model

behavior, so that multilevel interventions can subsequently be planned and implemented strategically (Bronfenbrenner 1979; NIH 2011; WHO 2002). While many health programs and interventions are implemented at the individual level (e.g., provider to patient), the SEM acknowledges that a person does not exist in isolation. People are influenced by their relationships; the organizations and communities they belong to; the places where they live, work, and play; and the societal forces that surround all of us. Of note, for providers who work with youth, research supports social ecological models in youth development and in risk behaviors such as youth violence and suicide prevention research and practice (Bowen et al. 2008; Umemoto et al. 2009; Williams et al. 2007). It is only with a strategically planned effort to better guide our collective movement that a coordinated, integrated, and comprehensive approach to health and wellness is possible.

There are five levels of influence described in the SEM (McLeroy et al. 1988; NIH 2011):

Level	Description	Examples of Interventions
Individual	Characteristics of the individual, including knowledge, attitudes, behaviors, self-concept, skills, etc.; includes the developmental/biological history of the individual	Education programs that help people prevent, control, and manage health conditions Individual clinical encounters, interventions, and treatment
Interpersonal	Formal and informal social networks and support systems, including the family, co-workers, and friends	Enhancing opportunities for interpersonal contact and connection (e.g., clubs, teams, groups) Group-based activities or interventions (e.g., family strengthening, peer groups)
Organizational/ institutional	Social organizations/institutions with organizational characteristics, as well as formal and informal rules and regulations for operation	Working with organizations to increase availability/access to health-promoting goods and services Ensuring appropriate training for those working for and/or being served by the organization
Community	Relationships among organizations, institutions, and informal networks	Strengthening communication and connection among organizations Interventions aiming to increase cohesion between individuals and groups within a community
Societal	Includes local, state, and national laws and policies; considers broader determinants such as culture, norms, and media	Advocacy for policies and resources Broad public campaigns to impact changes in culture and norms

Key Concepts in Changing Behaviors and Patterns

A key tenet of public health is the development of strategies to change the patterns and behaviors of individuals and organizations. Such interventions may take place in a variety of settings, such as schools, clinics, workplaces, homes, communities, and even via media outlets, including social media. They may address one, or a combination, of the prevention and social ecological model levels. They may also target entire communities (i.e., universal programming) or specific subgroups (e.g., by race/ethnicity, age group, occupation, risk status, community, etc.). As one can imagine, the development, implementation, and evaluation of such strategies are associated with a multitude of challenges. Considerations may include cultural/personal attitudes and beliefs, mixed and/or "competing" messages (e.g., sales pitches through the media for unhealthy foods), and social determinants of health (i.e., employment and work status, early life conditions/events, stress, social exclusion/support, addiction, food availability/choices, and transportation). In addition, health behavior change is different from traditional health promotion and education. Promotion and education can increase awareness and help enable people to adopt new behaviors. Health behavior change encompasses these tasks and also incorporates (1) one's personal behaviors, expectations, motives, values, and perceptions; (2) maintenance of the behavior change over time; and (3) how the change helps to maintain, restore, and improve overall health (Glanz et al. 2015).

Behavior change theories and models are useful when designing, implementing, and evaluating interventions. They provide guidance at all stages of the process and bring research- and evidence-based concepts that have been shown to contribute to attitude, intention, and behavior changes. Of course, it is important to build in evaluation processes when incorporating any theory or model, to ensure adequacy of fit to the target population as well as intervention effectiveness. While a comprehensive review of behavior change theories and models is beyond the scope of this chapter and probably best reviewed in a public health reference textbook, the pediatric consultation-liaison psychiatrist, when advocating for change on either an individual patient/family or broader systems level, should be aware that such a literature exists.

Public Health Assessment

A public health approach to addressing a specific health issue aims to answer questions such as "Where does the problem begin?" and "How could we prevent it from occurring in the first place?" A systematic, scientific approach to understanding and preventing an issue requires multiple steps, with each step informing the next (CDC n.d.). In addition, collaborations among multiple people, organizations, and systems are essential at each phase.

Assessment is an essential first step to building a strong foundation for a public health approach to prevention. During this phase, the following are assessed:

1. Needs: A "needs assessment" is the process of systematically identifying, defining, and assessing the needs of a target organization/ population, as well as any potential gaps between desired needs and current resources (Hodges and Videto 2011). Following a needs assessment, the program or organization should be able to adjust their focus and/or resources to better meet the needs of their target population.
2. Assets: Assessment methodologies are now focusing not only on gaps and deficiencies but also the existing services, research, connections, values, and strengths within communities. Youth programs grounded in a strengths-based model of positive youth development can promote healing and facilitate a sense of belonging to a valued community (Goebert et al. in press; Guerra and Bradshaw 2008; Kral et al. 2009; Trinidad 2009).
3. Risk and protective factors: The identification of risk and protective factors helps to elicit possible reasons why one person or community experiences a health condition, while another does not. Scientific research methods are used to identify the factors that increase the risk, as well as factors that may buffer against these risk factors (CDC n.d.). Ultimately, public health interventions aim to decrease risk factors and increase protective factors.
4. Readiness: In clinical practice, the concept of readiness has traditionally referred to the precondition necessary to maximize the likelihood that an intervention with an individual patient will succeed (e.g., transtheoretical model) (Prochaska et al. 2015). Application of readiness assessments has since expanded to community interventions (e.g., Parker et al. 2011; Sugimoto-Matsuda and Rehuher 2014). A community has varying degrees of readiness to change which can impact the likelihood that a program will be successful. Two widely applied models include:

   - The Community Readiness Model has been applied to various health issues and has relevance for native and indigenous communities (Plested et al. 2006). Nine stages of readiness are described along six dimensions: (1) existing efforts, (2) knowledge of the problem, (3) knowledge of alternatives, (4) leadership, (5) resources, and (6) community climate.
   - Communities That Care (CTC) employs a public health prevention model to helping communities prepare for introducing interventions that reduce risk factors and increase protective factors (Arthur et al. 2010; Hawkins et al. 2008). CTC is composed of five phases: (1) getting started; (2) organizing, introducing, and involving; (3) developing a community profile; (4) creating a community action plan; and (5) implementing and evaluating the action plan.

Public Health Evaluation

Evaluation is another cornerstone of public health research and practice. The importance of evaluation in any system, program, or intervention cannot be overstated. Far too often practices occur without strategic and systematic means of ensuring the intended outcomes are truly being achieved, instead relying on anecdotal stories or "gut instincts." Providers have a duty to ensure they are not causing harm, which cannot be systematically detected without evaluation. Additionally, employing a strategic and systematic evaluation cycle serves as the basis for continuous quality improvement of health programs, interventions, and treatments.

There are two major types of evaluation, outcome or "summative" and process or "formative." Many practitioners think only of outcome measures when designing an evaluation process. Outcome evaluation measures program effects and allows us to determine if program goals are being achieved. For example, a suicide prevention program would monitor outcome measures such as suicide attempts and deaths. This is important information to review and apply to program improvement processes. However, process measures are just as important to include in an evaluation plan. Process evaluation is the ongoing review of program operations and helps to determine if activities are being implemented as intended. For example, the suicide prevention program mentioned above may include training workshops for clinicians. In this case, process measures would include benchmarks such as the development and testing of a training curriculum, number of clinicians trained, and effectiveness of the training measured by a knowledge-based exam. Such process measures must also be incorporated into the feedback loop for program improvement.

Of relevance for health and the healthcare system are the processes of quality assurance (QA) and continuous quality improvement (CQI). Generally stated, QA is a system for evaluating the delivery of services or the quality of products. There are three components to a QA system (Environmental Protection Agency 2002):

1. Defining quality: Identifying inputs, processes, and outcome standards that a healthcare delivery system must meet for the population to achieve optimum health gains.
2. Measuring quality: Quantifying the current level of compliance with expected standards.
3. Improving quality: Engaging in appropriate methodologies to close the gap between current and expected level of quality. Use quality management tools and principles to understand and address system deficiencies and improve or redesign efficient and effective healthcare practices.

Specific to health systems and practices, there is now a movement toward continuous quality improvement (CQI). In contrast to traditional QA, which emphasizes correcting after-the-fact errors, CQI focuses on understanding and improving underlying work processes and systems. According to Armstrong (2009), there are six requirements for CQI:

1. Leadership: Individuals in this role provide the direction in which the organization is headed with regard to continuous improvement.
2. Shared organizational values: Examples of this include patient satisfaction, respect for people, trust, cooperation, and openness.
3. Structure: The structure of an organization should be open and flexible to improvement and change to support the concept of CQI.
4. Process: Effective processes lead to continuous improvement.
5. Personnel development: Individual growth and teamwork among staff are needed to implement CQI.
6. High-performance culture: An organization should strive to identify and meet the needs of the patient.

Further, Deming (1986) outlined the five principles of CQI:

1. Focus on underlying organizational processes and systems, rather than individuals.
2. Use structured problem solving based on statistical analyses as appropriate.
3. Use cross-disciplinary teams.
4. Encourage employee empowerment to identify problems and opportunities for improved care and to take necessary action.
5. Remember to include both internal and external stakeholders.

Importance of Data-Driven Planning and Action

Over the past several decades, the importance of "data-driven" and "evidence-based" strategies has been growing among healthcare practitioners. At the most basic level, public health evidence can be defined as: "…some form of data – including epidemiologic (quantitative) data, results of program or policy evaluations, and qualitative data – to use in making judgments or decisions" (Chambers and Kerner 2007). There are multiple sources of public health evidence, including the scientific literature, surveillance data, program evaluations, community and other stakeholder data, media and marketing data, word of mouth, and personal experience (Chambers and Kerner 2007). It has been widely recommended that public health evidence should always be incorporated in the selection and implementation of programs, policies, and evaluation plans (Brownson et al. 1999). For example, data and evidence permeate all four steps of CDC's public health approach to prevention: (1) describe the problem and perform surveillance; (2) identify causes and risk/protective factors; (3) develop, implement, and evaluate prevention strategies; and (4) disseminate and ensure widespread adoption (Mercy et al. 1993).

Data can be classified in several ways. First, one can refer to the type of data collected as either quantitative (numerical, discrete, using close-ended inquiries) or qualitative (words, statements, or narratives, using open-ended inquiries). Data can also be categorized by the source from which they are obtained. Primary data are those collected or obtained from people firsthand, for example, through interviews, focus groups, and surveys. Primary data takes time and proper permission to collect, but it provides the researcher control over the specific questions, instruments, and data collection methods utilized. On the other hand, secondary data are those gathered in the past or obtained from another party (i.e., does not involve direct contact with people or communities). Examples include medical records, law enforcement reports, population-based databases, and other archived quantitative or qualitative data. Data from different types and sources can be triangulated, or combined and compared, to provide a more comprehensive picture of the health issue and its determinants.

In public health and healthcare, it is essential that data inform practice to ensure a sound foundation for the programs, treatments, and policies that are implemented. This is achieved through translational research, in which proven scientific discoveries are successfully institutionalized into established practice and policy. The use of such approaches has been particularly useful in areas that are complex and multidimensional, such as youth development and risky behaviors (Bell et al. 2008).

However, challenges remain that impede translational research and actions. For example, many effective prevention programs have been identified, but few have gained wide acceptance, and little is known about the best ways to encourage their broader use (Spoth 2008). In addition, the broader challenge that remains is how to efficiently and effectively translate public health evidence not only to individual- and community-level interventions but also societal-level interventions such as public policy. To make an impact on health from a systems and population perspective, public health evidence must be generated, policies must be grounded in the evidence, interventions must be implemented as designed, and evaluation findings must be disseminated broadly.

Specific Tools for Public Health Assessment, Planning, and Evaluation

This final section discusses examples of specific tools that may be useful in health program assessment, planning, and evaluation and that may be helpful for the pediatric CL psychiatrist working on the systems levels as described in this chapter's vignettes. Again, the reader is referred to public health textbooks for potential further reading.

Tool 19.1: Logic Models The logic model is one of the most widely used tools in public health for both planning and evaluation. It provides a big picture graphic that maps out a program's resources, activities, and outcomes, in addition to showing the interactive relationships among these components. From a planning perspective, the mapping of resources and activities helps to ensure adequate infrastructure to support the planned activities. From an evaluation perspective, the mapping of activities and outcomes helps to ensure the activities are appropriate for the changes desired. Thus, it is important to clearly lay out these components ahead of time, as well as to continuously revisit and revise the components as implementation occurs.

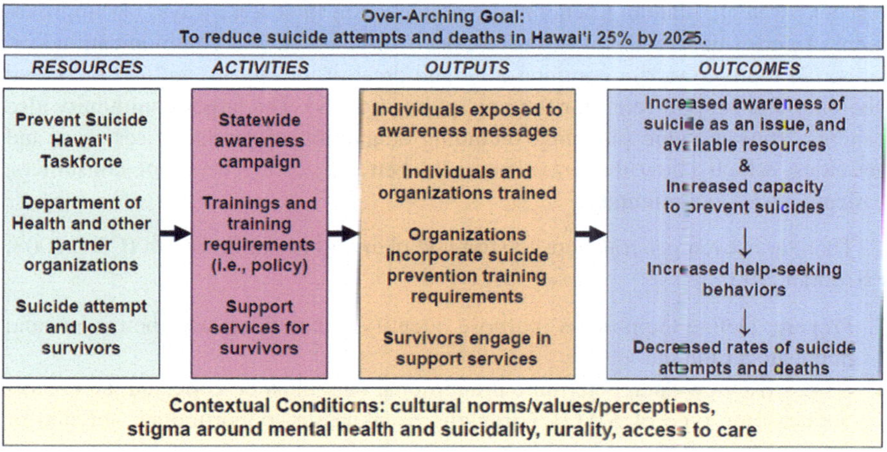

Fig. 19.3 Sample logic model

There are five major parts of a logic model: resources (sometimes referred to as "inputs"), activities, outputs, outcomes, and contextual conditions. Fig. 19.3 presents a sample logic model relating to suicide prevention.

1. Resources: Assumptions underlying a program and the necessary infrastructure for implementation (e.g., finances, human resources, technology, materials, space, key partnerships, etc.). Resources are interrelated and will influence one another in the implementation of the project.
2. Activities: Specific actions that will be implemented (i.e., what you will do with the resources to achieve the intended outcomes).
3. Outputs: Direct and measurable products of the program's activities and services, often expressed in terms of volume or units delivered.
4. Outcomes: Intended effects of cumulative program components (i.e., what changes would be seen if the program is successful).
5. Contextual conditions: Includes the values and/or theories behind the program, the conditions necessary for success, and the conditions beyond your control that must be considered (e.g., culture, rurality, health and service gaps, and socioeconomic conditions).

Tool 19.2: Strategic Planning Many professionals in health fields – including pediatric consultation-liaison psychiatrists involved in program leadership and healthcare system-level planning – are now being tasked with large-scale strategic planning processes to create a purposeful direction and set of activities for an organization or community. In broad terms, strategic planning refers to the collection of information and data, organizing and channeling that information to a stakeholder group, and building consensus to establish decisions and/or priorities (CDC 2008; Friedman 2011). The end goal for strategic planning is to design appropriate actions that will guide the program or organization, usually for an extended period. In this respect, strategic planning benefits the organization in several ways: (1) improvement of performance, use of resources, decision-making, and communication systems; (2) focus toward a common goal and creation of buy-in; and (3) increased visibility and support (e.g., for funding, policymakers). The larger community also benefits from strategic planning, including adaptation of products, services, and activities, which allow the organization to better meet the needs of consumers, patients, and the community.

There are seven general steps to strategic planning in public health (CDC 2008; Friedman 2011):

1. Prepare: Define the process' purpose, identify stakeholders and their roles, and delineate a timeline.
2. Assess: Review data, determine if additional data must be collected, and incorporate some type of SWOT (strengths, weaknesses, opportunities, threats) or similar analysis.
3. Create: Develop and write the objectives and activities (usually for a 5-year period), develop or revise your logic model, and draft annual work plans.
4. Communicate: Share plans with your stakeholders and community.
5. Implement: Put strategies into action.
6. Evaluate: Ensure both process and outcome evaluation of the strategic plan are conducted, and utilize results to inform annual work plans and future strategic plan revisions.

Tool 14.3: Advocacy Often, when health practitioners think about "advocacy," they usually associate this term with legislative testimony. While testimony is an important part of advocacy, there are many other ways to advocate. Advocacy is an umbrella term for actions and strategies aiming to garner public support or attention for policies or causes. Certain advocacy activities may specifically involve and/or target policymakers. Examples include providing formal oral or written testimony on proposed legislation, educating policymakers as a subject-matter expert, attending in-office visits, and participating in community meetings and forums. However, there are many other ways to advocate, such as mobilizing others around a cause, increasing public awareness of an issue, facilitating connections and collaborations via workgroups and task forces, helping to formulate a common message around an issue, establishing and maintaining relationships with key organizational and community leaders, participating in a workgroup with an advocacy arm including national or local chapters of professional organizations, and exploring and evaluating solutions to health issues through research and scholarship.

There are many strategies to raise awareness of an issue among the public. Personal engagement can be effective, such as going door-to-door in the community, tabling in public areas, conducting public polls or petitions, and arranging a town hall meeting or other large event. However, these strategies can be time- and resource-intensive. Most cost-efficient strategies include using printed information (e.g., newspaper or press release, flyers), offering editorials, and leveraging the various forms of media including television, radio, email, internet websites, and social media platforms. Advocacy groups have also developed relationships with key public figures including policymakers, local and national celebrities, and other respected community individuals or organizations. When engaging large groups, it is important to maintain consistent communication of a clear strategy and message and to create multiple opportunities for engagement.

There is a burgeoning field within public health that pertains to message development, framing, and marketing. In general, "messaging" refers to the pairing of an impactful message with a coordinated strategy. This activity allows the linking of an issue to a specific audience in an impactful way, changing people's perceptions relating to the value of a particular issue, and helping to gain social and political will to move the issue forward. Messaging techniques are being actively studied, given the many challenges that arise in public health communication.

Messaging experts offer the following guidelines when developing an awareness campaign (CDC 2010):

Things to do	Words of caution
1. Start with a strong statement about the problem	1. Don't dwell on the problem; people want to know about solutions
2. Use positive, action-oriented statements to present solutions	2. Don't provide exhaustive lists of statistics
3. Mention community-specific issues and programs	3. Use an uplifting tone
4. Underscore personal and community responsibility	4. Don't describe the problem using a single situation; instead, describe the broader context and long-term effects
5. Reinforce science/research involvement (but do not use jargon)	
6. Be specific on the "ask"	
7. End by reinforcing value and tangible actions	

"Social math," a specific messaging strategy, is the process of translating statistics to terms more meaningful to the audience (CDC 2010). Its use can help people to think about social and environmental contributors to behavioral choices. Examples of social math include comparing health statistics to (1) familiar numbers or costs (e.g., cost of car payment); (2) dramatic events (e.g., number of residents displaced by natural disaster); (3) costs that are smaller or more understandable (e.g., program costs less than a cup of coffee a day); and (4) numbers from other high-profile issues (e.g., more than what we spend on prescription medications each year). Two examples offered by the CDC (2010) are:

- "Every 35 minutes, an older adult dies from a fall-related injury."
- "Nationwide, implementation of effective school-based violence prevention programs could result in 187,000 less fight-related injuries among high school students. That's equivalent to nearly 7500 classrooms of students."

Many professionals can engage in another advocacy strategy, the contribution of opinions/editorials (op-eds) to media and professional publications. The Op-Ed Project (n.d.) offers sample outlines and guidelines for formulating op-eds:

Example Op-Ed outline	Tips for Op-Ed writing
1. "Hook"	1. Own your expertise: Know what you are an expert in and why, but don't limit yourself.
2. Thesis: Statement of argument	2. Stay current: Follow the news, both general and specific to your area, including local/community papers.
3. Arguments: 1st point with evidence and conclusion, 2nd point, etc. For a "simple" issue, arguments may be more straightforward (e.g., "policy X is bad, here's why"). In a more complex commentary, the 3rd point may expand on the bigger picture (e.g., historical context, global context, why a bad policy continues despite its failures, etc.).	3. "Perfection is the enemy of the good": In other words, write fast. You may have only a few hours to get your piece in before the moment is gone.
4. "To be sure" paragraph: Preempt your potential critics by acknowledging any flaws in your argument, and address any obvious counterarguments	4. Cultivate a flexible mind: A good idea may have more than one hook. Keep an eye out for surprising connections and new news hooks. The opportunity may come around again.
5. Conclusion: Circle back to your hook	5. Use plain language: Jargon serves a purpose, but can cloud your argument. Speak to your reader in straight talk.
	6. Respect your reader: Try not to underestimate your reader's intelligence or overestimate their level of expertise in your topic.

Summary and Conclusion

Healthcare and public health are complementary disciplines, yet tools of the trade from each discipline are not always shared and applied across aisles. The hope is that by familiarizing pediatric CL psychiatrists with general public health principles, approaches, and tools, they will begin to apply them in patient care. In sharing best practices, practitioners will be able to collaborate more effectively to bolster the health and wellness of patients, families, organizations, and communities.

References

American Academy of Pediatrics [AAP]. (2013). Community pediatrics: Navigating the intersection of medicine, public health, and social determinants of children's health. *Pediatrics, 131*, 623–628. https://doi.org/10.1542/peds.2012-3933.

American Association of Suicidology [AAS]. (n.d.). *Knowing the warning signs*. Washington, DC: American Association of Suicidology. Accessed from: http://www.suicidology.org/resources/warning-signs

Armstrong, M. (2009). *Armstrong's handbook of management and leadership: A guide for managing for results* (2nd ed.). Philadelphia: Kogan Page Limited.

Arthur, M. W., Hawkins, J. D., Brown, E. C., Briney, J. S., Oesterle, S., & Abbott, R. D. (2010). Implementation of the communities that care prevention system by coalitions in the community youth development study. *Journal of Community Psychology, 38*(2), 245–258.

Bell, E., Allen, R., Hogan, D., & Martinez, C. (2008). Why risk irrelevance? A translational research model for adolescent risk-taking data. *Journal of Youth Studies, 11*(4), 461–471.

Bowen, G. L., Rose, R. A., Powers, J. D., & Glennie, E. J. (2008). The joint effects of neighborhoods, schools, peers, and families on changes in the school success of middle school students. *Family Relations, 57*, 504–516.

Brennan-Ramirez, L. K., Baker, E. A., & Metzler, M. (2008). *Promoting health equity: A resource to help communities address social determinants of health*. Atlanta: Social Determinants of Health Workgroup, Centers for Disease Control and Prevention, Department of Health and Human Services. Accessed from: https://www.cdc.gov/nccdphp/dch/programs/healthycommunitiesprogram/tools/pdf/sdoh-workbook.pdf

Bronfenbrenner, U. (1979). *The ecology of human development: Experiments by nature and design*. Cambridge, MA: The Harvard University Press.

Brownson, R. C., Gurney, J. G., & Land, G. (1999). Evidence-based decision making in public health. *Journal of Public Health Management and Practice, 5*(5), 85–97.

Centers for Disease Control and Prevention [CDC]. (2008). *Using evaluation to improve programs: Strategic planning*. Atlanta: Centers for Disease Control and Prevention, Division of Adolescent and School Health, Evaluation Technical Assistance. Accessed from: https://www.cdc.gov/HealthyYouth/evaluation/pdf/sp_kit/sp_toolkit.pdf

Centers for Disease Control and Prevention [CDC]. (2010). *Adding power to our voices: A framing guide for communicating about injury*. Atlanta: Centers for Disease Control and Prevention, National Center for Injury Prevention and Control. Accessed from: https://www.cdc.gov/injury/pdfs/framing/CDCFramingGuide-a.pdf

Centers for Disease Control and Prevention [CDC]. (2012). *Web-based Injury Statistics Query and Reporting System (WISQARS)*. Atlanta: Centers for Disease Control and Prevention, National Center for Injury Prevention and Control. Accessed from: www.cdc.gov/injury/wisqars

Centers for Disease Control and Prevention [CDC]. (2014). *The 10 essential public health services*. Centers for Disease Control and Prevention, Office for State, Tribal, Local, and Territorial Support. Accessed from: https://www.cdc.gov/nphpsp/documents/essential-phs.pdf

Centers for Disease Control and Prevention [CDC]. (2015a). *National estimates of the ten leading causes of non-fatal injuries treated in hospital emergency departments, United States, 2015*. Atlanta: Centers for Disease Control and Prevention, National Center for Injury Prevention and Control. Accessed from: https://www.cdc.gov/injury/wisqars/pdf/leading_causes_of_non-fatal_injury_2015-a.pdf

Centers for Disease Control and Prevention [CDC]. (2015b). *Ten leading causes of death by age group highlighting unintentional injury deaths, United States, 2015*. Atlanta: Centers for

Disease Control and Prevention, National Center for Injury Prevention and Control. Accessed from: https://www.cdc.gov/injury/images/lc-charts/leading_causes_of_injury_deaths_unintentional_injury_2015_1050w760h.gif

Centers for Disease Control and Prevention [CDC]. (2015c). *Ten leading causes of death by age group, United States, 2015.* Atlanta: Centers for Disease Control and Prevention, National Center for Injury Prevention and Control. Accessed from: https://www.cdc.gov/injury/images/lc-charts/leading_causes_of_death_age_group_2015_1050w740h.gif

Centers for Disease Control and Prevention [CDC]. (n.d.). *The public health approach to violence prevention.* Atlanta: Centers for Disease Control and Prevention, National Center for Injury Prevention and Control, Division of Violence Prevention. Accessed from: https://www.cdc.gov/violenceprevention/pdf/PH_App_Violence-a.pdf

Chambers, D., & Kerner, J. (2007). *Closing the gap between discovery and delivery.* Rockville: Presentation at the "Harnessing Science to Maximize Health" Dissemination and Implementation Research Workshop.

Deming, W. E. (1986). *Out of the crisis.* Boston: Massachusetts Institute of Technology, Center for Advanced Engineering Study.

Environmental Protection Agency. (2002, December). *Guidance for quality assurance project plans.* Washington, DC: United States Environmental Protection Agency, Office of Environmental Information. Accessed from: https://nepis.epa.gov/Exe/ZyPDF.cgi/20011HPE.PDF?Dockey=20011HPE.PDF

Federal Bureau of Investigation. (2012). *Arrests by age, 2011.* Accessed from: http://www.fbi.gov/ucr/cius2011/arrests/index.html

Friedman, L. H. (2011). Strategic planning and marketing for public health managers. In R. E. Burke & L. H. Friedman (Eds.), *Essentials of management and leadership in public health* (pp. 39–52). Sudbury: Jones and Bartlett Learning.

Glanz, K., Rimer, B. K., & Viswanath, K. (2015). *Health behavior: Theory, research, and practice* (5th ed.). San Francisco: Jossey-Bass.

Goebert, D., Alvarez, A., Andrade, N. N., Balberde-Kamalii, J., Carlton, B. S., Chock, S., Chung-Do, J., Eckert, M. D., Hooper, K., Kaninau-Santos, K., Kaulukukui, G., Kelly, C., Pike M., Rehuher, D., & Sugimoto-Matsuda, J. (in press). Hope, help, and healing: Culturally-embedded approaches to suicide prevention, intervention and postvention services with Native Hawaiian youth. *Psychological Services.*

Guerra, N. G., & Bradshaw, C. P. (2008). Linking the prevention of problem behaviors and positive youth development: Core competencies to prevent problem behaviors and promote positive youth development. In N. G. Guerra & C. P. Bradshaw (Eds.), *Core competencies to prevent problem behaviors and promote positive youth development* (New directions for child and adolescent development, Vol. 122, pp. 1–17). San Francisco: Jossey-Bass.

Hawkins, J., Brown, E. C., Oesterle, S., Arthur, M. W., Abbott, R. D., & Catalano, R. F. (2008). Early effects of communities that care on targeted risks and initiation of delinquent behavior and substance use. *Journal of Adolescent Health, 43*(1), 15–22.

Hodges, B. C., & Videto, D. M. (2011). *Assessment and planning in health programs* (2nd ed.). Sudbury: Jones and Bartlett Learning.

Israel, B. A., Schulz, A. J., Parker, E. A., Becker, A. B., Allen, A. J., & Guzman, J. R. (2003). Critical issues in developing and following community based participatory research principles. In M. Minkler & N. Wallerstein (Eds.), *Community-based participatory research for health* (pp. 53–76). San Francisco: Jossey-Bass.

Johns Hopkins University. (2008). *Core functions and essential services.* Baltimore: Johns Hopkins University, Bloomberg School of Public Health. Accessed from: http://ocw.jhsph.edu/courses/publichealthpractice101/PDF/Session4.pdf

Kochanek, K. D., Xu, J., Murphy, S. L., Minino, A. M., & Kung, H. C. (2011). Deaths: Final data for 2009. *National and Vital Statistics Report, 60*(3), 1–116.

Kral, M. J., Wiebe, P. K., Nisbet, K., Dallas, C., Okalik, L., Enuaraq, N., & Cinotta, J. (2009). Canadian Inuit community engagement in youth suicide prevention. *International Journal of Circumpolar Health, 68*(3), 292–308.

Larkin, G. L., Smith, R. P., & Beautrais, A. L. (2008). Trends in US emergency department visits for suicide attempts, 1992-2001. *Crisis, 29*(2), 73–80.

McLeroy, K. R., Bibeau, D., Steckler, A., & Glanz, K. (1988). An ecological perspective on health promotion programs. *Health Education Quarterly, 15*(4), 351–377.

Mercy, J. A., Rosenberg, M. L., Powell, K. E., Broome, C. V., & Roper, W. L. (1993). Public health policy for preventing violence. *Health Affairs, 12*, 7–29.

National Institute on Alcohol Abuse and Alcoholism (NIAAA). (2017). *Underage drinking*. Bethesda: National Institutes of Health, National Institute on Alcohol Abuse and Alcoholism. Accessed from: https://pubs.niaaa.nih.gov/publications/UnderageDrinking/Underage_Fact.pdf

National Institutes of Health (NIH). (2011, June). *Principles of community engagement* (2nd ed.). Bethesda: National Institutes of Health, Clinical and Translational Science Awards Consortium Community Engagement Key Function Committee Task Force on the Principles of Community Engagement. Accessed from: https://www.atsdr.cdc.gov/communityengagement/pdf/PCE_Report_508_FINAL.pdf

Owen, A. L., Splett, P. L., & Owen, G. M. (1999). *Nutrition in the community: The art and science of delivering services* (4th ed.). New York: McGraw-Hill.

Parker, R. N., Alcaraz, R., & Payne, P. R. (2011). Community readiness for change and youth violence prevention: A tale of two cities. *American Journal of Community Psychology, 48*, 97–105.

Plested, B. A., Jumper-Thurman, P., & Edwards, R. W. (2006). *Community readiness: Advancing suicide prevention in native communities* (Community readiness model handbook). Fort Collins: Center for Applied Studies in American Ethnicity, Colorado State University.

Prochaska, J. O., Redding, C. A., & Evers, K. E. (2015). The trans-theoretical model and stages of change. In K. Glanz, B. K. Rimer, & K. Viswanath (Eds.), *Health behavior: Theory, research, and practice* (5th ed., pp. 125–148). San Francisco: Jossey-Bass.

Sallis, J. F., Owen, N., & Fisher, E. B. (2008). Ecological models of health behavior. In K. Glanz, B. K. Rimer, & K. Viswanath (Eds.), *Health behavior and health education* (4th ed., pp. 465–485). San Francisco: Wiley.

Schneider, M. J. (2006). *Introduction to public health* (2nd ed.). Sudbury: Jones and Bartlett Publishers.

Solar, O., & Irwin, A. (2010). *A conceptual framework for action on the social determinants of health*. Geneva: World Health Organization.

Spoth, R. (2008). Translating family-focused prevention science into effective practice: Toward a translational impact paradigm. *Current Directions in Psychological Science, 17*(6), 415–421.

Sugimoto-Matsuda, J. & Rehuher, D. (2014). Suicide prevention in diverse populations: A systems and readiness approach for emergency settings. *Psychiatric Times*, pp. 40G–40H.

The Op Ed Project (n.d.). *Op-ed writing: Tips and tricks*. New York: The Op Ed Project. Accessed from: https://www.theopedproject.org/oped-basics/

Thornton, T. N., Craft, C. A., Dahlberg, L. L., Lynch, B. S., & Baer, K. (2002). *Best practices of youth violence prevention: A sourcebook for community action (Rev.)*. Atlanta: Centers for Disease Control and Prevention, National Center for Injury Prevention and Control.

Ting, S. A., Sullivan, A. F., Boudreaux, E. D., Miller, I., & Camargo, C. A. Jr. (2012). Trends in US emergency department visits for attempted suicide and self-inflicted injury, 1993–2008. *General Hospital Psychiatry, 34*(5), 557–565. https://doi.org/10.1016/j.genhosppsych.2012.03.020.

Trinidad, A. M. O. (2009). Toward *kuleana* (responsibility): A case study of a contextually grounded intervention for native Hawaiian youth and young adults. *Aggression and Violent Behavior, 14*, 488–498.

Umemoto, K., Baker, C. K., Helm, S., Miao, T., Goebert, D. A., & Hishinuma, E. S. (2009). Moving toward comprehensiveness and sustainability in a social ecological approach to youth

violence prevention: Lessons from the Asian/Pacific islander Youth Violence Prevention Center. *American Journal of Community Psychology, 44*(3–4), 221–232.
United States Department of Health and Human Services [DHHS]. (2001). *Youth violence: A report of the Surgeon General*. Rockville: US Department of Health and Human Services, Centers for Disease Control and Prevention, National Center for Injury Prevention and Control, Substance Abuse and Mental Health Services Administration, Center for Mental Health Service; and National Institutes of Health, National Institute of Mental Health.
United States Department of Health and Human Services [DHHS], Office of the Surgeon General, and the National Action Alliance for Suicide Prevention. (2012). *2012 National strategy for suicide prevention: Goals and objectives for action*. Washington, DC: Department of Health and Human Services. Accessed from: http://www.ncbi.nlm.nih.gov/books/NBK109917/pdf/Bookshelf_NBK109917.pdf
Wallerstein, N., & Duran, B. (2003). The conceptual, historical and practice roots of community-based participatory research and related participatory traditions. In M. Minkler & N. Wallerstein (Eds.), *Community-based participatory research for health* (1st ed., pp. 27–52). San Francisco: Jossey-Bass.
Williams, K., Riveras, L., Neighbours, R., & Reznik, V. (2007). Youth violence prevention comes of age: Research, training and future directions. *Annual Review of Public Health, 28*, 195–211.
World Health Organization [WHO]. (1947). *Constitution*. New York: World Health Organization.
World Health Organization [WHO]. (2002). *World report on violence and health*. Geneva: World Health Organization.
World Health Organization [WHO]. (2014). *Preventing suicide: A global imperative*. Geneva: World Health Organization.
World Health Organization [WHO]. (2017). *Adolescent health epidemiology*. Geneva: World Health Organization. Accessed from: http://www.who.int/maternal_child_adolescent/epidemiology/adolescence/en/

Chapter 20
Addressing Healthcare Disparities

Diane Eckert and Deborah Goebert

Introduction

The prevalence of mental disorders varies significantly by race and ethnicity across the lifespan (Breslau et al. 2006; Breslau et al. 2005; Alegría et al. 2007; McGuire and Miranda 2008; Smedley et al. 2002; Williams and Earl 2007; World Health Organization 2014; US Department of Health and Human Services 2001). Minority groups experience greater numbers of risk factors that accrue incrementally over time, with differential effects, contributing to mental health and healthcare disparities (Alegría et al. 2015; Gee and Payne-Sturges 2004). This chapter aims to illustrate the important role that the well-informed and culturally humble pediatric psychosomatic medicine practitioner can play in identifying and addressing mental health disparities in children and adolescents.

Race, Ethnicity, and Culture

Race, ethnicity, and culture are often ill-defined, controversial, and ambiguous. As social concepts, they have many different meanings, and those meanings continue to change over time. Race is often considered a biological category – as a way to divide and label groups by skin pigmentation or other physical characteristics. However, genetic variation within a putative racial group is overwhelmingly greater than genetic variation across putative racial groups. Thus, race is given meaning – albeit non-scientifically – as a social category, especially when certain social groups are separated, treated as inferior or superior, or provided differential access to power

D. Eckert (✉) · D. Goebert
Department Psychiatry, John A Burns School of Medicine, University of Hawaii at Manoa, Honolulu, HI, USA
e-mail: deckert@dop.hawaii.edu; goebertd@dop.hawaii.edu

A. P. S. Guerrero et al. (eds.), *Pediatric Consultation-Liaison Psychiatry*,
https://doi.org/10.1007/978-3-319-89488-1_20

and resources. Ethnicity refers to a common heritage shared by a particular group. Heritage includes similar history, language, rituals, practices, and preferences for music, diet, and foods. Though less common, ethnicity can also include a geographical connection. Culture is a system of shared meanings obtained from a common heritage or set of beliefs, norms, and values. Yet, culture can be experienced uniquely by different members of the same cultural group.

Case Vignette #1
You are a psychiatrist working in a community-based, integrated primary care/behavioral health clinic. During a weekly team meeting to review cases that screen positive for mental health concerns, the primary care provider presents the first case.

A first-generation immigrant Chinese couple with two older daughters gave birth to an infant, now 13 years of age, with ambiguous genitalia. Initially, the physicians wanted to run further tests, and they recommended that the family wait until the test results were completed in order to make a gender assignment. However, the family made the immediate decision to assign the gender of male to this infant and refused any further testing. The child was raised as a boy; however, early on, he exhibited effeminate mannerisms and preferred wearing female clothing and playing with dolls with his sisters. These behaviors led to significant parent-child conflict, which only escalated as he approached adolescence.

The team seeks your advice on how they can best help the family. You begin to organize your thoughts into a matrix to guide further inquiry and assessment, and you highlight for the team the importance of further inquiring into cultural identity issues:

Facts	Hypotheses	Information needed	Learning issues
First-generation Chinese-American parents	Female gender preference	Context of gender selection	Gender identity
Child, now 12 years old, born with ambiguous genitalia	Role of cultural conflict	Context of family conflict	Gender expression
		Child's cultural identity, parents' cultural identity, and expectations for their children	**Cultural identity (discussed further below)**

Cultural Identity

Cultural identity refers to the totality of a person's cultural self-definition, including ethnicity, race, country of origin, language, age, marital status, gender, sexual orientation, religious/spiritual beliefs, acculturation, individualism, and collectivism (Schwartz et al. 2007). Acculturation is the process by which foreign-born individuals and their families learn and adopt the language, values, beliefs, and behaviors of the new sociocultural environment (Sam and Berry 2010). It refers to orientations toward both heritage and host cultural contexts and practices (Tadmor and Tetlock 2006). Historically, acculturation has been operationalized as a unidimensional continuum ranging from retention of heritage-culture values and practices to acquisition of host-culture values and practices (Flannery et al. 2001). It is increasingly recognized as a bidimensional model in which orientations toward heritage and host values and practices are considered separate dimensions (Ryder et al. 2000). This process takes place over time, and it involves cultural groups with different characteristics.

For many ethnic minority youths, this may entail changes in values, beliefs, and norms such as shifting from a more collectivistic to a more individualistic orientation. This type of emphasis on independence, autonomy, and self-determination is characteristic of Western cultural values. Triandis et al. (1988) explore the concepts of individualism and collectivism as a major dimension of cultural variation in identity formation, providing a list of characteristics related to notions of the self, activities, attitudes, values, and behaviors. Oetting and Beauvais's (1990) cultural identification theory also implies that lower levels of cultural identification are associated with adverse psychosocial characteristics, including lower self-esteem, poor school performance, negative personal adjustment, and fewer personal and social resources. Such characteristics are likely to increase the vulnerability to mental illness among ethnic minority children.

Risk and Protective Factors

Alegría et al. (2015) present a model that is useful in examining the risk and protective factors associated with disparities in the prevalence of mental health disorders. Their model focuses on four risk categories as minority children and adolescents transition into adulthood: (i) socioeconomic status, (ii) adverse childhood events, (iii) family structure across development (e.g., single and/or early motherhood, divorce, paternal involvement), and (iv) neighborhood characteristics (e.g., residential composition, stability, and segregation). It also includes individual- and neighborhood-level protective factors (e.g., social support, religiosity, neighborhood stability). These sociocultural factors and the resultant life experiences of youth have a profound impact on their rapidly developing biological systems that also influence their mental health trajectories (Mistry et al. 2012) (Fig. 20.1).

Case Vignette #1 (Conclusion)

You accompany the primary care provider to a follow-up meeting with the family. The primary care provider conducts the interview in both Chinese (a language understood by and primarily spoken by the parents and understood by but not primarily spoken by the child) and English (a language fairly understood by but not primarily spoken by the parents, though primarily spoken by the child). The family describes the various adversities – including poverty and discrimination – they have

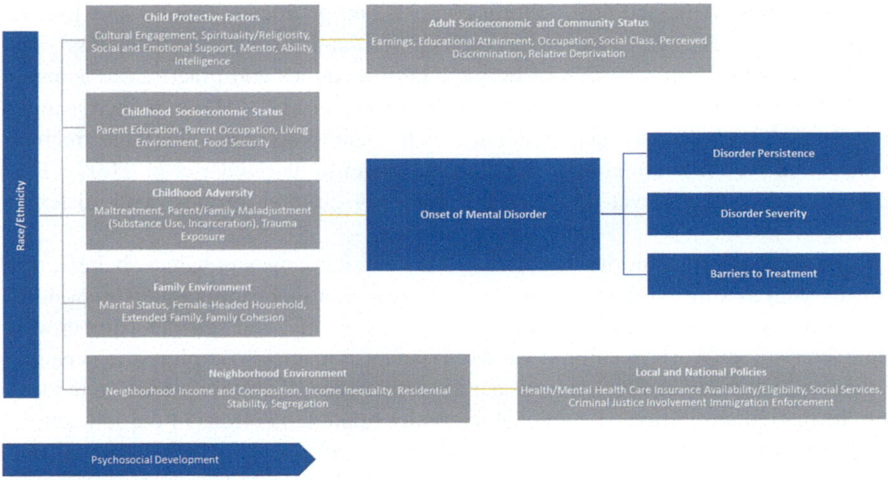

Fig. 20.1 Conceptual model of risk and protective factors for child mental health and mental health service disparities. (Adapted from Alegría et al. 2015)

overcome in raising their children in the USA. The parents work long hours to provide for their children and to send money to various relatives.

In an individual meeting with the child, he conveys that he loves his parents very much but is disappointed with their decision to "raise me as the boy that they always wanted… why can't I be more free like all of my friends are?" Likewise, in a meeting with the parents, they convey that they love their child very much but lament the fact that "he is growing closer to his 'rebel' friends than he is to us… he seems to hate being at home." They admit that the diagnosis of ambiguous genitalia had been a surprise to them, as they had not previously been familiar with such a condition. However, they trust the primary care physician, who has cared for the child since age 2 years, and are open to learning more about how they can best help their child and understand his development.

It has been a while since they have spoken to their child about this condition, and they all agree that establishing a more open and positive line of communication with their child is an important first step, as they plan further follow-up, as recommended, with medical specialists.

This first vignette illustrates the importance, in all consultations, of collaboration with primary care providers and others who may know the patient/family well, who may have the patient/family's trust, who may have skills (e.g., multilingualism) in effectively engaging the patient/family, and who may otherwise have important insights into the patient/family's culture and cultural dynamics. It also illustrates the importance of addressing acculturative stressors and other socioeconomic factors that might adversely health.

Case Vignette #2

You are called as a consultant to the emergency department to see a 14-year-old female who is brought by her grandmother, a first-generation immigrant from American Samoa, because the granddaughter has not been behaving like her "normal self." For the last several days, she has been talking to herself, refusing to eat, and only occasionally drinking a few sips of water. The patient's grandmother has been using prayer, massage, and healing herbs without success. The teenager's teacher encouraged this grandmother to bring her to the hospital.

On physical examination, the patient is pale and slightly overweight. She appears her stated age. She is afebrile with a pulse of 105 and blood pressure of 100/68. Her lips appear dry and chapped. Her examination is otherwise unremarkable. Laboratory findings are significant for ketones in her urine. Her urine drug screen is negative, and her blood counts, chemistry profile, and thyroid-stimulating hormone are all within normal limits.

On mental status examination, the patient is mildly disheveled and appears anxious. She can make eye contact and is cooperative with the evaluation. She is noted at times to be responding to internal stimuli and mumbling to herself. Her speech is mostly coherent except for the mumbling. She appears frightened and refuses to elaborate on what she has just said. She admits to believing that her food is being poisoned and that she is being "punished for bad behavior" but refuses to clarify. She describes seeing "a woman in white" at various times throughout the day. She denies suicidal and homicidal ideation. She is oriented to year and month but incorrectly identifies the date and day of the week. She understands that she is in the hospital and desperately wants help. She can register three out of three objects but is only able to recall two of the three after five minutes, and her remote memory is intact. When asked about similarities between a bike and a plane, she responds with "ways to get places." She can provide an abstract interpretation of the saying "don't cry over spilled milk" but does not understand what is meant by "a rolling stone gathers no moss."

The patient is admitted to an acute psychiatric inpatient unit for further evaluation and management. The grandmother initially refuses to allow her granddaughter to be admitted, but when faced with the possibility of the legal system becoming involved, she concedes.

During the hospitalization, additional history is obtained. The patient has never used any substances and does not have any history of sexual or physical abuse. There is no known family psychiatric history. At the age of three, the patient and her father moved to Hawai'i to live with her grandparents. Her mother remained in Samoa with her 5-year-old and 1-year-old brothers. Her father was unable to find employment and returned to Samoa a year later. She has visited her family once since that time. Her grandfather died 6 months ago, and since then, there has been increased financial stress. Up until that time, she had been doing well at home and school. Over the last several months, the patient has become increasingly isolated from friends, and she spends her free time with her grandmother.

Following completion of the diagnostic evaluation, the patient is started on an antipsychotic and an antidepressant. After a few days, she eats again. Her grandmother angrily approaches the medical staff and states that her granddaughter is being treated badly, is "out of balance," and is now constipated. She wants to take her granddaughter out of the hospital, even though the psychiatric symptoms are not yet resolved. In your mind, you quickly review the current facts, your hypotheses, and your working formulation. You reflect on the patient's likely diagnosis of a mood disorder with psychotic features and are worried about what may happen if inpatient care were terminated prematurely. You ask the grandmother to meet with you.

Facts	Hypotheses	Information needed	Learning issues
A 14-year-old Samoan girl presents with psychotic features to ER	Samoan cultural beliefs and practices	Cultural context of child and family including beliefs about illness and traditional healing methods	DSM-5 cultural outline for formulation
Use of Samoan cultural beliefs and practices	Possible alternate view of the etiology of the psychiatric symptoms		
Evidence for mild dehydration and malnutrition	Possible distrust/lack of familiarity with western cultural practices		
Early losses and recent loss of grandfather	Cultural differences between clinician and patient/caregiver may pose barriers		
Grandmother's concern over constipation	Potential compromise of care if trust is lost and treatment is discontinued		

Effect on Help Seeking

Several factors impact whether individuals access or seek care. These factors include perception of illness and its causes, structural components (e.g., lack of transportation and limited access to care), familiarity with services and providers, mental health literacy, mental health stigma, and perceptions of mental healthcare providers (Alegría et al. 2010; Chow et al. 2003; Kilbourne et al. 2006; Raguram et al. 2002; Saravanan et al. 2007).

Globally, there is a sizable gap between individuals who need mental healthcare and those receiving them, with the most dramatic differences in lower-income countries and racial/ethnic minority groups (Barnett et al. 2017; McGuire and Miranda 2008). Furthermore, when underserved communities have available mental health services, affective disorders are more likely to be underdiagnosed and undertreated, while psychotic disorders are overdiagnosed and overtreated (Holden et al. 2014). The Institute of Medicine (2002) identified more than 175 studies documenting racial/ethnic disparities in the diagnosis and treatment of various conditions, even when analyses were controlled for socioeconomic status, insurance status, site of care, stage of disease, comorbidity, age, and other potential confounders. Minorities are also less likely to receive evidence-based, high-quality, newer, and more comprehensive treatment modalities. Making evidence-based treatments and evidence-informed practices accessible in underserved communities has been a major focus of international policies as a strategy to reduce the global burden of mental disorders (Barry and Huskamp 2011; Becker and Kleinman 2013; Dua et al. 2011).

Case Vignette #2 (Conclusion)
You quickly review your notes on the DSM-5 outline for cultural formulation.

You then meet with the grandmother and learn that, in their culture, constipation is a serious condition. The grandmother has always made sure to keep her family members in good health. You ask the grandmother about her methods for relieving constipation. She reports that she makes a paste out of a plant and massages this paste into the umbilicus. The grandmother is encouraged to participate in the treatment of her granddaughter by providing this care. She does so with good results. The patient's mood continues to improve, and her psychosis resolves. Her eating and bowel patterns return to baseline. Her grandmother is very pleased with the outcome and provides the unit with a home-cooked Samoan meal to express her gratitude.

Cultural Humility

As illustrated in the two preceding vignettes, cultural competence is the ability of providers and systems to respond respectfully and effectively to people of all cultures, affirming the worth and preserving the dignity of individuals, families, and communities (Betancourt et al. 2016). Cultural competency implies that better care is provided with a thorough knowledge of the mores and beliefs of another culture. While cultural competency is an ongoing process, more recently the term cultural humility has been taking root. Cultural humility encourages individuals to identify their own biases and to acknowledge that those biases must be recognized. It concedes that it is impossible to be adequately knowledgeable about cultures other than one's own. It also implies an openness to new ideas, advice, and contradictory information. By approaching each encounter with the knowledge that one's perspective may be full of assumptions and prejudices, providers will be more open to the seeking the involvement of the patient.

Case Vignette #3
A 15-year-old Mexican girl is admitted to the pediatric ward for "medical evaluation of possible new onset psychosis." She is "boarding in the children's hospital pending psychiatric bed availability within a drivable radius." The attending

physician requests, from your team, a psychiatric consultation. Her primary language is Spanish. She is reportedly experiencing visual hallucinations and making bizarre statements since being placed in child protective custody after her parents were incarcerated for drug-related charges 6 days prior to admission.

Although you have basic command of the Spanish language, you believe that a psychiatric interview requires a higher fluency level. Therefore, an interview was performed with a native Spanish-speaking interpreter. As she gazes around the room, the patient states, "the angels are protecting me." She reports that she can see these angels: "I sometimes see shadows or movement out of the corners of my eyes, and I know that it is them!" She denies seeing the angels currently but appears to be actively looking for them. She admits to worrying about her and her family's situation, as her father's distant cousin is her only family contact in the USA. The worry has been keeping her awake at night, so she tends to be fatigued during the day. She has cried most of the day since her parents' incarceration. She has always been a picky eater but has not been very hungry at all in the past week. The patient reports that she has always been in good health, and she denies any history of trauma or sexual or physical abuse. The patient and her family arrived in the USA illegally from Mexico a little over a year ago. Prior to arriving in the USA, they lived in a small village and lived a very simple life, helping on a farm. The patient's father became disabled and could no longer engage in manual labor, and the family soon lost their home. Her mother was adopted, and her father was the last alive in his line except for a distant cousin in the USA. The family was assisted in obtaining illegal transportation to the USA; however, upon arrival, they discovered that they were required to engage in drug trafficking to pay off their debt. The patient states that she and her parents did not engage in drug use. She has not attended school in the USA but has been receiving tutoring from a neighbor in exchange for looking after that woman's infant daughter and helping to clean her house. The patient would like to one day "be a teacher, get married, and have children."

Other than the patient's father, who "worries a lot," and a now deceased elderly uncle who became confused and forgetful as he aged, there is no other known family psychiatric history.

Her vital signs and physical exam are unremarkable. Her urine drug screen is negative, and her blood counts, chemistry profile, thyroid-stimulating hormone, and urinalysis are all within normal limits.

On mental status examination, the patient is a slender female with good hygiene and grooming. She constantly frowns and wrings her hands. She is cooperative and has good eye contact. Her mood is anxious and dysphoric with a congruent affect. She speaks in a rapid but non-pressured manner, with low volume. Her thought process is goal directed. She denies any suicidal or homicidal ideations. She is abstract in her interpretation of similarities and a Spanish proverb that roughly translates to "the shrimp that sleeps gets carried by the current." She is alert and oriented to person, place, and time.

She points toward a glass of water and asks if you and the interpreter understand the importance of that glass of water. When the provider asks the patient to explain what she thinks is the importance, the patient expresses her disappointment and refuses to elaborate. She becomes tearful and insists, "no one understands." She then terminates the interview.

You apologize and reflect on what may have happened.

Facts	Hypotheses	Information needed	Learning issues
A 15-year-old Mexican girl with "visual hallucinations" and "bizarre statements"	Bipolar disorder with psychosis?	Patient's perception of problem/fears for future	DSM-5 cultural concepts of distress
	Substance-induced psychosis?		
	Major depressive disorder with psychosis?		
	Anxiety disorder? Adjustment disorder?		
Immigrated within last year from a small rural environment to an urban city with different language and culture	Inadequate support system?	Timeline of symptoms	**DSM-5 cultural formulation interview**
		Cultural context	
Parents incarcerated less than 1 week ago, and now the patient is in temporary custody of CPS	Culture or language barrier with current foster family	Information about foster family's language and culture	Effective/appropriate use of interpreters/translators
Language barrier		Contact with case manager to obtain information on options/support available	

Case Vignette #3 (Conclusion)

Following the interview, the interpreter informed that provider that in the Mexican culture, it is believed that placing a glass of water over the refrigerator or some other conspicuous area helps to absorb any bad spirits and prevents harm or evil to the family there. The patient feels validated when this issue was later discussed with her, as she reported previously feeling isolated and misunderstood when she attempted to discuss her beliefs with her foster family, who spoke only a little Spanish and had limited knowledge of the Mexican culture and traditional belief systems. They also regarded her "seeing angels" as visual hallucinations. In the context of her anxiety, tearfulness, lack of sleep, poor appetite, and fatigue they were worried about her mental health.

You observe her over the next couple of days, and you conclude that the likely diagnosis is an anxiety disorder, exacerbated by significant social stress, rather than a psychotic disorder or mood disorder with psychotic features.

Cultural Formulation Interview

The cultural formulation interview (CFI) can guide providers to explore four areas in which culture can impact the assessment of the clinical presentation. These include (1) cultural definition of the problem; (2) cultural perceptions of cause, context, and support (including cultural identity); (3) cultural factors that affect self-coping and past help seeking; and (4) cultural factors that affect current help seeking (American Psychiatric Association 2013). There are 12 modules that supplement the core CFI, aiding clinicians in conducting a more comprehensive cultural assessment (American Psychiatric Association 2013). Eight of the supplementary modules explore the CFI in greater depth including (1) explanatory model; (2) level of functioning; (3) social network; (4) psychosocial stressors; (5) spirituality, religion, and moral traditions; (6) cultural identity; (7) coping and help seeking; and (8) clinician-patient relationship. Three modules focus on specific populations, including children and adolescents, older adults, and immigrants and refugees. The last module explores the caregiver experiences and views in order to clarify the nature and cultural context of support they provide.

Such an interview allows the patient and family to provide their own illness narrative and information about the community context, and it encourages the patient and family to engage in the treatment process. The CFI can be used by all clinicians and with all patients, not just in clinical encounters with cultural minorities or in situations where there are obvious cultural differences between clinicians and patients. In all clinical encounters, providers bring their own cultures, values, and expectations, which influence how specific aspects of care are approached.

Conclusion

Advancing our understanding of cultural issues is critical for good patient care, particularly as we practice in a shortage specialty and work in settings where there may only be a small window of opportunity to engage a patient and family. A focus on culture clarifies that one cannot consider cultural influences separate from the influence of other social factors including cultural identity, gender ideologies, generational experience, racial discrimination, and socioeconomic status. As we continue to understand how culture influences mental illness, health, and well-being, we enhance our ability to reduce stigma, optimize screening, and design more effective interventions for all groups.

References

Alegría, M., Mulvaney-Day, N., Torres, M., Polo, A., Cao, Z., & Canino, G. (2007). Prevalence of psychiatric disorders across Latino subgroups in the United States. *American Journal of Public Health, 97*(1), 68–75.

Alegría, M., Vallas, M., & Pumariega, A. J. (2010). Racial and ethnic disparities in pediatric mental health. *Child and Adolescent PsychiatricClinics of North America, 19*, 759–774. https://doi.org/10.1016/j.chc.2010.07.001.

Alegría, M., Green, J. G., McLaughlin, K. A., & Loder, S. (2015). *Disparities in child and adolescent mental health and mental health services in the U. S.* New York: William T Grant Foundation.

American Psychiatric Association. (2013). Cultural formulation. In *Diagnostic and statistical manual of mental disorders* (5th ed., pp. 749–759). Washington, DC: American Psychiatric Association.

Barnett, M. L., Gonzalez, A., Miranda, J., Chavira, D. A., & Lau, A. S. (2017). Mobilizing community health workers to address mental health disparities for underserved populations: A systematic review. *Administration and Policy in Mental Health and Mental Health Services Research, 45*, 1–17.

Barry, C. L., & Huskamp, H. A. (2011). Moving beyond parity—Mental health and addiction care under the ACA. *New England Journal of Medicine, 365*(11), 973–975.

Becker, A. E., & Kleinman, A. (2013). Mental health and the global agenda. *New England Journal of Medicine, 369*(1), 66–73.

Betancourt, J. R., Green, A. R., Carrillo, J. E., & Owusu Ananeh-Firempong, I. I. (2016). Defining cultural competence: A practical framework for addressing racial/ethnic disparities in health and health care. *Public Health Reports, 118*(4), 293–302.

Breslau, J., Kendler, K. S., Su, M., Gaxiola-Aguilar, S., & Kessler, R. C. (2005). Lifetime risk and persistence of psychiatric disorders across ethnic groups in the United States. *Psychological Medicine, 35*(03), 317–327.

Breslau, J., Aguilar-Gaxiola, S., Kendler, K. S., Su, M., Williams, D., & Kessler, R. C. (2006). Specifying race-ethnic differences in risk for psychiatric disorder in a USA national sample. *Psychological Medicine, 36*(01), 57–68.

Chow, J. C. C., Jaffee, K., & Snowden, L. (2003). Racial/ethnic disparities in the use of mental health services in poverty areas. *American Journal of Public Health, 93*, 792–797. https://doi.org/10.2105/AJPH.93.5.792.

Dua, T., Barbui, C., Clark, N., Fleischmann, A., Poznyak, V., van Ommeren, M., et al. (2011). Evidence-based guidelines for mental, neurological, and substance use disorders in low- and middle-income countries: Summary of WHO recommendations. *PLoS Medicine, 8*(11), e1001122.

Flannery, W. P., Reise, S. P., & Yu, J. (2001). An empirical comparison of acculturation models. *Personality and Social Psychology Bulletin, 27*(8), 1035–1045.

Gee, G. C., & Payne-Sturges, D. C. (2004). Environmental health disparities: A framework integrating psychosocial and environmental concepts. *Environmental Health Perspectives, 112*, 1645–1653.

Holden, K., McGregor, B., Thandi, P., Fresh, E., Sheats, K., Belton, A., et al. (2014). Toward culturally centered integrative care for addressing mental health disparities among ethnic minorities. *Psychological Services, 11*(4), 357.

Institute of Medicine. (2002). *Unequal treatment: Confronting racial and ethnic disparities in health care*. Washington, DC: National Academies Press.

Kilbourne, A. M., Switzer, G., Hyman, K., Crowley-Matoka, M., & Fine, M. J. (2006). Advancing health disparities research within the health care system: A conceptual framework. *American Journal of Public Health, 96*, 2113–2121. https://doi.org/10.2105/AJPH.2005.07762821.

McGuire, T. G., & Miranda, J. (2008). Racial and ethnic disparities in mental health care: Evidence and policy implications. *Health Affairs (Project Hope), 27*(2), 393–403. https://doi.org/10.1377/hlthaff.27.2.393.

Mistry, K. B., Minkovitz, C. S., Riley, A. W., Johnson, S. B., Grason, H. A., Dubay, L. C., & Guyer, B. (2012). A new framework for childhood health promotion: The role of policies and programs in building capacity and foundations of early childhood health. *American Journal of Public Health, 102*(9), 1688–1696.

Oetting, E. R., & Beauvais, F. (1990). Orthogonal cultural identification theory: The cultural identification of minority adolescents. *International Journal of the Addictions, 25*, 655–685.

Raguram, R., Venkateswaran, A., Ramakrishna, J., & Weiss, M. G. (2002). Traditional community resources for mental health: A report of temple healing from India. *BMJ: British Medical Journal, 325*, 38–40.

Ryder, A. G., Alden, L. E., & Paulhus, D. L. (2000). Is acculturation unidimensional or bidimensional? A head-to-head comparison in the prediction of personality, self-identity, and adjustment. *Journal of Personality and Social Psychology, 79*(1), 49.

Sam, D. L., & Berry, J. W. (2010). Acculturation when individuals and groups of different cultural backgrounds meet. *Perspectives on Psychological Science, 5*(4), 472–481.

Saravanan, B., Jacob, K. S., Johnson, S., Prince, M., Bhugra, D., & David, A. S. (2007). Belief models in first episode schizophrenia in South India. *Social Psychiatry and Psychiatric Epidemiology, 42*, 446–451. https://doi.org/10.1007/s00127-007-0186-z.

Schwartz, S. J., Zamboanga, B. L., Rodriguez, L., & Wang, S. C. (2007). The structure of cultural identity in an ethnically diverse sample of emerging adults. *Basic and Applied Social Psychology, 29*(2), 159–173.

Smedley, B., Stith, A. Y., & Nelson, A. R. (2002). *Unequal treatment: Confronting racial and ethnic disparities in health care*. Washington, DC: Institute of Medicine of the National Academie.

Tadmor, C. T., & Tetlock, P. E. (2006). Biculturalism: A model of the effects of second-culture exposure on acculturation and integrative complexity. *Journal of Cross-Cultural Psychology, 37*(2), 173–190.

Triandis, H. C., Brislin, R., & Hui, C. H. (1988). Cross-cultural training across the individualism-collectivism divide. *International Journal of Intercultural Relations, 12*(3), 269–289.

U.S. Department of Health and Human Services. (2001). *Mental Health: Culture, race, and ethinicity-A supplement to mental health: A report of the surgeon general*. Rockville: U.S. Department of Health and Human Services, Substance Abuse and Mental Health Services Administration, Center for Mental Health Services.

Williams, D. R., & Earl, T. R. (2007). Commentary: Race and mental health—More questions than answers. *International Journal of Epidemiology, 36*(4), 758–760.

World Health Organization. (2014). *Social determinants of mental health*. Geneva: World Health Organization.

Chapter 21
Complementary and Alternative Approaches to Improving Comfort and Access

Asad Ghiasuddin

Case Vignette 21.1

You are the attending child psychiatrist on the pediatric consultation-liaison service at the children's hospital in an urban, cosmopolitan city. As part of your duties you routinely round with the hematology-oncology service to introduce yourself to the new patients and their families, and you follow up with established patients who may be hospitalized.

Paul is an 8-year-old little boy who has been newly diagnosed with acute lymphoblastic leukemia (ALL). He is originally from a small island in Micronesia. He and his parents have moved to your city to receive chemotherapy for ALL, which is not available on their island. The family is very appreciative of the outstanding care they have received so far, but they ask whether you and the rest of the team would allow Paul to take some of their "medicine from back home" to help decrease his vomiting and sleep better. They also say that Paul misses his family's home cooking, and they have been bringing in their own food for him to eat instead of the hospital food that is served.

As you continue to get to know Paul and his family and their psychosocial needs, you recall what you previously learned about complementary and alternative medicine (CAM) use in the pediatric hematology-oncology population, how different remedies interact with conventional chemotherapy, and which CAM treatments might be available in hospitals to alleviate treatment side effects and improve patients' comfort.

A. Ghiasuddin (✉)
Department of Psychiatry, University of Hawaii, John A. Burns School of Medicine, Honolulu, HI, USA
e-mail: ghiasuddina@dop.hawaii.edu

A. P. S. Guerrero et al. (eds.), *Pediatric Consultation-Liaison Psychiatry*,
https://doi.org/10.1007/978-3-319-89488-1_21

What Is CAM?

The National Institutes of Health's (NIH) National Center for Complementary and Integrative Health (NCCIH) defines CAM as a "group of diverse medical and health care systems, practices, and products that are not presently considered to be part of conventional Western medicine" (NCCIH). "Complementary" refers to treatments that are used *in conjunction with* conventional medicine (e.g., using aromatherapy alongside chemotherapy), while "alternative" refers to treatments that are used *in place of* conventional medicine (e.g., using herbal remedies instead of chemotherapy).

"Traditional medicine" is defined by the World Health Organization as "the sum total of knowledge, skills, and practices based on the theories, beliefs and experiences indigenous to different cultures, whether explicable or not, used in the maintenance of health, as well as in the prevention, diagnosis, improvement or treatment of physical and mental illnesses" (World Health Organization). When traditional medicine is used in populations in which it is not indigenous, it may then come to be known as CAM in that culture. An example of this would be the use of acupuncture in Western societies. In this chapter, the term CAM is used to refer to any treatments not routinely used in conventional Western medicine.

The use of CAM is very common in the general population worldwide (TCM, Ayuverda) (WHO), and its use has been rising in Western cultures in recent years. One third of adults in the United States have used CAM, and it is a $20 billion-per-year industry. According to the National Health Interview Survey, 12% of children in the United States use some form of CAM (Perrin et al. 2012), and other estimates are as high as 20–40% (Kemper et al. 2008). A 2013 Canadian study revealed that 42–71% of parents report that their children are using some sort of CAM therapy (Adams et al. 2013).

The use of CAM in children with chronic illnesses and special healthcare needs is even more common (Kemper et al. 2008), with reports in the literature for the following conditions:

- Asthma
- Attention-deficit/hyperactivity disorder
- Autism spectrum disorder
- Cancer
- Cerebral palsy
- Cystic fibrosis
- Inflammatory bowel disease
- Juvenile rheumatoid arthritis

Caregivers may use multiple CAM modalities simultaneously to treat their children with chronic conditions. In one study, the families of children with autism spectrum disorder reported using an average of seven CAM therapies (Perrin et al. 2012).

CAM use seems to vary by country. A 2012 review of CAM use showed varying prevalence rates around the world: Great Britain at 10–13%, Australia at 20–26%, and South Korea at 74% (Frass et al. 2012).

A 2013 study involving two large pediatric samples revealed that the most commonly used CAM products were (1) multivitamins, (2) herbal preparations, and (3) homeopathy, while the top methods of CAM practices were (1) massage, (2) chiropractic care, (3) relaxation, and (4) aromatherapy (Adams et al. 2013).

Given CAM use is prevalent and on the rise in the pediatric population, and even higher among children who are hospitalized frequently with chronic conditions such as asthma, cancer, and rheumatic illnesses, it is important for the pediatric consultation-liaison (C-L) psychiatrist to know how to talk to patients and families about these therapies. Becoming familiar with common CAM therapies and understanding the potential medical ethical considerations of using CAM in children will allow for optimal care for the patient.

Overview of Common CAM Therapies

CAM can be divided into biochemical, lifestyle, biomechanical, and bioenergetic modalities (Kemper et al. 2008). Biochemical includes herbs, vitamins, minerals, and dietary supplements. Lifestyle includes nutrition, exercise, music, meditation, and hypnosis. Biomechanical includes massage, bodywork, and chiropractic adjustment. Bioenergetic includes acupuncture, magnets, Reiki, healing touch, prayer, and homeopathy.

Case Vignette 21.2
His family reports that prior to developing ALL, Paul was a healthy, active youngster who enjoyed school and playing outside with his friends. Since becoming ill, he has tried to maintain his usual upbeat attitude, but at times it seems like he is worried. His mother asks if there is anything you can do to ease his (and her) worries. She wants to give him the kiup plant from back home as she thinks it will make him stronger and heal faster.

You look up what the kiup plant might be (this is the local name for Crinum asiaticum, which is used for bone pain and other conditions) (Ling 2016) *to determine if it contains any active substances that may potentially interact with his treatment regimen and discuss with the primary oncology team.*

Biochemical

Herbal preparations are among the most common type of CAM used in the pediatric population. In the United States, herbs are not regulated by the Food and Drug Administration and, as such, do not need to demonstrate any safety or efficacy

(Kemper et al. 2008) before being made available to the public. St. John's wort (*Hypericum perforatum)* is used by children and adolescents for depression and anxiety; it has been shown to improve mild depression in some open studies (Soh and Walter 2012). However, it can interact with many other drugs, including prescription serotonergic antidepressants (Soh and Walter 2012). Kava (*Piper methysticum*) and valerian (*Valeriana officinalis*) are used for anxiety, and both have shown some small benefits in adults in open studies, but no improvement in randomized control trials (Soh and Walter 2012; Andreatini et al. 2002). Kava has been associated with hepatotoxicity as well as an intoxication state when taken in larger quantities described as a "tranquil relaxation," somewhat like alcohol (Norton 1998). Neither has evidence to support their use in children. In 2009, the *Canadian Pharmacists Journal* published a tool for rapid identification of natural health product-drug interactions which is freely available online at https://www.ncbi.nlm.nih.gov/pmc/articles/PMC4813519/figure/fig2-1715163516629156/.

Dietary supplements are widely used by families because of their availability and perceived safety compared to prescription medications. Omega 3 fatty acids have been promoted as beneficial in a variety of conditions including depression and attention-deficit/hyperactivity disorder (ADHD); there seems to be some slight improvement with the latter (Derbyshire 2017), but the effect size does not approach that of stimulants. Additionally, at high doses, omega 3 fatty acids can increase the risk of bleeding (Soh and Walter 2012).

Probiotics are another example of a dietary supplement. Their use has become commonplace in the pediatric population. Currently, it is an almost mainstream treatment for children with inflammatory bowel conditions (Kostic et al. 2014).

Dietary therapies for autism spectrum disorder (ASD), including elimination diets, do not have reliable evidence to support their use and can place young children at risk for nutritional deficiencies depending on the type of diet. Most elimination diets focus on the removal of gluten and casein, which could lead to deficiencies in vitamin B, vitamin D, calcium, iron, fiber, and protein. (Ly et al. 2017) The ketogenic diet does have evidence of benefit for certain types of seizure disorders and has been accepted in conventional medicine (Kemper et al. 2008).

Aromatherapy uses essential oils derived from different plant sources (e.g., lavender, rosemary, eucalyptus, chamomile). These oils can be applied topically, with or without massage, or added to an atomizer, humidifier, or bathwater (Boehm et al. 2012). It has been used to treat nausea and insomnia.

Case Vignette 21.3

After meeting with Paul and his family, it appears that he has some developmentally appropriate anxiety around his current diagnosis, the chemotherapy, and being in a new environment without the support of his extended family and friends, but that he does not meet criteria for a major mood or anxiety disorder. His mom reports that when Paul receives his chemotherapy, he experiences nausea and gastrointestinal distress. She massages his abdomen to ease the pain. Paul smiles and says he likes it when his mom massages him, stating "it helps me to relax."

Biomechanical Therapies

Massage is a common type of CAM practice that is used by parents in the home and in the hospital (Ghiasuddin et al. 2015) and can serve as a therapeutic activity time for both child and caregiver. Massage is also sanctioned in many children's hospitals, with infant massage being offered to babies in neonatal intensive care units (Kemper et al. 2008; Ghiasuddin et al. 2015). Chiropractic care is another type of CAM used by some children and teens for a variety of conditions, though the evidence for its benefit is limited (Kemper et al. 2008).

Bioenergetic Therapies

Also known as biofield therapies, these techniques purport to manipulate an energy in and around a patient's body (Kemper et al. 2008). Acupuncture, with originates from the field of traditional Chinese medicine, is one of the best known biofield therapies. It involves the placement of needles into acupressure points in the body. Acupuncture is the most common CAM used in children with ASD in Hong Kong (Cheuk et al. 2011). It has also been shown to be helpful for headaches and is used to treat nausea and chronic pain (NIH consensus 1997). Adverse effects appear to be rare (Brittner et al. 2016).

Healing touch and therapeutic touch are popular energy modalities that have been developed by nurses in the past several decades and purport to balance patients' energy fields by the laying of a practitioner's hands on or near these patients' bodies. Practitioners go through formal training and are certified prior to working with patients. Like many CAM modalities, the evidence base for their effectiveness is limited, though recent work has shown that it can reduce parents' perceptions of their children's pain and anxiety (Wong et al. 2013). Given the low potential risk of harm to patients with these interventions, several children's hospitals have been offering these services, along with other fairly benign interventions such as aromatherapy.

Lifestyle Therapies

Lifestyle therapies include optimizing daily habits (e.g., exercise, sleep, nutrition), incorporating relaxation activities into mental health practice (e.g., guided imagery, progressive muscle relaxation, diaphragmatic breathing), and engaging in nonmedical health and relaxation practices (e.g., meditation, tai chi, prayer). These practices have some evidence of benefit for some aspect of overall health, usually alleviating stress, modifying the pain experience, or addressing insomnia. Some studies include prayer as a type of CAM, while others do not; if included, prayer appears to be the most prevalent type of CAM used in the United States (NCCIH 2004).

Case Vignette 21.4
You praise Paul's parents for their loving attention. You discuss with them that massage is something that many children with cancer find helpful. You let Paul and his family know that the hospital also provides aromatherapy, which sometimes helps with sleep, as well as healing touch, which many patients find helpful in lowering stress and anxiety. Both the child and the parents are interested in taking advantage of what the hospital has to offer.

Case Vignette 21.5
You are now doing your medical mission work as a child psychiatrist in Cameroon. Unlike your home hospital in the United States, the major childhood malignancy is not ALL but Burkitt lymphoma. Most children are diagnosed very late in their illness, if they can obtain conventional Western medical care at all. In Cameroon, most children are typically seen in their village by the local traditional healer, who may provide some concoction, perform a ritual with incantations, or cut/burn the skin as a form of treatment. You recognize that traditional medicine in some parts of the world has not been studied for its effectiveness or safety yet is the primary treatment provided, rather than evidence-based medicine. You learn that the traditional healer has a higher status than physicians in certain villages, and gaining the trust of the patients and families to go to a hospital for conventional treatment can be a challenge.

Ethical Considerations in Working with Patients

In most Western countries, CAM modalities are truly used in a complementary way. They are used alongside the conventional treatments physicians prescribe and recommend. In other parts of the globe, traditional healing practices and medical systems have been used for generations; they are the more trusted and utilized method of healing, sometimes to the point of being the sole treatment (Afungchwi et al. 2017). How should a physician respond when parents refuse conventional treatments in favor of CAM therapies that may have little efficacy?

A good starting point to evaluate any CAM treatment is as follows (Kemper and Cohen 2004):

	Effective	Not effective
Safe	Recommend	Tolerate
Unsafe	Monitor or discourage	Discourage

Some CAM techniques such as guided imagery and relaxation are safe and effective. Many others, including prayer, bioenergy methods, and aromatherapy, are most likely safe but lack a robust evidence base for efficacy. It may be appropriate to recommend or tolerate their use, as most people who utilize CAM seek out and use these methods because they align with their personal values and beliefs (McFadden et al. 2010). However, conventional treatment continues to be the dominant therapeutic approach utilized in most Western countries.

A smaller number of CAM treatments, such as St. John's wort or kava, are potentially unsafe but may have some efficacy in the pediatric population and should either be closely monitored or more commonly, discouraged. The last groups of CAM methods are both unsafe and ineffective, such as the use of traditional healing or prayer in lieu of established lifesaving treatments, such as chemotherapy for pediatric cancer.

Case Vignette 21.6
You meet with the local oncologist, who tells you about initiatives the medical staff have been undertaking, going into villages and meeting with families, local leaders, and healers. Your colleague describes some of the challenges they have faced in their outreach program: variable levels of engagement from the traditional healers of different communities and distrust from the villagers, who have seen children go to the hospital only to succumb to their illness. However, there are also several experiences of healers who want to work alongside the hospital team and are receptive to the bilateral sharing of knowledge. They gain a better understanding of the signs and symptoms of Burkitt lymphoma, and at what point it is imperative to send children to the hospital, while the local medical staff gain a better understanding of the traditional approaches that are important to the villagers.

The first step for the physician wishing to assist families in making safe decisions around the use of CAM is to become comfortable engaging in discussions on the topic. Inquiring about alternative treatments, home remedies, and the family's beliefs about what is making their child sick, and what more could be done to help, should all be routine parts of the medical history (Kemper et al. 2008; Kemper 2012; Hwang et al. 2008). Discussing a family's health practices with a nonjudgmental attitude and exploring the alignment with their beliefs and values can pay dividends.

The next step is to become knowledgeable about the types of CAM commonly utilized in your practice setting and their potential benefits and risks. Additionally, it can be helpful to become familiar with the traditional remedies of your patients if their cultural backgrounds differ from your own. Allowing families to continue using safe traditional treatments shows respect for their backgrounds, values, and beliefs. It may also encourage compliance with conventional treatment and strengthen the doctor-patient relationship.

The C-L psychiatrist should also be aware of which CAM modalities are offered by local hospitals. Many US children's hospitals offer patients and families a variety of CAM treatments including infant massage, aromatherapy, Reiki, and healing touch, as well as the use of a prayer room and chaplain services.

While having an open, accepting attitude toward CAM is valuable, it is vital to also be thorough in your review of the available evidence on safety and efficacy of those treatments. It is also essential to be clear when educating patients and their families about any potential harm that is known about the treatment. In the United States, when the reliance on CAM interferes with the treatment of a condition for which effective conventional medical care exists, child protective services should be consulted as this may represent medical abuse or neglect on the part of the parent. Typically, courts will allow parental choice of care unless the situation is life threatening (Mears 2010). In other regions of the world, it is best to consult with local providers on what might constitute abuse or neglect, as local standards will vary. For example, in Cameroon, receiving care from a traditional healer in lieu of conventional treatment is not necessarily considered abusive or neglectful.

Case Vignette 21.7
As you make rounds at the hospital with your host medical staff, you meet a little boy diagnosed with Burkitt lymphoma. He is with his family, and they share with you their experience of being frightened when their son first became ill and sought out treatment from their local traditional healer. When the healer recommended they go to the hospital, at first they were a little dubious. However, after meeting with the team and learning about what was making their son sick, they went forward with treatment. They are happy that they are still able to use some local remedies in the hospital, after first checking with their doctor to make sure they didn't interfere with his other treatments. You reflect on the similarities of patient experiences with CAM in such different parts of the world and realize that its use in medicine today is truly global.

In Summation

- CAM treatments have been adopted from common traditional practices from around the world, and their use in the United States is increasing.
- Most CAM treatments in the Western world are used alongside conventional treatments.
- Children with chronic illnesses such as asthma, cancer, ASD, inflammatory bowel disease (IBD), and juvenile rheumatoid arthritis (JRA) use CAM more often than the general pediatric population.
- It is important to maintain a nonjudgmental perspective when talking with patients about types of CAM they might use.
- It is useful to become familiar with the types of CAM most commonly used in your locale. Be aware that CAM supplements do NOT undergo rigorous testing for safety and efficacy.
- As most CAM currently have a limited evidence base, be aware of reliable resources which provide up-to-date evidence on CAM (NHP drug interaction grid, PedCAM network, NCCAM).
- When advising patients and families about CAM use, follow the four basic principles of biomedical ethics: respect patients'/families' autonomy, avoid harm,

prioritize patients' interests and well-being, and ensure fairness in providing access to essential care.

– In the United States, if the safety of the child is at risk because of CAM use interfering with the delivery of lifesaving conventional treatment, then child protective services should be notified.

References

Adams, D., Dagenais, S., Clifford, T., Baydala, L., King, W. J., Hervas-Malo, M., Moher, D., & Vohra, S. (2013). Complementary and alternative medicine use by pediatric specialty outpatients. *Pediatrics*, Peds-2012. http://pediatrics.aappublications.org/content/pediatrics/early/2013/01/08/peds.2012-1220.full.pdf

Afungchwi, G. M., Hesseling, P. B., & Ladas, E. J. (2017). The role of traditional healers in the diagnosis and management of Burkitt lymphoma in Cameroon: Understanding the challenges and moving forward. *BMC Complementary and Alternative Medicine, 17*(1), 209.

Andreatini, R., Sartori, V., Seabra, M., & Leite, J. (2002). Effect of valepotriates (valerian extract) in generalized anxiety disorder: A randomized placebo-controlled pilot study. *Phytotherapy Research, 16*(7), 650–654.

Boehm, K., Büssing, A., & Ostermann, T. (2012). Aromatherapy as an adjuvant treatment in cancer car—A descriptive systematic review. *African Journal of Traditional, Complementary and Alternative Medicines, 9*(4), 503–518. http://scholar.google.com/scholar?hl=en&q=Aromatherapy+as+an+adjuvant+treatment+in+cancer+car%E2%80%94A+descriptive+systematic+review&btnG=&as_sdt=1%2C5&as_sdtp=.

Brittner, M., Le Pertel, N., & Gold, M. (2016). Acupuncture in pediatrics. *Current Problems in Pediatric and Adolescent Health Care, 46*(6), 179–183.

Cheuk, D., Wong, V., & Chen, W. (2011). Acupuncture for autism spectrum disorders (ASD). *Cochrane Database of Systematic Reviews, 9*. https://doi.org/10.1002/14651858.CD007849.pub2.

Derbyshire, E. (2017). Do omega-3/6 fatty acids have a therapeutic role in children and young people with ADHD? *Journal of Lipids, 2017*(2), 1–9. https://doi.org/10.1155/2017/6285218.

Frass, M., Strassl, R. P., Friehs, H., Müllner, M., Kundi, M., & Kaye, A. D. (2012). Use and acceptance of complementary and alternative medicine among the general population and medical personnel: A systematic review. *The Ochsner Journal, 12*(1), 45–56. http://www.ochsnerjournal.org/doi/pdf/10.1043/1524-5012-12.1.45.

Ghiasuddin, A., Wong, J., & Siu, A. M. (2015). Ethnicity, traditional healing practices, and attitudes towards complementary medicine of a pediatric oncology population receiving healing touch in Hawai'i. *Asia-Pacific Journal of Oncology Nursing, 2*(4), 227–231. https://doi.org/10.4103/2347-5625.158015.

Hwang, W. C., Myers, H. F., Abe-Kim, J., & Ting, J. Y. (2008). A conceptual paradigm for understanding culture's impact on mental health: The Cultural Influences on Mental Health (CIMH) model. *Clinical Psychology Review, 28*(2), 211–227. https://doi.org/10.1016/j.cpr.2007.05.001.

Kemper, K. (2012). *Pediatric integrative medicine: A view from North America*. Columbus: Center for Integrative Health and Wellness, Ohio State University. https://www.aap.org/en-us/Documents/soim_presentation_pim.pdf

Kemper, K., & Cohen, M. (2004). Ethics meets complementary and alternative medicine: New light on old principles. *Contemporary Pediatrics, 21*(65).

Kemper, K. J., Vohra, S., & Walls, R. (2008). The use of complementary and alternative medicine in pediatrics. *Pediatrics, 122*(6), 1374–1386. https://pdfs.semanticscholar.org/9?9d/d8801be40ad1a43380a13185757cc953b1ca.pdf.

Kostic, A. D., Xavier, R. J., & Gevers, D. (2014). The microbiome in inflammatory bowel diseases: Current status and the future ahead. *Gastroenterology, 146*(6), 1489–1499. https://doi.org/10.1053/j.gastro.2014.02.009.

Ling, D. L. (2016). *Micronesian ethnobotany, a course companion*. College of Micronesia-Federated States of Micronesia. (Edition 4.1) [2016–6–23, date of last access]. http://www.comfsm.fm/~dleeling/ethnobotany/text/ethnobotany.html

Ly, V., Bottelier, M., Hoekstra, P., Arias Vasquez, A., Buitelaar, J., & Rommelse, N. (2017). Elimination diets' efficacy and mechanisms in attentions deficit hyperactivity disorder and autism spectrum disorder. *European Child & Adolescent Psychiatry*. https://doi.org/10.1007/s00787-017-0959-1. [Epub ahead of print].

McFadden, K. L., Hernández, T. D., & Ito, T. A. (2010). Attitudes towards complementary and alternative medicine influence its use. *Explore, 6*(6), 380–388. https://doi.org/10.1016/j.explore.2010.08.004.

Mears, B. J. (2010). Ethics for the pediatrician. *Pediatrics in Review, 31*(7) e49-e51. doi:https://doi.org/10.1542/pir.31-7-e49. https://nccih.nih.gov/news/2004/052704.htm. Last accessed 9 Sep 2017.

NIH Consens Statement. (1997, November 3–5). Acupuncture, *15*(5), 1–34.

Norton, S. (1998). Herbal medicines in Hawaii from tradition to convention. *Hawaii Medical Journal, 57*(1), 382–386.

Perrin, J. M., Coury, D. L., Hyman, S. L., Cole, L., Reynolds, A. M., & Clemons, T. (2012). Complementary and alternative medicine use in a large pediatric autism sample. *Pediatrics, 130*(Supplement 2), S77–S82. http://pediatrics.aappublications.org/content/pediatrics/130/Supplement_2/S77.full.pdf

Soh, N. L., & Walter, G. (2012). Traditional and alternative medicine treatments in child and adolescent mental health. *IACAPAP e-Textbook of Child and Adolescent Mental Health*. http://www.iacapap.org/wp-content/uploads/J.2-ALTERNATIVE-072012.pdf

Wong, J., Ghiasuddin, A., Kimata, C., Patelesio, B., & Siu, A. (2013). The impact of healing touch on pediatric oncology patients. *Integrative Cancer Therapies*, *12*(1), 25–30. doi:https://doi.org/10.1177/1534735412446864. http://who.int/medicines/areas/traditional/en/. Last accessed 19 Sep 2017.

Chapter 22
Pediatric Consultation-Liaison Psychiatry Approach to Optimize Global Access to Child and Adolescent Mental Healthcare

Olurotimi Adejumo, Patricia Ibeziako, and Myron Belfer

There is much evidence pointing to significant gaps in the availability of mental healthcare for youth all over the world (Belfer 2008; Kieling et al. 2011; Patel et al. 2013; Paula et al. 2014). In addition to the general scarcity of specially tailored mental health programs for children and adolescents, several factors are responsible for reduced access to children's mental health services where these exist. Some of these factors include a general lack of awareness in some settings, stigma ascribed to mental ill-health, unavailability of trained providers, and infrastructural barriers such as difficult-to-access mental health facilities, as well as challenges with cost and payment for health services (Remschmidt and Belfer 2005).

A significant proportion of mental health problems in children are identified by nonmental health professionals, including pediatricians, general practitioners, and other primary care workers. Consequently, there is an opportunity and a challenge to provide mental health services in a setting where these problems are first identified. In addition, children with primary medical problems on medical, surgical, and emergency wards may also experience psychiatric symptoms, presenting a need for liaison care with psychiatry teams. Liaison psychiatry services have evolved over the years to address mental health problems that frequently occur in pediatric settings. In this chapter, we examine the role of pediatric psychosomatic medicine and psychiatric consultation-liaison services in improving access to mental healthcare on a global scale.

O. Adejumo (✉)
Hertfordshire Partnership University NHS Foundation Trust, Hertfordshire, UK

P. Ibeziako
Department of Psychiatry, Harvard Medical School, Boston, MA, USA
e-mail: Patricia.Ibeziako@childrens.harvard.edu

M. Belfer
Department of Psychiatry, Boston Children's Hospital/Harvard Medical School, Boston Children's Hospital, Boston, MA, USA
e-mail: myron_belfer@hms.harvard.edu

A. P. S. Guerrero et al. (eds.), *Pediatric Consultation-Liaison Psychiatry*,
https://doi.org/10.1007/978-3-319-89488-1_22

It has been recognized that children with medical conditions are at increased risk of mental health problems. Such problems often manifest in pediatric inpatient settings, where children with acute or chronic medical conditions receive care. Pediatric treatment settings therefore present an important platform for identification and management of mental health problems among a significant population of children and adolescents.

Many challenges exist to pediatric psychosomatic medicine services in low-resource settings, including lack of trained personnel, competition between professionals, stigma, and difficulties with funding these services. In the context of these challenges, mental healthcare for medically ill children and adolescents is often provided by adult psychiatrists or pediatricians, and inpatient treatment often must be provided on adult psychiatric or pediatric wards. Payment for mental healthcare in these settings is often made out-of-pocket, presenting a challenge in impoverished low-income settings.

To utilize the important platform of pediatric care, psychiatric skills need to be included in training for pediatricians, psychiatrists, hospital-based psychologists, nurses, and social workers all over the world. At the same time, collaborative care models may be effective in ensuring that mental health services are not left out in the provision of holistic care for children and adolescents at various levels of care.

Background

Global Challenges to Mental Healthcare Access

According to the World Health Organization (WHO) *Atlas: Child and Adolescent Mental Health Resources*, there is a global shortage of child mental health services, and the greatest lack of mental health policy and services exists in countries having the highest percentage population of children (World Health Organization et al. 2005). A wide range of interventions have been explored to address the inequalities in access to mental healthcare for children and adolescents. These have ranged from focused policy and program formulations to improved funding for mental health for youth (World Health Organization 2005; Harper 2012), to training nonspecialist healthcare workers in the identification and management of mental conditions in children and adolescents (Divan et al. 2015; Woods-Jaeger et al. 2017).

Given the limited number of mental health specialists globally, a potentially effective approach to addressing the existing inequalities may be the introduction of mental healthcare into existing general health services. A significant proportion of children and adolescents who present in pediatric clinics are known to have associated emotional or behavioral problems (Garralda and Bailey 1989; Glazebrook et al. 2003; Sayal 2006), and both acute and chronic pediatric conditions are frequently associated with high rates of psychopathology, which could impact the course or outcome of the other medical condition (Bernstein et al. 2013; Myrvik et al. 2013; Sztein and Lane 2016). The interrelationships between mental health and other medical problems have long been recognized and are largely responsible for the perceived need for collaborative care between mental health and pediatric services. The collaborative care approach (Unützer et al. 2002; Katon et al. 2010; Huijbregts et al. 2013; Bauer et al. 2014; Solberg et al. 2015), which utilizes a unified strategy of healthcare provision, enables mental health services to be integrated into comprehensive care involving other medical specialties and potentially provides for structured, holistic care while ensuring that attention to mental healthcare needs is not left out. This approach may be particularly important in low- and middle-income countries (LMIC) where a system of integrated psychiatric and pediatric services may be the first and most acceptable form of mental health intervention for children and adolescents. An advantage of this strategy is the improved efficiency of simultaneous attention to mental and other health needs when these coexist, as well as a reduction in mental health stigma. The pediatric setting is less stigmatized, and the challenge of evaluating and managing complex medical problems that may have a psychological component calls for an inclusive approach to care. Such coordinated care has been demonstrated to yield better outcomes for both the psychiatric and other medical conditions (World Health Organization and World Organization of Family Doctors 2008).

Psychosomatic Medicine

With the increased understanding of the interrelationships between mental health and other medical conditions in youth, professional alliances between pediatric and psychiatric specialists have evolved within the discipline of pediatric psychosomatic medicine. Pediatric psychosomatic medicine focuses on psychiatric issues affecting medically ill children and adolescents in the context of their development, cognition, communication, family and social interactions, and drug metabolism (Pao and Raza 2006). The practice has gradually grown in prominence over the past few decades in response to a recognized need for psychological support in children with chronic medical conditions and in children undergoing surgery, dialysis, organ transplants, or other medical procedures; and it has resulted in more holistic and efficient care for this group of at-risk children and adolescents. In a world coming to grasp the burden of mental health problems among children and adolescents, pediatric psychosomatic medicine presents a potential opportunity to increase access to much-needed mental health services.

Pediatric psychosomatic medicine and child psychiatry consultation-liaison services are relatively poorly developed in several parts of the developing world. This lack of development is a consequence of the nonexistence of child psychiatric services in many of these locations. As pointed out earlier, a prevailing shortage of mental health professionals in most low-resource settings implies that access to mental health services is considerably limited and often not available for children and adolescents. The implications of this shortage are that mental health problems occurring in the context of medical illness are frequently missed. However, where these problems are identified, a range of interventions may be taken to address them.

Mental Health Problems Presenting in Pediatric Care Settings Throughout the World

Emergency

One of the most common sources of child psychiatry consultations is the pediatric emergency department. There is evidence to suggest that there has been a disproportionate increase in pediatric emergency room presentations for mental health concerns, compared to other chronic medical conditions, over the past few decades in the United States and Canada (Sills and Bland 2002; Grupp-Phelan et al. 2007; Mapelli et al. 2015). Some possible reasons for this increase include a rise in prevalence of mental health problems, including an increase in psychoactive substance use in several societies, amidst limited access to community mental health services (Cooper and Masi 2007; Caradang et al. 2012).

Given the shortage of mental health practitioners in most settings, emergency departments have become an important entry point into mental healthcare and provide an important safety net for families in need of mental healthcare (Caradang et al. 2012; Ali et al. 2012). It is believed that the acuteness of this shortage in some regions of the United States was partly responsible for a disproportionate rise in mental health presentations to pediatric emergency departments among nonwhite, female adolescents in the North-East or Midwest United States between 1993 and 1999 (Sills and Bland 2002). In these settings in the United States, the most common emergency room diagnoses made using the *Diagnostic and Statistical Manual of Mental Disorders, Fourth Edition*, were substance-related disorders, anxiety disorders, and attention deficit and disruptive disorders (24.2%, 16.6%, and 11.3%, respectively) (Sills and Bland 2002).

Reflecting similar trends, emergency departments in Alberta, Canada, saw a 15% rise in pediatric mental health presentations between 2002 and 2006. A significant majority of this increase occurred in adolescents aged 13–17 years (Newton et al. 2009). Patterns of presenting concerns were also similar to those reported in the United States. In the Canadian review, substance misuse accounted for 41.3% of mental health presentations, and anxiety/stress-related disorders accounted for 32.5%, while mood disorders accounted for 21.4% (Newton et al. 2009). Overall, types of mental health conditions seen in hospital emergency departments vary, but those commonly encountered include violence-related problems, aggressive behaviors, emotional disturbance, suicidal ideation or attempts, substance and alcohol abuse, depression and other mood disorders, anxiety disorders, and cases of child abuse or neglect (Christodulu et al. 2002).

Mental healthcare may be provided by a variety of professionals in the emergency department. A survey conducted in two tertiary care emergency departments in the United States between 2004 and 2006 revealed two distinct scenarios. In one facility, mental healthcare was provided by general emergency medicine-trained physicians about 55% of the time, with a visiting psychiatric crisis team providing care 45% of the time. In the other facility, practically 100% of emergency mental healthcare was provided by emergency medicine-trained pediatricians, with no regular input from psychiatry personnel. As might be expected, significantly less psychiatric consultation, assessment, and intervention occurred at the latter pediatric setting, where recommendations for subsequent management were more likely to be incomplete (Newton et al. 2011). Routine mental health screening in emergency departments is likely to aid identification and management of problems where they exist and is more likely to be carried out in settings with dedicated child mental health expertise (Cooper and Masi 2007).

It is crucial to pay attention to emergency psychiatric presentations of children and adolescents, especially as these account for between 1.6% and 5% of pediatric emergency room visits (Sills and Bland 2002; Grupp-Phelan et al. 2007; Case et al. 2011). Given the risk of suboptimal psychiatric care being offered in the emergency situation, recommendations have been made for emergency room personnel to be trained to appropriately screen, intervene for, and refer children and adolescents with mental health problems (Cooper and Masi 2007). This training may allow for effective interventions in the absence of a dedicated psychiatric team.

In many low-income settings, pediatric services may not be distinguished from adult services. Emergency departments in such settings may cater to both adult and pediatric needs, creating a challenging arrangement for mental health emergencies when these present. In several of these facilities, children may be referred to better-equipped centers if the emergency staff does not feel confident of their capacity to manage the symptoms. In centers where there are facilities for emergency pediatric services, liaison with psychiatric services sometimes exists, whether these are child and adolescent or general psychiatric services. Consultations may be requested where there are emotional or behavioral symptoms, such as psychosis or depression, or when such symptoms preceded the presenting medical symptoms. Adolescent presentations involving problems such as suicidal ideation, aggression, deliberate self-harm, or psychoactive substance use may be causes for early psychiatric consultation requests.

Children or adolescents whose presenting symptoms result from, or are suggestive of, abuse may also be reasons for an early psychiatric consultation request in LMIC, especially when abuse is of a physical or sexual nature. In some cases, children who have experienced acute trauma may be referred for a mental health evaluation, for example, if selective mutism or withdrawal follows a major stressor, such as witnessing the loss of a loved one or surviving a natural disaster.

Consultation requests are usually to request some form of collaborative management, but pediatric practitioners may request a complete transfer to psychiatric services if there are no clear indications for continued pediatric involvement. These situations may pose a dilemma in settings where there are no inpatient psychiatric facilities for children or adolescents. Psychiatrists in this situation may be faced with the options of (1) admitting to an adult psychiatric ward, (2) admitting to the pediatric ward for continued psychiatric care, or (3) providing psychiatric treatment on an outpatient basis. While none if these options may be ideal, a temporary admission for inpatient treatment on an adult psychiatry ward or pediatric ward may need to be arranged to provide necessary care in the acute stages of a challenging mental health crisis.

Case Vignette 22.1

S.M., a 17-year-old female high school student, was referred to a tertiary care facility in Chandigarh, North India, after having ingested approximately 35mls of a liquid insecticide. She was the first of five children in a single-parent family that was undergoing considerable financial hardship. Collateral history obtained later indicated that S.M.'s mother had been diagnosed with a depressive disorder several years before, but her treatment had been irregular. Three and a half years before S.M.'s current incident, her mother had died unexpectedly of complications suspected to have resulted from a deliberate medication overdose. Since then, S.M. had to work at a tailoring outfit after school to support the family income and had to care for her younger siblings in her mother's absence. Recently, her academic performance had markedly declined, and she had become withdrawn, unhappy, and reluctant to carry out her regular activities.

S.M. received immediate care from the hospital emergency team, who later requested involvement of the hospital's consultation-liaison (CL) psychiatry service, which provided care for patients of all ages. When her medical condition became stable, S.M. was transferred to the general adult psychiatry ward, where she received treatment for a depressive disorder over the next few weeks.

Inpatient Settings

One important source of child psychiatric consultations is children and adolescents admitted on pediatric, surgical, or other inpatient wards. In a 2003 survey of US hospitals with child psychiatric consultation services, the participating units reported an average patient census of six, representing a 61% increase in consult requests over the preceding 5 years (Shaw et al. 2006). Overall, inpatient consultations averaged approximately 7.5 weekly and reflect the highest source of liaison requests (Shaw et al. 2006).

Inpatient liaison services typically constitute an important part of pediatric psychosomatic team activities. Most pediatric and general hospital settings can only support consultations, but where possible the development of a liaison relationship between the child psychiatrist and the pediatric clinical team is beneficial and has rewards for both the child psychiatrist and the pediatric clinicians caring for the patient. It can be a stimulating educational experience. Consultations usually cover a broad range of requests, from requests for assessment of children with specific symptoms or diagnoses, such as delirium or procedural anxiety, to requests requiring decisions for disposition and referral. Some of the most commonly reported reasons for consultation include difficult psychological adjustment to illness manifesting as depression or anxiety, or assessment for suicidality, and treatment nonadherence, especially in children and adolescents with chronic illnesses (Shaw et al. 2006).

In several parts of the developing world, the need for child psychiatry liaison services may be most frequently recognized on pediatric wards when children have acute behavioral problems that constitute a challenge to pediatric care providers and that may impair management. Hence, psychiatrists may be requested to evaluate youth with disruptive or aggressive behavior or sleep disturbances as part of a picture that may be seen in delirium. Restlessness, disruptive behavior, disturbed sleep, and cognitive disturbances are typical features of delirium and may occur in the presence of electrolyte derangement, infection, pain, or other acute physiologic disturbances. Similarly, challenges to management in the form of medication and treatment refusal or nonadherence may lead to requests for psychiatric consultation. A consultation may also be requested if mental health problems are suspected in a caregiver. In these cases, the psychiatric consultant is required to evaluate the situation and provide some intervention for the difficulties. The focus is usually the challenging symptoms, and psychiatric care is typically provided through repeat bedside consultations and thorough treatment advice communicated to the pediatric managing team.

In many developing countries, mental healthcare for children and adolescents may be provided by general adult psychiatrists, where these are present. In some settings, mental health professionals may be completely unavailable, and pediatric practitioners are forced to manage such symptoms to the best of their ability. The busy pediatrician may consider a psychiatric referral unnecessary if there is no challenge to medical management, and may prefer to refer the child for outpatient psychiatric services, where these exist, after other medical problems have resolved.

Case Vignette 22.2

A.Y., a 12-year-old boy in a lower middle-income country, presented at the only tertiary healthcare center in the region because of swelling of the face, abdomen, and lower limbs after a febrile episode that had been unsuccessfully managed with herbal concoctions. He was admitted for management of nephrotic syndrome and commenced on increasing doses of diuretic agents. There was only minimal improvement in the generalized edema, and after about 3 more weeks on inpatient treatment, prednisolone was added to his medications.

A.Y. started to have a resolution of edema after a week of prednisolone, but he then began to have visual hallucinations. He would also leave his bed abruptly, roll on the floor, intermittently shout uncontrollably for no apparent reason, and sleep poorly at night. The on-call adult psychiatry team was consulted. They diagnosed possible steroid-induced psychosis, prescribed oral risperidone, and advised that the steroid be gradually withdrawn, since the renal symptoms appeared to have resolved. A.Y.'s mental state improved drastically, and he was back to his normal state within 3 days.

Unfortunately, a week after discontinuing steroids, generalized edema began to recur, and the pediatric team began to consider a diagnosis of steroid-dependent nephrotic syndrome. Symptoms remained resistant to all medications until prednisolone was reintroduced. Within a few days of steroid recommencement, A.Y. again developed psychotic symptoms, and the dose of risperidone had to be increased. A.Y. had to be maintained on both steroids and antipsychotics and was followed up by the adult psychiatry team until discharge.

Chronic Illnesses in Childhood and Adolescence

Recent scientific discoveries and consequent improvements in healthcare for life-threatening conditions have resulted in increased survival for children with chronic congenital or acquired disease (Stiller 2002; van der Veen 2003; Van Cleave et al. 2010). The effect of this improved survival has been an increase in prevalence of chronic pediatric conditions in developed settings, with between 10% and 20% of children and adolescents in Western settings estimated to be living with a chronic disorder (van der Lee et al. 2007; Janse et al. 2005). Chronic illnesses are known to be associated with risk for emotional and behavioral problems (Hysing et al. 2007; Pinquart and Shen 2011; Erhart et al. 2011; Gómez-Restrepo et al. 2016), and this risk frequently informs psychiatric referrals (Blancquaert et al. 1992).

In several cases, children or adolescents may be hospitalized because of illness complications, and psychiatric consultation may be requested because of a history of poor treatment adherence. Nonadherence to treatment regimens is a frequently encountered challenge, resulting in medical complications, reduced quality of life, and increased healthcare costs (World Health Organisation 2003; Alvarez et al. 2009; Shemesh et al. 2010). In examining the role of the child's perceptions and family functioning in situations of nonadherence, it is important to understand the nature of the family's interrelationships, their understanding of the child's illness, and the impact of the illness on members individually and the family. Family therapy may be targeted at improving problem-solving strategies to improve adherence (DeMaso et al. 2009). In LMIC, while financial limitations and restricted access to care are often primary considerations in the assessment of nonadherence, religious and cultural influences on the understanding of medical and psychiatric intervention and on expectations of outcome should also be considered. Where pertinent, language barriers may require the services of an interpreter, who ideally should be well trained to work in the medical care setting (DeMaso et al. 2009).

An area of concern is the disclosure of the nature of illness. It is a sensitive issue that poses a concern for several families with youth living with chronic disease. Negative stereotypes associated with certain illnesses sometimes make caregivers withhold details about the nature and implications of the diagnosis from a child for as long as possible. In several parts of the developed and developing world, a diagnosis of human immunodeficiency virus (HIV) infection is associated with considerable stigma, and caregivers act to "protect" the child and family by avoiding a disclosure of the diagnosis to the child and other acquaintances for as long as possible (Spiegel 2011; Vreeman et al. 2013). Unfortunately, nondisclosure has been associated with suboptimal treatment adherence in adolescents living with HIV (Vreeman et al. 2008; Haberer et al. 2011; Nabukeera-Barungi et al. 2015).

The process of disclosing HIV diagnosis to a teenager is ideally done in several stages, with information presented as the youth can understand it, process it, and seek clarification (Krauss et al. 2011; National Department of Health South Africa

2016). This process may involve multiple meetings at different time points, but the family may be allowed to determine who does the actual disclosing. Working with the pediatric or medical team and the family, the psychiatrist may have the task of modifying information to suit the child's level of development and managing the interactions between the child, the family, and the healthcare teams.

The process of adjusting to a chronic disorder is also eased by social support for the child and family. In some situations, effective treatment depends on interventions within external agencies such as the school. Mental health professionals can work to collaborate with school services to facilitate reentry of children after a period of hospitalization or illness and can provide valuable support and advice for children needing special services or exemptions from certain activities. Community-based resources, such as religious groups and nongovernmental organizations, sometimes can provide valuable support for a child with a chronic illness or their family. Additional resources in the form of support groups, special educational services, and camps or rehabilitative groups for individuals living with specific disorders may be helpful in managing the challenges experienced as children grow into adolescence (Gillard et al. 2011; Moola et al. 2014; McCarthy 2015). Through these resources, families may be able to access respite care, educational literature, contacts with other families, and even financial or material aid (Neil-Urban and Jones 2002; Sharma et al. 2012).

It is important for the mental health professional to have a working knowledge of the local legal and forensic issues guiding care provision in children and adolescents. Such knowledge could prove invaluable in helping the pediatric team and child's family to successfully work through challenges of medical decision making, but it may be necessary to involve an ethics committee or child protection services in difficult or controversial life-threatening cases.

Because of the crucial contribution of psychosocial issues to the overall quality of life of children and youth with chronic physical conditions, it has been advocated that child psychiatric services be included as a component in management teams for such conditions (Bergman and Fritz 1981; Turkel and Pao 2007). To this end, a variety of outpatient arrangements may enable an effective and efficient role for psychiatric outpatient care, without additional burden to the child and family.

Glbal Challenges in the Development of Psychiatry Liaison Services in Pediatric Settings

One of the consequences of the different ways in which pediatric/psychiatric liaison services have developed in different parts of the world is the absence or inconsistency of standards that guide the practice. Therefore, psychiatrists may be uncertain of how to address mental health challenges in pediatric patients, especially in non-specific presentations.

Training

Surveys conducted among pediatric practitioners in both high- and low-income settings have reported a need for training in psychological aspects of pediatric care, with a view of improving their capacities to recognize and intervene upon mental health problems (Anders 1977; Vandvik 1994; Henderson 2013). Exposure to child mental health training varies significantly in different medical schools and pediatric training programs globally. This variability in exposure results in disparate levels of understanding of mental health problems, particularly in children with comorbid medical conditions. Given that a large proportion of countries do not currently have child and adolescent psychiatry training programs, considerably fewer countries would be expected to have formal subspecialty training provisions for liaison psychiatry within child and adolescent psychiatry training.

Professional Competition

The care of pediatric patients with coexisting psychiatric and other medical problems requires collaboration between pediatric and psychiatry professionals. However, for as long as such collaborations have existed, there have been conflicts regarding practice boundaries in the care of children with mental and other healthcare needs.

Several authors throughout the world have proposed interventions to improve the collaboration between pediatricians and child psychiatrists. A survey conducted in Norway revealed a desire by both pediatricians and child psychiatrists for more training in consultation/liaison, interprofessional assessments, and therapeutic interventions for children with medical illnesses (Vandvik 1994). In an earlier survey of directors of pediatric training programs in the United States, a general need was expressed for child mental health experience for pediatric trainees in the form of "behavioral pediatrics" (Anders 1977). It has also been recommended that the establishment of well-defined subspecialty groups within both child psychiatry and pediatrics, such as "pediatric psychiatry" and "behavioral pediatrics," may be beneficial. It is proposed that these subspecialties could constitute a "behavioral" team that serves a well-defined patient population and that role models, for future specialists, interdisciplinary collaboration, dialogue, and research (Anders 1977).

Financing of Care

An important challenge to the provision of optimal pediatric liaison services is the source of funding for the care offered. Despite evidence of significant cost benefits through reduction in medical complications, length of stay (Bujoreanu et al. 2015), and the subsequent number of hospitalizations (Aoki et al 2004), funding consultation-liaison services in pediatrics remains a challenge in many countries.

The first consultation-liaison units in the United States were set up on institutional funds, but in the 1970s, the National Institutes of Health began to provide funding through training grants for consultation-liaison programs (Martin et al. 2007). In the United Kingdom, a survey of liaison psychiatry services in 30 general hospitals revealed that services were managed by mental health trusts under the National Health Service. Among these services, 55% were directly funded by these mental health trusts, 21% by an acute trust, and 24% by joint funding (Naidu et al. 2015). In some well-resourced settings, government healthcare funding supports psychiatry liaison services. However, it has been pointed out that separate funding for mental healthcare and other healthcare is unhelpful for psychosomatic/consultation-liaison psychiatry services, which typically serve as a bridge between these two areas (Sharpe 2014). It has therefore been recommended that governments fund psychiatry liaison services for the added value provided over traditional medical and psychiatry services (Sharpe 2014).

Child and adolescent liaison and pediatric psychosomatic services are typically funded, like pediatric services, separately from adult services. However, like adult psychiatric services, child psychiatry liaison services are very poorly funded. In a survey of child healthcare practitioners in London, up to 89% of pediatricians thought that mental health was an important area to target for pediatric resources, even though 87% of existing child mental health services was being funded by sources other than pediatric resources (Woodgate and Elena Garralda 2006).

Case Vignette 22.3

L.P. was an 8-year-old boy who had been taken off the streets of Kathmandu, Nepal, by a small nongovernmental organization (NGO). The whereabouts of his family were not known, as he had survived by begging on the streets for as long as he could remember until he was picked up by the NGO, who housed him in a home with other children and who provided for his upkeep. L.P. was very inattentive, restless, and "playful," and he would frequently sneak out of the home to play on the streets when his caregivers were not watching.

One afternoon, L.P. fell into a deep ditch while playing vigorously. He sustained a tibial fracture and was rushed first to a nearby private hospital and then to a tertiary health facility in Nepal. He received care from the orthopedic and trauma team, but all payments had to be made out-of-pocket and borne by the NGO. As L.P. had to remain on inpatient care for several months, the cost of treatment gradually accumulated, constituting a major burden to the NGO.

A month after admission on the orthopedic ward, the psychiatry team was consulted because L.P. would not keep still and kept attempting to get out of bed to play, bearing weight on his healing fractured limb. After a detailed assessment, the psychiatry team recommended that stimulants be prescribed to manage the hyperactivity. However, given the already-incurred healthcare costs, the NGO caregivers expressed doubts that they would be able to bear the additional cost of these medications in the long term.

Because reduced mobility was crucial to the healing of L.P.'s fractured tibia, the nurses and doctors on the pediatric ward all made personal cash contributions toward purchasing stimulant medications over the course of L.P.'s inpatient admission. The NGO was very grateful. He was eventually discharged with his injury almost completely healed.

The NGO financially struggled to maintain L.P.'s stimulants after discharge. During outpatient visits, the psychiatry team decided to reduce his medication dose and to prioritize his in-school hours. A few weeks afterward, a private pharmacy was discovered to have a less expensive generic formulation of the same psychostimulant. At L.P.'s reduced dose, this medication was now much easier to afford, and the NGO was able to sustain his medication supply for long afterward. LP's hyperactivity and "playfulness" reduced significantly, and he subsequently had no serious injuries.

Models and Strategies for Integrating Mental Healthcare into Pediatric Care

With the advancement of pediatric care, there is a global move to integrate mental health into primary care. Optimizing the primary care setting for mental healthcare provision may involve increasing the number and types of professionals who can provide preventive and treatment services in these settings (Wissow et al. 2016). Because primary care is provided by various professionals with different skill sets and levels of training around the world, there may be a need for flexibility in the degrees and forms of child mental health integration. An example of such differences is the relative emphasis on integration around primary healthcare sites in the United States, compared to integration around a combination of primary care, school-based, and other community services (Wissow et al. 2016). In these various approaches, a broad focus on children's healthy development creates the opportunity for child mental health integration (Wissow et al. 2016).

Challenges in the Global Implementation of Collaborative Mental Healthcare Models

Financial and Administrative Challenges

The pressure for primary care providers (PCPs) to generate revenue in some developed settings has sometimes produced situations in which these practitioners are unable to conduct the thorough evaluations necessary for mental healthcare needs to be identified and addressed through either a collaborative or traditional model. In countries where costs are covered by managed care, the reluctance of insurance companies to pay for the extra effort and time required for these interventions may serve as a challenge to the evolution of collaborative models (Power et al. 2013). In countries where costs are covered mostly out-of-pocket, the cost of multiple collaborating care teams could be difficult to afford for low-income families without access to insurance or other financial support (Foy et al. 2010).

Differences in Professional Approach

Differences in conceptual approach to illness and management and in terminologies used may create barriers between psychiatrists and other primary care providers. These differences may lead to uncomfortable working relationships, distrust in extreme situations, and reluctance to maintain collaborative arrangements. Unfortunately, there are limited opportunities – especially in low-resource settings – for these different professional teams to undergo common educational experiences to improve understanding and communication (Power et al. 2013). These conceptual differences may also lead to a restriction of focus – for example, medication prescription to the neglect of educational or psychological interventions – and, ultimately, fragmentation of care.

Task Shifting

Task shifting is currently regarded as an essential response to global shortages in human resources for mental healthcare (Kakuma et al. 2011). Defined as "delegating tasks to new or existing cadres with less training or narrowly tailored training" (Fulton et al. 2011), task shifting or task "sharing" may involve the employment of mental health professionals in nonmental health sectors, and intersectoral collaboration with other professionals, such as primary care providers, to improve awareness, identification, and management of mental health conditions (Kakuma et al. 2011). The move to transfer mental health provision skills to nonspecialist health workers has been attempted with some success in several parts of both the developed and the developing world (Lancet Global Mental Health Group et al. 2007; Eaton et al. 2011). In adopting this strategy, mental health professionals assume roles beyond a pure clinical focus and become broadly involved in training and providing support, supervision, and occasional clinical expertise (Eaton et al. 2011). There is, however, anecdotal evidence that care provided by "less trained" workers is sometimes not well received by the recipients of such care, who feel that they are being discriminated against and that they will receive lower-quality care that may lack confidentiality.

Challenges of Task Shifting

Case Vignette 22.4

J is a 16-year-old boy who was just accepted into a local university in South West Nigeria. J was considered a hero in his local community for his academic success; however, he was younger than most students in his class at the university, and he experienced some bullying. He became increasingly depressed, socially withdrawn, and isolated. He began to skip classes because he preferred to stay in his room, where he would smoke marijuana. J, a previous "honors" student, started failing classes in his first year at the university. His poor performance came under scrutiny, and he was referred to the university mental health clinic. The history of the development of this clinic was as follows:

A primary care clinic serving the large university community identified a significant need for mental health services. Although alcohol and substance use problems among the university staff had been recognized as a problem, increasing awareness about mental health conditions led to the identification of psychiatric problems during routine health screening of new university intakes, who were often teenagers and young adults. The clinic had addressed such problems in the past by referring them to a nearby teaching hospital. However, a psychiatrist in the teaching hospital's psychiatry department proposed setting up a mental health clinic to bring services closer to the university community and to reduce the stigma of mental health problems.

Student attendance at the university mental health clinic grew steadily in the subsequent years, and university referrals to the teaching hospital declined drastically. However, the increasing demand for services presented a challenge to the psychiatry department in the teaching hospital. Consultation periods at the university stretched from a half-day to full-day clinic, and the "visiting" psychiatrist had to be supported by a senior trainee from the teaching hospital to cope with the steadily expanding caseload. Like for other health services, students paid greatly subsidized rates for mental healthcare; however, there was no university funding set aside for this clinic. Sustaining these specialist services became an increasing challenge, especially as other psychiatrists in the understaffed teaching hospital resented having to extend beyond their already high caseloads to provide care at the university clinic.

These problems were discussed at a number of management meetings, and some potential solutions were considered. A series of training sessions, focused on identifying and managing common mental health problems and appropriately triaging more serious cases for specialist review, were organized for the university clinic's primary care doctors, nurses, and social workers.

The training sessions were well attended but were received with much more interest by the social workers than by the doctors and nurses. Over the subsequent weeks, the psychiatrist attended the mental health clinics to provide supervision and noticed that, while more patients with mental health conditions were being identified, the university doctors and nurses were making no effort to manage them and preferred instead to continue sending them to the psychiatrist. When inquiries were made, the predominant reason given was a lack of confidence in the ability to manage psychiatric conditions.

While this situation was being evaluated, the university finally approved some funds to support the clinics, which helped to dedicate hospital specialists' time to the university clinic. The clinic services were also subsumed under a new child and adolescent liaison/outreach team in the Department of Psychiatry and therefore recognized as a routine part of the teaching hospital services. This reorganization helped to sustain the university mental health clinic, while discussions continued about designing a suitable task-shifting model for this unique setting.

J received services at the university mental health clinic during his first 2 years at the university. He was prescribed an antidepressant by the visiting psychiatrist and received counseling from the social work staff. Over time, his functioning improved, and he had made both social and academic progress at the university by the time he turned 18 years old.

Communication Barriers

One important barrier to effective task shifting is problems with communication. Professional training and expertise manifest in the use of terminologies and technical approaches to mental healthcare delivery that may be difficult to communicate to nonmental health professionals who are required to provide mental health services at the primary care level. In some developing communities, marked linguistic and cultural diversity makes it challenging for psychiatric consultants to communicate with primary care workers and may present a challenge to scaling up mental health services (Swartz et al. 2014).

Funding Challenges for Mental Health Integration

In low-income countries, insufficient funding has been a barrier to integration, across age groups, of mental health into primary care. Government funding is often insufficient to establish and sustain mental health task-shifting initiatives. Public health experts have attributed this situation to multiple factors, including weak policy support for mental health services due to ineffective lobbying by mental health advocates, inaccurate perception of the burden of mental health problems, and in some cases, social stigma (Saraceno et al. 2007).

Reluctance to Decentralize Mental Healthcare

In several countries, mental healthcare is largely confined to tertiary health facilities. In many settings of low- and middle-income, most of these centers are situated in or around large cities and account for most of the available mental health resources in terms of staff, beds, and allocated funds. The changes in mental healthcare administration required for task shifting would necessitate a significant modification in these arrangements. These changes have been met with resistance from healthcare administrators and mental health specialists themselves in low- and middle-income settings. A potential loss of control and funding, as well as general reluctance to change established approaches to mental health delivery, may be responsible for this resistance.

Logistical Challenges

Within already stretched existing primary care services, it may be difficult for staff to accommodate new responsibilities relating to mental healthcare provision. This is the case in several low-income countries where primary care staff often have large patient caseloads and limited time to devote to individual patients. These constraints are an even bigger problem in settings where there are low primary care staff retention rates (Labhardt et al. 2010), often related to inadequate incentives attached to working in remote or rural primary care settings. The degree of detail required in even basic mental health assessments and the need for frequent visits within stipulated periods may be challenging, given existing primary care practitioner constraints (Wissow et al. 2016).

Issues Related to Mental Health Specialists

In some low-resource settings where there are shortages in mental healthcare practitioners, training of nonspecialists may be restricted to one or just a few contact sessions with mental health experts and may be followed by inadequate supervision, resulting in a lack of confidence in primary care capacity for managing mental health problems (Saraceno et al. 2007).

It is also possible that specialist physicians may be reluctant to transfer skills to nonspecialist and non-physician staff for fear of gradually losing status or relevance (Munga et al. 2012; Gilbert 2013). Where this is not the case, mental health specialists may themselves have inadequate public health training and may have more experience in providing care rather than in training and supervising other professionals (Saraceno et al. 2007). Specialists may also be overburdened in their primary hospital roles involving demanding clinical and administrative responsibilities and may therefore have difficulty in prioritizing task shifting for primary care.

Conclusion

Amidst shortages of child and adolescent mental health personnel in countries of low and middle income globally, the need to address co-occurring psychiatric and other medical problems among pediatric populations is considerable. It is important for psychiatry practitioners and healthcare planners to begin to consider the potential contributions of child and adolescent psychiatry to meeting the needs of medical wards, surgical wards, emergency departments, primary care centers, and other settings where children present with general and mental healthcare needs. Skills in assessing and intervening for psychosocial challenges in the child and family are important and should be integrated in training for pediatric practitioners. There is also a need to create more avenues for collaboration between child psychiatrists and pediatricians and to improve communication between these groups of practitioners. Furthermore, the existing shortage of mental health practitioners globally can be addressed through collaboration with non-mental health professionals. It is important to develop strategies to address existing challenges in both well-resourced and low- and middle-income settings to improve these collaborations given their potential impact on the mental health outcomes of large proportions of the world's children and adolescents.

References

Ali, S., Rosychuk, R. J., Dong, K. A., McGrath, P. J., & Newton, A. S. (2012). Temporal trends in pediatric mental health visits: Using longitudinal data to inform emergency department health care planning. *Pediatric Emergency Care, 28*, 620–625. https://doi.org/10.1097/PEC.0b013e31825cf93b.

Alvarez, O., Rodriguez-Cortes, H., Robinson, N., Lewis, N., Pow Sang, C. D., Lopez-Mitnik, G., et al. (2009). Adherence to deferasirox in children and adolescents with sickle cell disease during 1-year of therapy. *Journal of Pediatric Hematology Oncology, 31*, 739–744. https://doi.org/10.1097/MPH.0b013e3181b53363.

Anders, T. F. (1977). Child psychiatry and pediatrics: The state of the relationship. *Pediatrics, 60*, 616–620.

Aoki, T., Sato, T., & Hosaka, T. (2004). Role of consultation-liaison psychiatry toward shortening of length of stay for medically ill patients with depression. *International Journal of Psychiatry in Clinical Practice, 8*, 71–76. https://doi.org/10.1080/13651500310004957.

Bauer, A. M., Thielke, S. M., Katon, W., Unützer, J., & Areán, P. (2014). Aligning health information technologies with effective service delivery models to improve chronic disease care. *Preventive Medicine, 66*, 167–172. https://doi.org/10.1016/j.ypmed.2014.06.017.

Belfer, M. L. (2008). Child and adolescent mental disorders: The magnitude of the problem across the globe. *Journal of Child Psychology and Psychiatry, 49*, 226–236. https://doi.org/10.1111/j.1469-7610.2007.01855.x.

Bergman, A. S., & Fritz, G. K. (1981). Psychiatric and social work collaboration in pediatric chronic illness hospital. *Social Work in Health Care, 7*, 45–55.

Bernstein, C. M., Stockwell, M. S., Gallagher, M. P., Rosenthal, S. L., & Soren, K. (2013). Mental health issues in adolescents and young adults with type 1 diabetes: Prevalence and impact on glycemic control. *Clinical Pediatrics (Philadelphia), 52*, 10–15. https://doi.org/10.1177/0009922812459950.

Blancquaert, I. R., Zvagulis, I., Gray-Donald, K., & Pless, I. B. (1992). Referral patterns for children with chronic diseases. *Pediatrics, 90*, 71–74.

Bujoreanu, S., White, M. T., Gerber, B., & Ibeziako, P. (2015). Effect of timing of psychiatry consultation on length of pediatric hospitalization and hospital charges. *Hospital Pediatrics, 5*, 269–275. https://doi.org/10.1542/hpeds.2014-0079.

Caradang, C., Gray, C., Marval-Ospino, H., & MacPhee, S. (2012). In J. M. Rey (Ed.), *Child and adolescent psychiatric emergencies*. Geneva: IACAPAP E-Textb. Child Adolesc. Ment. Health.

Case, S. D., Case, B. G., Olfson, M., Linakis, J. G., & Laska, E. M. (2011). Length of stay of pediatric mental health emergency department visits in the United States. *Journal of the American Academy of Child and Adolescent Psychiatry, 50*, 1110–1119. https://doi.org/10.1016/j.jaac.2011.08.011.

Christodulu, K. V., Lichenstein, R., Weist, M. D., Shafer, M. E., & Simone, M. (2002). Psychiatric emergencies in children. *Pediatric Emergency Care, 18*, 268–270.

Cooper, J. L., & Masi, R. (2007). *Child and youth emergency mental health care: A national problem*. New York: Columbia University Academy Commons.

DeMaso, D. R., Martini, D. R., & Cahen, L. A. (2009). Practice parameter for the psychiatric assessment and management of physically ill children and adolescents. *Journal of the American Academy of Child & Adolescent Psychiatry, 48*, 213–233. https://doi.org/10.1097/CHI.0b13e3181908bf4.

Divan, G., Hamdani, S. U., Vajartkar, V., Minhas, A., Taylor, C., Aldred, C., et al. (2015). Adapting an evidence-based intervention for autism spectrum disorder for scaling up in resource-constrained settings: The development of the PASS intervention in South Asia. *Global Health Action, 8*, 27278.

Eaton, J., McCay, L., Semrau, M., Chatterjee, S., Baingana, F., Araya, R., et al. (2011). Scale up of services for mental health in low-income and middle-income countries. *Lancet London England, 378*, 1592–1603. https://doi.org/10.1016/S0140-6736(11)60891-X.

Erhart, M., Weimann, A., Bullinger, M., Schulte-Markwort, M., & Ravens-Sieberer, U. (2011). Psychological comorbidity in children and adolescents with chronic somatic diseases. *Bundesgesundheitsblatt Gesundheitsforschung Gesundheitsschutz, 54*, 66–74. https://doi.org/10.1007/s00103-010-1190-0.

Foy, J. M., Kelleher, K. J., Laraque, D., & American Academy of Pediatrics Task Force on Mental Health. (2010). Enhancing pediatric mental health care: Strategies for preparing a primary care practice. *Pediatrics, 125*, S87–S108. https://doi.org/10.1542/peds.2010-0788E.

Fulton, B. D., Scheffler, R. M., Sparkes, S. P., Auh, E. Y., Vujicic, M., & Soucat, A. (2011). Health workforce skill mix and task shifting in low income countries: A review of recent evidence. *Human Resources for Health, 9*(1). https://doi.org/10.1186/1478-4491-9-1.

Garralda, M. E., & Bailey, D. (1989). Psychiatric disorders in general paediatric referrals. *Archives of Disease in Childhood, 64*, 1727–1733.

Gilbert, L. (2013). "Re-Engineering the Workforce to meet service needs": Exploring "Task-Shifting" in South Africa in the Context of Hiv/Aids and antiretroviral therapy. *South African Review of Sociology, 44*, 54–75. https://doi.org/10.1080/21528586.2013.802537.

Gillard, A., Witt, P. A., & Watts, C. E. (2011). Outcomes and processes at a camp for youth with HIV/AIDS. *Qualitative Health Research, 21*, 1508–1526. https://doi.org/10.1177/1049732311413907.

Glazebrook, C., Hollis, C., Heussler, H., Goodman, R., & Coates, L. (2003). Detecting emotional and behavioural problems in paediatric clinics. *Child: Care, Health and Development, 29*, 141–149.

Gómez-Restrepo, C., Ramirez, S., Tamayo Martínez, N., Rodriguez, M. N., Rodríguez, A., & Rengifo, H. (2016). Probable mental health disorders prevalence in children with chronic conditions. Results from the national mental health survey of Colombia 2015. *Revista Colombiana Psiquiatria, 45*(Suppl 1), 135–140. https://doi.org/10.1016/j.rcp.2016.08.005.

Grupp-Phelan, J., Harman, J. S., & Kelleher, K. J. (2007). Trends in mental health and chronic condition visits by children presenting for care at U.S. emergency departments. *Public Health Reports, 122*, 55–61.

Haberer, J. E., Cook, A., Walker, A. S., Ngambi, M., Ferrier, A., Mulenga, V., et al. (2011). Excellent adherence to antiretrovirals in HIV+ Zambian children Is compromised by disrupted routine, HIV Nondisclosure, and Paradoxical income effects. *PLoS ONE, 6*. https://doi.org/10.1371/journal.pone.0018505.

Harper, G. (2012). Child and adolescent mental health policy. In J. Rey (Ed.), *IACAPAP E-textbook of child and adolescent mental health*. Geneva: International Association for Child and Adolescent Psychiatry and Allied Professions.

Henderson, T. (2013). *Pediatric consultation-liaison psychiatry: A description of the consultation-liaison service offered by a tertiary level children's hospital in Cape Town, South Africa*. Cape Town: University of Cape Town.

Huijbregts, K. M. L., de Jong, F. J., van Marwijk, H. W. J., Beekman, A. T. F., Adèr, H. J., Hakkaart-van Roijen, L., et al. (2013). A target-driven collaborative care model for major depressive disorder is effective in primary care in the Netherlands. A randomized clinical trial from the depression initiative. *The Journal of Affective Disorders, 146*, 328–337. https://doi.org/10.1016/j.jad.2012.09.015.

Hysing, M., Elgen, I., Gillberg, C., Lie, S. A., & Lundervold, A. J. (2007). Chronic physical illness and mental health in children. Results from a large-scale population study. *Journal of Child Psychology and Psychiatry, 48*, 785–792. https://doi.org/10.1111/j.1469-7610.2007.01755.x.

Janse, A. J., Uiterwaal, C. S. P. M., Gemke, R. J. B. J., Kimpen, J. L. L., & Sinnema, G. (2005). A difference in perception of quality of life in chronically ill children was found between parents and pediatricians. *Journal of Clinical Epidemiology, 58*, 495–502. https://doi.org/10.1016/j.jclinepi.2004.09.010.

Kakuma, R., Minas, H., van Ginneken, N., Dal Poz, M. R., Desiraju, K., Morris, J. E., et al. (2011). Human resources for mental health care: Current situation and strategies for action. *Lancet London England, 378*, 1654–1663. https://doi.org/10.1016/S0140-6736(11)61093-3.

Katon, W., Unützer, J., Wells, K., & Jones, L. (2010). Collaborative depression care: History, evolution and ways to enhance dissemination and sustainability. *General Hospital Psychiatry, 32*. https://doi.org/10.1016/j.genhosppsych.2010.04.001.

Kieling, C., Baker-Henningham, H., Belfer, M., Conti, G., Ertem, I., Omigbodun, O., et al. (2011). Child and adolescent mental health worldwide: Evidence for action. *The Lancet, 378*, 1515–1525. https://doi.org/10.1016/S0140-6736(11)60827-1.

Krauss, B., Letteney, S., de Baets, A., Murugi, J., Okero, F. A., & World Health Organization. (2011). *Guideline on HIV disclosure counselling for children up to 12 years of age*. Geneva: World Health Organization.

Labhardt, N. D., Balo, J.-R., Ndam, M., Grimm, J.-J., & Manga, E. (2010). Task shifting to non-physician clinicians for integrated management of hypertension and diabetes in rural Cameroon: A programme assessment at two years. *BMC Health Services Research, 10*, 339. https://doi.org/10.1186/1472-6963-10-339.

Lancet Global Mental Health Group, Chisholm, D., Flisher, A. J., Lund, C., Patel, V., Saxena, S., et al. (2007). Scale up services for mental disorders: A call for action. *Lancet London England, 370*, 1241–1252. https://doi.org/10.1016/S0140-6736(07)61242-2.

Mapelli, E., Black, T., & Doan, Q. (2015). Trends in pediatric emergency department utilization for mental health-related visits. *The Journal of Pediatrics, 167*, 905–910. https://doi.org/10.1016/j.jpeds.2015.07.004.

Martin, A., Volkmar, F. R., & Lewis, M. (2007). *Lewis's child and adolescent psychiatry: A comprehensive textbook*. Philadelphia: Lippincott Williams & Wilkins.

McCarthy, A. (2015). Summer camp for children and adolescents with chronic conditions. *Pediatric Nursing, 41*, 245–250.

Moola, F. J., Faulkner, G. E. J., White, L., & Kirsh, J. A. (2014). The psychological and social impact of camp for children with chronic illnesses: A systematic review update. *Child: Care, Health and Development, 40*, 615–631.

Munga, M. A., Kilima, S. P., Mutalemwa, P. P., Kisoka, W. J., & Malecela, M. N. (2012). Experiences, opportunities and challenges of implementing task shifting in underserved remote settings: the case of Kongwa district, central Tanzania. *BMC International Health and Human Rights, 12*, 27. https://doi.org/10.1186/1472-698X-12-27.

Myrvik, M. P., Burks, L. M., Hoffman, R. G., Dasgupta, M., & Panepinto, J. A. (2013). Mental health disorders influence admission rates for pain in children with sickle cell disease. *Pediatric Blood & Cancer, 60*, 1211–1214. https://doi.org/10.1002/pbc.24394.

Nabukeera-Barungi, N., Elyanu, P., Asire, B., Katureebe, C., Lukabwe, I., Namusoke, E., et al. (2015). Adherence to antiretroviral therapy and retention in care for adolescents living with HIV from 10 districts in Uganda. *BMC Infectious Diseases, 15*. https://doi.org/10.1186/s12879-015-1265-5.

Naidu, S., Bolton, J., & Smith, J. (2015). London's liaison psychiatry services: Survey of service provision. *BJPsych Bulletin, 39*, 65–69. https://doi.org/10.1192/pb.bp.114.046862.

National Department of Health South Africa. (2016). *Disclosure guidelines for children and adolescents in the context of HIV, TB and non-communicable diseases*. Republic of South Africa: National Department of Health South Africa.

Neil-Urban, S., & Jones, J. B. (2002). Father-to-father support: Fathers of children with cancer share their experience. *Journal of Pediatric Oncology Nursing, 19*, 97–103. https://doi.org/10.1177/104345420201900304.

Newton, A. S., Ali, S., Johnson, D. W., Haines, C., Rosychuk, R. J., Keaschuk, R. A., et al. (2009). A 4-year review of pediatric mental health emergencies in Alberta. *CJEM, 11*, 447–454.

Newton, A. S., Ali, S., Hamm, M. P., Haines, C., Rosychuk, R. J., Warron, L., et al. (2011). Exploring differences in the clinical management of pediatric mental health in the emergency department. *Pediatric Emergency Care, 27*, 275–283. https://doi.org/10.1097/PEC.0b013e31821314ca.

Pao, M., & Raza, H. (2006). Essential issues in pediatric psychosomatic medicine. *Psychiatric Times*. http://www.psychiatrictimes.com/articles/essential-issues-pediatric-psychosomatic-medicine. Accessed 25 Mar 2017.

Patel, V., Kieling, C., Maulik, P. K., & Divan, G. (2013). Improving access to care for children with mental disorders. Medscape. http://www.medscape.com/viewarticle/802929. Accessed December 20, 2015.

Paula, C. S., Bordin, I. A. S., Mari, J. J., Velasque, L., Rohde, L. A., & Coutinho, E. S. F. (2014). The mental health care gap among children and adolescents: Data from an Epidemiological Survey from four Brazilian Regions. *PLOS ONE, 9*, e88241. https://doi.org/10.1371/journal.pone.0088241.

Pinquart, M., & Shen, Y. (2011). Behavior problems in children and adolescents with chronic physical illness: A meta-analysis. *Journal of Pediatric Psychology, 36*, 1003–1016. https://doi.org/10.1093/jpepsy/jsr042.

Power, T. J., Blum, N. J., Guevara, J. P., Jones, H. A., & Leslie, L. K. (2013). Coordinating mental health care across primary care and schools: ADHD as a case example. *Advances in School Mental Health Promotion, 6*, 68–80. https://doi.org/10.1080/1754730X.2013.749089.

Remschmidt, H., & Belfer, M. (2005). Mental health care for children and adolescents worldwide: A review. *World Psychiatry, 4*, 147–153.

Saraceno, B., van Ommeren, M., Batniji, R., Cohen, A., Gureje, O., Mahoney, J., et al. (2007). Barriers to improvement of mental health services in low-income and middle-income countries. *Lancet London England, 370*, 1164–1174. https://doi.org/10.1016/S0140-6736(07)61263-X.

Sayal, K. (2006). Annotation: Pathways to care for children with mental health problems. *Journal of Child Psychology and Psychiatry, 47*, 649–659. https://doi.org/10.1111/j.1469-7610.2005.01543.x.

Sharma, A., Prematta, T., & Fausnight, T. (2012). A pediatric food allergy support group can improve parent and physician communication: Results of a parent survey. *Journal of Allergy, 2012*, 168053. https://doi.org/10.1155/2012/168053.

Sharpe, M. (2014). Psychological medicine and the future of psychiatry. *British Journal of Psychiatry, 204*, 91–92. https://doi.org/10.1192/bjp.bp.113.132894.

Shaw, R. J., Wamboldt, M., Bursch, B., & Stuber, M. (2006). Practice patterns in pediatric consultation–liaison psychiatry: A national survey. *Psychosomatics, 47*, 43–49. https://doi.org/10.1176/appi.psy.47.1.43.

Shemesh, E., Annunziato, R. A., Arnon, R., Miloh, T., & Kerkar, N. (2010). Adherence to medical recommendations and transition to adult services in pediatric transplant recipients. *Current Opinion in Organ Transplantation, 15*, 288–292. https://doi.org/10.1097/MOT.0b013e32833984a5.

Sills, M. R., & Bland, S. D. (2002). Summary statistics for pediatric psychiatric visits to US emergency departments, 1993–1999. *Pediatrics, 110*, e40–e40. https://doi.org/10.1542/peds.110.4.e40.

Solberg, L. I., Crain, A. L., Maciosek, M. V., Unützer, J., Ohnsorg, K. A., Beck, A., et al. (2015). A stepped-wedge evaluation of an initiative to spread the collaborative care model for depression in primary care. *Annals of Family Medicine, 13*, 412–420. https://doi.org/10.1370/afm.1842.

Spiegel, H. M. L. (2011). Nondisclosure of HIV status in adolescence. *Adolescent Medicine: State of the Art Reviews, 22*, 277–282. x.

Stiller, C. (2002). Epidemiology of cancer in adolescents. *Medical and Paediatric Oncology, 39*, 149–155. https://doi.org/10.1002/mpo.10142.

Swartz, L., Kilian, S., Twesigye, J., Attah, D., & Chiliza, B. (2014). Language, culture, and task shifting – An emerging challenge for global mental health. *Global Health Action, 7*. https://doi.org/10.3402/gha.v7.23433.

Sztein, D. M., & Lane, W. G. (2016). Examination of the comorbidity of mental illness and somatic conditions in hospitalized children in the United States using the kids' inpatient database, 2009. *Hospital Pediatrics, 6*, 126–134. https://doi.org/10.1542/hpeds.2015-0117.

Turkel, S., & Pao, M. (2007). Late consequences of pediatric chronic illness. *Psychiatric Clinics of North America, 30*, 819–835. https://doi.org/10.1016/j.psc.2007.07.009.

Unützer, J., Katon, W., Callahan, C. M., Williams, J. W., Hunkeler, E., Harpole, L., et al. (2002). Collaborative care management of late-life depression in the primary care setting: A randomized controlled trial. *JAMA, 288*, 2836–2845.

Van Cleave, J., Gortmaker, S. L., & Perrin, J. M. (2010). Dynamics of obesity and chronic health conditions among children and youth. *JAMA, 303*, 623–630. https://doi.org/10.1001/jama.2010.104.

van der Lee, J. H., Mokkink, L. B., Grootenhuis, M. A., Heymans, H. S., & Offringa, M. (2007). Definitions and measurement of chronic health conditions in childhood: A systematic review. *JAMA, 297*, 2741–2751. https://doi.org/10.1001/jama.297.24.2741.

van der Veen, W. J. (2003). The small epidemiologic transition: Further decrease in infant mortality due to medical intervention during pregnancy and childbirth, yet no decrease in childhood disabilities. *Nederlands Tijdschrift Voor Geneeskunde, 147*, 378–38[illegible].

Vandvik, I. H. (1994). Collaboration between child psychiatry and paediatrics: The state of the relationship in Norway. *Acta paediatrica Oslo, Norway : 1992, 83*, 884–887.

Vreeman, R. C., Wiehe, S. E., Pearce, E. C., & Nyandiko, W. M. (2008). A systematic review of pediatric adherence to antiretroviral therapy in low- and middle-income countries. *The Pediatric Infectious Disease Journal, 27*, 686–691. https://doi.org/10.1097/INF.0b013e31816dd325.

Vreeman, R. C., Gramelspacher, A. M., Gisore, P. O., Scanlon, M. L., & Nyandiko, W. M. (2013). Disclosure of HIV status to children in resource-limited settings: A systematic review. *Journal of the International AIDS Society, 16*, 18466.

Wissow, L. S., van Ginneken, N., Chandna, J., & Rahman, A. (2016). Integrating children's mental health into primary care. *Pediatric Clinics of North America, 63*, 97–113. https://doi.org/10.1016/j.pcl.2015.08.005.

Woodgate, M., & Elena Garralda, M. (2006). Paediatric liaison work by child and adolescent mental health services. *Child and Adolescent Mental Health, 11*, 19–24. https://doi.org/10.1111/j.1475-3588.2005.00373.x.

Woods-Jaeger, B. A., Kava, C. M., Akiba, C. F., Lucid, L., & Dorsey, S. (2017). The art and skill of delivering culturally responsive trauma-focused cognitive behavioral therapy in Tanzania and Kenya. *Psychological Trauma: Theory, Research, Practice, and Policy, 9*, 230–238. https://doi.org/10.1037/tra0000170.

World Health Organisation. (2003). *Adherence to long-term therapies - Evidence for action*. Geneva: World Health Organisation.

World Health Organization. (2005). *Child & adolescent mental health policy and plans*. Geneva: World Health Organisation.

World Health Organization and World Organization of Family Doctors. (2008). *Integrating mental health into primary health care a global perspective*. Geneva: World Health Organization: Wonca.

World Health Organization, World Psychiatric Association and International Association for Child and Adolescent Psychiatry and Allied Professions. (2005). *Child and adolescent mental health resources: Global concerns – implications for the future*. Geneva/Herndon: World Health Organization Stylus Pub., LLC [distributor].

Correction to: Administrative and Financing Models

Claire De Souza

Correction to:
Chapter 16 in: A. P. S. Guerrero et al. (eds.), *Pediatric Consultation-Liaison Psychiatry*, https://doi.org/10.1007/978-3-319-89488-1_16

The name of the author of this chapter has been inadvertently mentioned Claire Souza without his middle name. The correct name is Claire De Souza. We are moving the particle "De" into the last name as "De Souza".

The updated online version of this chapter can be found at
https://doi.org/10.1007/978-3-319-89488-1_16

A. P. S. Guerrero et al. (eds.), *Pediatric Consultation-Liaison Psychiatry*,
https://doi.org/10.1007/978-3-319-89488-1_23

Appendices

Appendix 1: Screening Tools

Flávio Dias Silva

Screening tools are useful standardized questionnaires to gather important diagnostic information in child and adolescent evaluations. These instruments may enable general healthcare professionals to efficiently obtain information, to make a provisional diagnosis, and to determine the need for further specialized assessment. There are many well-developed screening tools worldwide, of varied types. Practical tools in nonspecialized clinical settings are frequently in a questionnaire form. This section presents some instruments that may be helpful in pediatric consultation-liaison psychiatry. They were chosen based on several criteria, including ease of administration by general health professionals, availability in several languages, relevant for the most common clinical conditions seen in pediatric healthcare services, and preferably free of charge and Internet-accessible.

Types of Assessment Tools

Type of assessment tool	Example
Questionnaires	*Children's Eating Attitudes Test (ChEAT)* (1): screening for eating disorders
	Spence Children's Anxiety Scale (SCAS) (2): screening, diagnosis, and monitoring of anxiety disorders
	Children's Yale-Brown Obsessive-Compulsive Scale (CY-BOCS) (3): screening and monitoring of obsessive-compulsive disorders
Structured/semi-structured interviews (SSI's)	*Diagnostic Interview Schedule for Children (DISC-IV)* (4): a fully structured diagnostic instrument that assesses 34 common psychiatric diagnoses of children and adolescents
Observational protocols	*Autism Diagnostic Observation Schedule (ADOS)* (5): a semi-structured assessment of communication, social interaction, and play (or imaginative use of materials) for individuals suspected of having autism spectrum disorders

A. P. S. Guerrero et al. (eds.), *Pediatric Consultation-Liaison Psychiatry*
https://doi.org/10.1007/978-3-319-89488-1

Aspects to Consider When Choosing a Rating Scale

Aspect	Comments
Purpose	Elect a scale that was tested for the objective you need – screening, diagnosis, or monitoring (6). Consider using general screening tools first and then tools to evaluate for specific problems based on the screening results
Language, culture, and context	Search for a tool that has been psychometrically validated for the language, culture, and context (e.g., general population, healthcare setting, specific age range) relevant for the clinical situation (7,8). Self-rating tools are more appropriate for some situations and parent/guardian rating for others (9)
Scoring	Insure that you are using the tools in agreement with the author's instructions

General Screening Tools

	Age range	No. of items
Strengths and Difficulties Questionnaire (SDQ)	2–17 year	25
Goodman 1997 (11)		
Evaluates prosocial behavior and problems in emotions, peer relationships, hyperactivity, and conduct		
Tools available from www.sdqinfo.com		
Pediatric Symptom Checklist (PSC) and Pediatric Symptom Checklist-Youth (PSC-Y)	3–18 year	35
Jellnek et al. 1988 (12)		
Besides the original parent report form, there are many other forms: a youth self-report, a pictorial version, and a briefer 17-item version for both the parent and youth forms		
Tools available from http://www.massgeneral.org/psychiatry/services/psc_home.aspx		

Specific Screening Tools

Autism	Age range	No. of items
Modified Checklist for Autism in Toddlers, Revised with Follow-Up (M-CHAT-R/F)	16–30mo	20
Robins et al. 2013 (13)		
Reduces the false-positive rate and detects more autism spectrum disorders (ASD) cases than the original tool		
Tools available from http://mchatscreen.com/		

Childhood Autism Spectrum Test (CAST)	4–11 year	39
Willians et al. 2005 (14)		
Developed by University of Cambridge Autism Research Centre among several other tests for ASD detection		
Tools available from https://www.autismresearchcentre.com/arc_tests		
Depressive symptoms	Age range	No. of items
Center for Epidemiologic Studies Depression Scale for Children (CES-DC)	6–23 year	20
Weissman et al. 1980 (15)		
Self-rating scale about depressive symptomatology in the last week		
Tools available (in English) from https://www.brightfutures.org/mentalhealth/pdf/professionals/bridges/ces_dc.pdf		
Depression Self Rating Scale for Children (DSRSC)	8–14 year	18
Birleson 1978 (16)		
Similar to the CES-DC and widely used in the United States, Japan, China, and Europe		
Tools available from http://www.childrenandwar.org/measures/depression-self-rating-scale-for-children-birleson/		
Kutcher Adolescent Depression Scale (KADS)	12–22 year	6- and 11-item versions
LeBlanc et al. 2002 (17)		
The briefer version is especially useful in schools or primary care, where it can help to identify risk for depression		
Tools available from http://teenmentalhealth.org/care/health-professionals/clinical-tools/		
Edinburgh Postnatal Depression Scale (EPDS)	Mothers	10
Cox et al. 1987 (18)		
Useful tool to screen for maternal depression		
Tools available from http://www.fresno.ucsf.edu/pediatrics/downloads/edinburghscale.pdf		
Attention deficit hyperactivity disorder (ADHD) and oppositional defiant disorder (ODD)	Age range	No. of items
Swanson, Nolan, and Pelham-IV Questionnaire (SNAP IV)	6–12 year	26- and 90-item versions
Swanson 1992 (19)		
The longer version allows a better general view of a child's behavior. The 26-item scale focuses on ADHD and ODD		
Tools available (in English) from http://www.caddra.ca/pdfs/caddraGuidelines2011SNAP.pdf		
ADHD Rating Scale (ADHD-RS)	5–17 year	18
DuPaul et al. 1998 (20)		
Based on DSM ADHD criteria, it includes 9-question inattention and 9-question hyperactivity/impulsivity subscales		
Tools available (in English, home version) from http://www2.sanfordhealth.org/health-plan-providers/content/cms-quality-child_adhd_rating_scale_screener.pdf		

Vanderbilt Assessment Scales	6–12 year	43 (teacher version) 55 (parent version)
Wolraich 1998 (21); Wolraich et al. 2003 (22)		
Teacher- and parent-rated versions, including screening and follow-up forms		
Toole available (in English) from https://www.nichq.org/resource/nichq-vanderbilt-assessment-scales		
Suicide risk evaluation	Age range	No. of items
Columbia Suicide Severity Risk Scale (CSSR-S)	From 7 year	It depends on the version
Columbia Lighthouse Project (CLP), 2009 (23)		
Comprehensive set of tools for different settings and populations		
Tools available from http://cssrs.columbia.edu/		
Anxiety symptoms	Age range	No. of items
Spence Children's Anxiety Scale (SCAS)	7–19 year	39 (parent version); 45 (child version)
Spence 1998 (24)		
Assesses six domains, including generalized anxiety, panic/agoraphobia, social phobia, separation anxiety, obsessive compulsive disorder, and physical injury fears		
Tools available from http://www.scaswebsite.com/		
Preschool Anxiety Scale, Revised	3–6 year	28
Spence et al. 2001 (25)		
Preschool version of SCAS designed for parent rating, including subscales for separation anxiety		
Tools available from https://www.scaswebsite.com/1_5_.html		
Revised Children's Anxiety and Depression Scale, Youth and Parent Versions (RCADS/RCADS-P)	6–18 year	47
Chorpita et al. 2000 (26)		
Tool composed of subscales on anxiety and major depressive disorder		
Tools available from http://www.childfirst.ucla.edu/Resources.html		
Screen for Child Anxiety Related Emotional Disorders (SCARED)	6–18 year	41
Birmaher et al. 1997 (27)		
Assesses anxiety disorders, including specific school phobia		
Tools available from http://pediatricbipolar.pitt.edu/resources/instruments		
Children's Yale-Brown Obsessive-Compulsive Scale (CY-BOCS)	6–17 year	10
Scahill et al. 1997 (3)		
Evaluates numerous obsessions or compulsions and measures the impact of the symptoms on child's life		
Tools available (in English) from https://iocdf.org/wp-content/uploads/2016/04/05-CYBOCS-complete.pdf		

Child Anxiety Life Interference Scale (CALIS) and CALIS Preschool Version (CALIS-PV)	3–5 year (PV) 6–17 year	18 (PV) 9
Lynehan et al. 2013 (28). Kennedy et al. (2009) (CALIS-PV) (27)		
Measures the impact of anxiety symptoms on a child's life, helpful in formulating treatment		
Tools available from https://www.mq.ecu.au/research/research-centres-groups-and-facilities/healthy-people/centres/centre-for-emotional-health-ceh/resources		
Delirium	Age range	No. of items
Cornell Assessment of Pediatric Delirium	0–21 year	8
Silver et al. 2012 (29)		
Aid to identify delirium diagnosis in an intensive care unit setting		
Free original paper available from https://pdfs.semanticscholar.org/c14e/0102f5a45849f3b23c97764c3edf8bb51282.pdf		
Eating disorders	Age range	No. of items
Eating Attitudes Test (EAT)/Children's Eating Attitudes Test (ChEAT)	8–13 year (ChEAT); From 14 year (EAT)	26
Garner and Garfinkel 1982 (30)/Maloney et al. 1988 (1)		
Easy-to-use screening tool for use in primary care or schools		
Tools available (in English) from http://www.eat-26.com/ and http://www.1000livesplus.wales.nhs.uk/sitesplus/documents/1011/ChEAT.pdf		
SCOFF Questionnaire	From 11 year	5
Morgan et al. 1999 (31)		
An acronym of five questions addressing core features of anorexia nervosa and bulimia nervosa in women		
Tools available from http://cedd.org.au/wordpress/wp-content/uploads/2015/04/SCOFF-Questionnaire.pdf		
Bulimic Investigatory Test of Edinburgh (BITE)	From 12 year	33
Henderson and Freeman 1987 (32)		
A self-rating scale validated in many countries		
Tools available (in English) from www.wales.nhs.uk/sitesplus/866/opendoc/224740		
Mania	Age range	No. of items
Parent Version of the Young Mania Rating Scale (P-YMRS)	5–17 year	11
Gracious et al. (33)		
Differentiates bipolar spectrum disorders from other diagnoses like ADHD or unipolar depression		
Tools available (in English) from https://www.healthyplace.com/images/stories/bipolar/p-ymrs.pdf		

Substance abuse	Age range	No. of items
CRAFFT Test	Less than 21 year	6
Knight et al. 1999 (34)		
Acronym of six points (Car, Relax, Alone, Forget, Friends, Trouble) to evaluate misuse of alcohol or drugs		
Tools available from http://www.ceasar-boston.org/CRAFFT/index.php		
Trauma	Age range	No. of items
Child Stress Disorders Checklist Short Form (CSDC-SF)	2–18 year	4
Bosquet et al. 2010 (35)		
SF comes from the original 36-item CSDC but maintains its power to detect stress-/trauma-related disorders		
Tools available (in English) from https://www.healthcaretoolbox.org/images/pdf/CSDC_SF.pdf		
Children's Revised Impact of Event Scale (CRIES-8)	From 8 year	8
Yule et al. (1997) (36)		
Based on *Impact of Event Scale,* CRIES-8 evaluates risk for trauma or stress-related disorder		
Tools available from http://www.childrenandwar.org/measures/children%E2%80%99s-revised-impact-of-event-scale-8-%E2%80%93-cries-8/		

Beidas, R. S., Stewart, R. E., Walsh, L., Lucas, S., Downey, M. M., Jackson, K., et al. (2015). Free, brief, and validated: Standardized instruments for low-resource mental health settings. *Cognitive and Behavioral Practice, 22*(1), 5–19. https://doi.org/10.1016/j.cbpra.2014.02.002.

Birleson, P. (1981). The validity of depressive disorder in childhood and the development of a self-rating scale: A research report. *Journal of Child Psychology and Psychiatry, 22*, 73–88.

Birmaher, B., Khetarpal, S., Brent, D., Cully, M., Balach, L., Kaufman, J., et al. (1997). The Screen for Child Anxiety Related Emotional Disorders (SCARED): Scale construction and psychometric characteristics. *Journal of the American Academy of Child and Adolescent Psychiatry, 36*, 545–553.

Chorpita, B. F., Yim, L. M., Moffitt, C. E., Umemoto, L. A., & Francis, S. E. (2000). Assessment of symptoms of DSM-IV anxiety and depression in children: A revised child anxiety and depression scale. *Behaviour Research and Therapy, 38*, 835–855.

Cox, J.L., Holden, J.M., & Sagovsky, R. (1987). Detection of postnatal depression: Development of the 10-item Edinburgh Postnatal Depression Scale. *British Journal of Psychiatry, 150*, 782–786. 435. [PubMed: 728692].

DuPaul, G. J., Power, T. J., Anastopoulos, A. D., & Reid, R. (1998). *ADHD rating scale IV: Checklists, norms, and clinical interpretation*. New York: Guilford.

Enlow, M. B., Kassam-Adams, N., & Saxe, G. (2010). The child stress disorders checklist-short form: A 4-item scale of traumatic stress symptoms in children.

General Hospital Psychiatry, 32(3), 321–327. https://doi.org/10.1016/j.genhosppsych.2010.01.009.

Garner, D. M., Olmsted, M. P., Bohr, Y., & Garfinkel, P. E. (1982, November). The eating attitudes test: Psychometric features and clinical correlates. *Psychological Medicine, 12*(4), 871–878.

Goodman, R. (1997). The strengths and difficulties questionnaire: A research note. *Journal of Child Psychology and Psychiatry, 38*, 581–586.

Gracious, B. L., et al. (2002). Discriminative validity of a parent version of the Young Mania rating scale. *Journal of the American Academy of Child & Adolescent Psychiatry, 41*(11), 1350–1359.

Henderson, M., & Freeman, C. P. (1987). A self-rating scale for bulimia. The BITE. *British Journal of Psychiatry, London, 150*, 18–24.

Jellinek, M. S., Murphy, J. M., Robinson, J., Feins, A., Lamb, S., & Fenton, T (1988). The pediatric symptom checklist: Screening school-age children for psychological dysfunction. *Journal of Pediatrics, 112*(2), 201–209. https://doi.org/10.1016/S0022-3476(88)80056-8. [PubMed: 3339501].

Kennedy, S. J., Rapee, R. M., & Edwards, S. L. (2009). A selective intervention program for inhibited preschool-aged children of parents with an anxiety disorder: Effects on current anxiety disorders and temperament. *Journal of the American Academy of Child and Adolescent Psychiatry, 48*(6), 602–609.

Knight J. R., Shrier, L. A., Bravender, T. D., Farrell, M., Vander Bilt, J., & Shaffer, H. J. (1999, June). A new brief screen for adolescent substance abuse. *Archives of Pediatrics and Adolescent Medicine, 153*(6), 591–596.

Kohrt B. A, Jordans, M. J. D., Tol, W. A., Luitel, N. P., Maharjan, S. M , & Upadhaya, N. (2011). Validation of cross-cultural child mental health and psychosocial research instruments: Adapting the depression self-rating scale and child PTSD symptom scale in Nepal. *BMC Psychiatry, 11*, 127. https://doi.org/10.1186/1471-244X-11-127.

LeBlanc, J. C., Almudevar, A., Brooks, S. J., & Kutcher, S. (2002). Screening for adolescent depression: Comparison of the Kutcher adolescent depression scale with the Beck depression inventory. *Journal of Child and Adolescent Psychopharmacology, 12*, 113–126.

Lord, C., Risi, S., Lambrecht, L., Cook, E. H., Jr., Leventhal, B. L., DiLavore, P. C., et al. (2000). The autism diagnostic observation schedule—generic: A standard measure of social and communication deficits associated with the spectrum of autism. *Journal of Autism and Developmental Disorders, 30*(3), 205–223.

Lyneham, H. J., Sburlati, E. S., Abbott, M. J., Rapee, R. M. Hudson, J. L., Tolin, D. F., & Carlson, S. E. (2013, October). Psychometric Properties of the Child Anxiety Life Interference Scale (CALIS). *Journal of Anxiety Disorders, 27*(7), 711719.

Michel, C., Schultze-Lutter, F., & Schimmelmann, B. G. (2014). Screening instruments in child and adolescent psychiatry: General and methodological considerations. *European Child & Adolescent Psychiatry, 23*, 725. https://doi.org/10.1007/s00787-014-0608-x.

Morgan J. F., Reid, F., & Lacey, J. H. (1999, December 4). The SCOFF questionnaire: Assessment of a new screening tool for eating disorders. *British Medical Journal, 319*(7223), 1467–1468.

Robins, D. L., Casagrande, K., Barton, M. L., Chen, C., Dumont-Mathieu, T., & Fein, D. (2014). Validation of the modified checklist for autism in toddlers-revised with follow-up (M- CHAT-R/F). *Pediatrics, 133*(1), 37–45. PMCID: PMC3876182.

Scahill, L., Riddle, M. A., McSwiggin-Hardin, M., Ort, S. I., King, R. A., Goodman, W. K., & Leckman, J. F. (1997). Children's Yale-Brown obsessive compulsive scale: Reliability and validity. *Journal of the American Academy of Child & Adolescent Psychiatry, 36*(6), 844–852. https://doi.org/10.1097/00004583-199706000-00023.

Shaffer, D., Fisher, P., Lucas, C. P., Dulcan, M. K., & Schwab-Stone, M. E. (2000). NIMH Diagnostic Interview Schedule for Children Version IV (NIMH DISC-IV): Description, differences from previous versions, and reliability of some common diagnoses. *Journal of the American Academy of Child and Adolescent Psychiatry, 39*(1), 28–38.

Smith, S. R. (2007). Making sense of multiple informants in child and adolescent psychopathology: A guide for clinicians. *Journal of Psychoeducational Assessment, 25*(2), 139–149.

Spence, S. H. (1998). A measure of anxiety symptoms among children. *Behaviour Research and Therapy, 36*(5), 545–566. S0005-7967(98)00034-5.

Spence, S. H., Rapee, R., McDonald, C., & Ingram, M. (2001). The structure of anxiety symptoms among preschoolers. *Behaviour Research and Therapy, 39*, 1293–1316.

Swanson, J. M., Schuck, S., Porter, M. M., et al. (2012). Categorical and dimensional definitions and evaluations of symptoms of ADHD: History of the SNAP and the SWAN rating scales. *The International Journal of Educational and Psychological Assessment, 10*(1), 51–70.

The Columbia Lighthouse Project. Columbia-Suicide Severity Rating Scale (C-SSRS). Available from http://cssrs.columbia.edu/. Last accessed Dec 2017

Traube, C., Silver, G., Kearney, J., Patel, A., Atkinson, T. M., Yoon, M. J., Halpert, S., Augenstein, J., Sickles, L. E., Li, C., & Greenwald, B. (2014, March). Cornell Assessment of Pediatric Delirium: A valid, rapid, observational tool for screening delirium in the PICU*. *Critical Care Medicine, 42*(3), 656–663. https://doi.org/10.1097/CCM.0b013e3182a66b76.

Weissman, M. M., Orvaschel, H., & Padian, N. (1980). Children's symptom and social functioning self-report scales: Comparison of mothers' and children's reports. *Journal of Nervous & Mental Disease, 168*(12), 736–740.

Williams, J., Scott, F., Stott, C., Allison, C., Bolton, P., Baron-Cohen, S., & Brayne, C. (2004). The CAST (Childhood Asperger Syndrome Test): Test accuracy. *Autism, 9*(1), 45–68.

Wolraich, M. L., et al. (1998). Obtaining systematic teacher reports of disruptive behavior disorders utilizing DSM-IV. *Journal of Abnormal Child Psychology, 26*, 141–152.

Wolraich, M. L., et al. (2003). Psychometric properties of the Vanderbilt ADHD diagnostic parent rating scale in a referred population. *Journal of Pediatric Psychology, 28*, 559–567.

Yule, W. (1997). Anxiety, depression and post-traumatic stress in childhood. In I. Sclare (Ed.), *Child psychology portfolio*. Windsor: NFER-Nelson.

Appendix 2: Teaching Tools

Flávio Dias Silva

Family doctors, pediatricians, and other general health professionals are in a privileged position to prevent and detect mental health disorders in children and adolescents. This appendix section provides tools that the pediatric consultation-liaison psychiatrist can use in optimally preparing their primary care colleagues for these important roles. It also includes a list of worldwide Internet resources for additional information that can guide team capacity building.

Potential Educational Activity to Introduce the Pediatric Consultation-Liaison Perspective

As noted in Chap. 10, the biopsychosocial approach is a key tool in insuring successful consultation and liaison, and as noted in Chap. 17, the psychosomatic model is essential in optimizing patient experience and safety and quality of care. The following group activity may be helpful in teaching colleagues about the pediatric consultation liaison perspective and how to think "psychosomatically":

> *Ask to a member present one real case in your field of pediatrics and try to apply, using the figures below, a comprehensive psychosomatic approach. Include discussion of how the physician-patient relationship can be improved with this approach.*

Case formulation tool

Identify problems that have contributed to the present clinical situation. Besides understanding the chronology of facts, try to understand the role of each problem as a **predisposing, protective, precipitating,** and/or **perpetuating factor.** After you complete that task, go to the next figure.

Perspective	Problems (including diagnosis / therapies used)
Biological • Genetics • Family history • Prenatal/perinatal history • Critical and sensitive periods • Physical development • Constitution • Intelligence • Temperament • Medical conditions	
Psychological • Information processing • Language and communication • Emotional development • Behavior patterns	
Social • Family constellation • Neighborhood • Peer relationships • School • Culture • Ethnic influences • Economic issues	

Birth → Present consultation

Timeline

Formulation-based treatment plan

Summarize the problems identified in case formulation in the left column of the box below. Then, write the plan of care in the left column. This may include additional investigation and/or any of the interventions shown in the graphic. Remember to be patient-centered and family/community-oriented. Avoid excessive interventions that may cause harm.

	Problems list	Plan of care
1		
2		
3		
4		
5		
6		
7		
8		
9		
10		

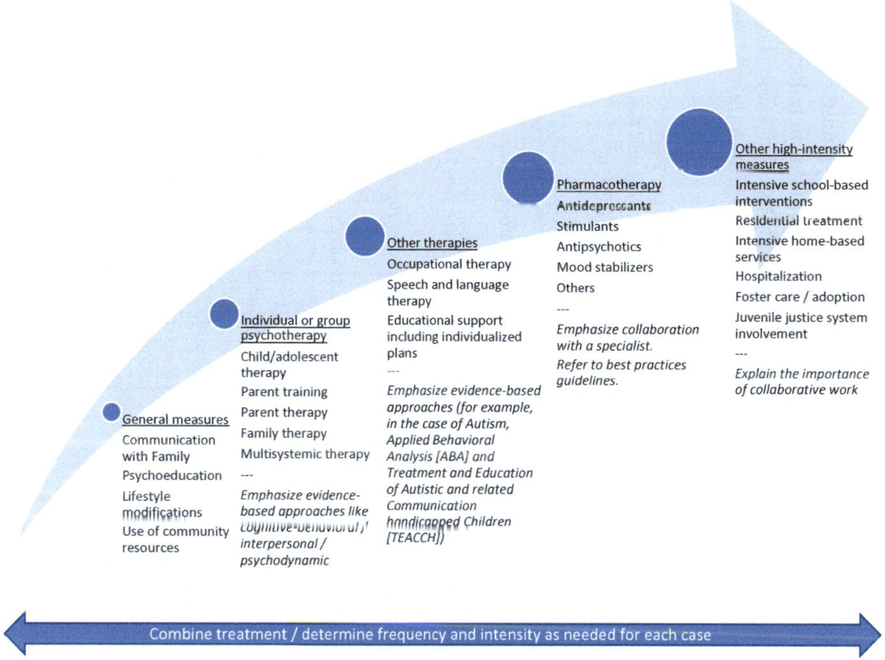

Potential Educational Activity to Introduce the Psychiatric Diagnostic Perspective

As reviewed in Chap. 3, there are several types of psychiatric conditions that referring pediatricians will ideally become familiar with through their work with pediatric consultation-liaison psychiatrists. Guided by the table below of DSM-5 categories, the following group activity may be helpful in introducing colleagues to the psychiatric diagnostic approach.

Discuss what are the main problems seen in each colleague's practice. Based on the group's interest, provide additional readings on DSM-5 categories and discuss the potential benefits of accurately identifying psychiatric conditions in pediatric practice.

DSM-5 categories of disorders	Examples of subcategories
Neurodevelopmental disorders	*Intellectual disability, autistic spectrum disorders, ADHD, tic disorders*
Spectrum of schizophrenia and other psychotic disorders	*Delusional disorder, brief psychotic disorder, schizophrenia*
Bipolar disorder and related disorders	*Bipolar I disorder, bipolar II disorder, cyclothymic disorder*
Depressive disorders	*Disruptive mood dysregulation disorder, major depressive disorder, persistent depressive disorder (dysthymia), premenstrual dysphoric disorder*
Anxiety disorders	*Separation anxiety disorder, selective mutism, specific phobia, social anxiety disorder, panic disorder, agoraphobia, generalized anxiety disorder*
Obsessive-compulsive disorder and related disorders	*Obsessive-compulsive disorder, trichotillomania (hair-pulling disorder)*
Trauma and stressor-related disorders	*Reactive attachment disorder, disinhibited social engagement disorder, post-traumatic stress disorder, acute stress disorder, adjustment disorders*
Dissociative disorders	*Dissociative identity disorder, dissociative amnesia, other specified dissociative disorder*
Disorder of somatic symptoms and related disorders	*Somatic symptom disorder, illness anxiety disorder, conversion disorder, factitious disorder*
Feeding and eating disorders	*Pica, anorexia nervosa, bulimia nervosa, binge eating disorder*
Disorders of elimination	*Enuresis, encopresis*
Sleep-wake disorders	*Insomnia disorder, narcolepsy, breathing-related sleep disorders, parasomnias*
Sexual dysfunctions	*Erectile disorder, female orgasmic disorder, premature (early) ejaculation*
Gender dysphoria	*Gender dysphoria*
Disruptive, impulse control, and conduct disorders	*Oppositional defiant disorder, intermittent explosive disorder, conduct disorder, antisocial personality disorder, pyromania, kleptomania*

DSM-5 categories of disorders	Examples of subcategories
Disorders related to substances	*Alcohol, caffeine, cannabis, hallucinogen, inhalant, opioid, sedative, hypnotic or anxiolytic, stimulant, or tobacco-related disorders, gambling disorder*
Neurocognitive disorders	*Delirium, major and mild neurocognitive disorders*
Personality disorders	*General personality disorder, Cluster A, B, or C personality disorders*
Paraphilic disorders	*Voyeuristic disorder, exhibitionistic disorder, frotteuristic disorder, sexual masochism disorder, sexual sadism disorder, pedophilic disorder, fetishistic disorder, transvestic disorder*
Other mental disorders	*Other specified/unspecified mental disorders due to another medical condition*
Medication-induced movement disorders and other adverse effects of medications	*Neuroleptic-induced and other medication-induced Parkinsonism, neuroleptic malignant syndrome, medication-induced acute dystonia and akathisia, tardive dyskinesia, tardive dystonia, tardive akathisia*
Other conditions that may be clinical attention focus	*Relational problems, abuse and neglect, educational and occupational problems*
	Housing and economic problems, problems related to crime or interaction with the legal system

Important Resources That Contain Helpful Information for Pediatric Colleagues

We close this section with a list of available resources that address global child and adolescent mental health concerns that are written for broad audiences (including primary care providers) and that are freely and readily accessible. They may be valuable resources not only for primary pediatric providers themselves but also for pediatric consultation-liaison psychiatrists who teach primary pediatric providers.

IACAPAP Textbook of Child and Adolescent Mental Health

– http://iacapap.org/iacapap-textbook-of-child-and-adolescent-mental-health

American Academy of Child and Adolescent Psychiatry Resources for Primary Care:

– http://www.aacap.org/aacap/Resources_for_Primary_Care/Home.aspx

World Health Organization mhGAP Training Manuals:

– http://www.who.int/mental_health/mhgap/training_manuals/en/

References and Suggested Readings

American Psychiatric Association. (2013). *Diagnostic and statistical manual of mental disorders: DSM* (5th ed.). Arlington: American Psychiatric Publishing.

Chiles, C., & Wise, T. N. (2008). Consultation–Liaison Psychiatry. In *Current diagnosis & treatment: Psychiatry* (2nd ed.). New York: McGraw-Hill Medical.

Christensen, J. F. (2014). Stress & disease. In *Current behavioral medicine: A guide for clinical practice* (4th ed.). New York: McGraw-Hill Education.

Fiertag, O., Taylor, S., Tareen, A., & Garralda, E. (2012). Somatoform disorders. In J. M. Rey (Ed.), *IACAPAP e-textbook of child and adolescent mental health*. Geneva: International Association for Child and Adolescent Psychiatry and Allied Professions.

Guerra, N. G., Williamson, A. A., & Lucas Molina, B. (2012). Normal development: Infancy, childhood, and adolescence. In J. M. Rey (Ed.), *IACAPAP e-textbook of child and adolescent mental health*. Geneva: International Association for Child and Adolescent Psychiatry and Allied Professions.

Henderson, S. W., & Martin, A. (2014). Case formulation and integration of information in child and adolescent mental health. In J. M. Rey (Ed.), *IACAPAP e-textbook of child and adolescent mental health*. Geneva: International Association for Child and Adolescent Psychiatry and Allied Professions.

Nurcombe, B. (2008). Psychological reactions to acute & chronic systemic illness in pediatric patients. In *Current diagnosis & treatment: psychiatry* (2nd ed.). New York: McGraw-Hill Medical.

Shaw, R. J., & DeMaso, D. R. (2010). *Textbook of psychosomatic medicine* (1st ed.). Washington, DC: American Psychiatric Publishing.

Stubbe, D. (2007). *Child and adolescent psychiatry: Practical guides in psychiatry* (1st ed.). Philadelphia: Lippincott Williams and Wilkins.

Trivedi, H. K., & Kershner, J. D. (2009). *Practical child and adolescent psychiatry for pediatrics and primary care*. Göttingen: Hogrefe & Huber Publishers.

Volkmar, F. R., & Martin, A. (2011). *Essentials of Lewis's child and adolescent psychiatry*. Philadelphia: Lippincott Williams and Wilkins.

Appendix 3: "Talking Points" for Justifying the Value of Pediatric Psychosomatic Medicine Services

Raissa Tanqueco

We hope that the knowledge presented in this textbook will not only improve individual patient care but also stimulate interest in developing pediatric psychosomatic medicine services wherever they may be needed in the world. We close by presenting a concise summary of "talking points" and references that the reader can readily access when advocating for this specialty.

We are more connected than ever before and so must be the care provided to our patients. Pediatric consultation-liaison (CL) psychiatry serves not only as the interface between psychiatry and other fields but also between providers, patients, and families. No matter where you happen to be in the world, pediatric and psychiatric settings should be considered non-mutually exclusive to provide comprehensive medical care.

Here are several bullet points a practicing CL psychiatrist can offer in describing the value of a pediatric CL service:

- Reduced long-term costs for coordinated and collaborative care: Muskin et al. discussed reduction in hospital length of stay in a comanaged care model, and Hall et al. reviewed these savings not only in relation to length of stay but also through timely transfers from psychiatric to medical floor and vice versa.
  - Muskin, P., et al. (2016). Comanaged care for medical inpatients, C-L versus C/L psychiatry. *Psychosomatics, 57*(3), 258–263. https://doi.org/10.1016/j.psym.2016.02.001.
  - Tadros, G., et al. (2013). Impact of an integrated rapid response psychiatric liaison team on quality improvement and cost savings The Birmingham RAID model. *The Psychiatrist Online, 37*(1), 4–10. https://doi.org/10.1192/pb.bp.111.037366.
  - Hall, R. C., et al. (1996). The value of consultation-liaison interventions to the general hospital. *Psychiatric Services, 47*(4), 418–420. https://doi.org/10.1176/ps.47.4.418.
- Improved well-being for the child, noted by Asamow et al., comparing integrated care with usual care:
  - Asamow, J. R., et al. (2015). Integrated medical-behavioral care compared with usual primary care for child and adolescent behavioral health: A meta-analysis. *JAMA Pediatrics, 169*(10), 929–937. https://doi.org/10.1001/jamapediatrics.2015.1141.
- Improved medical prognosis by better diagnosis, noted by Yellowlees et al., while Kramer et al. noted identification of psychiatric disorders in primary care usually for the most severe patients:
  - Kramer, T., et al. (1998). Psychiatric disorders in adolescents in primary care. *The British Journal of Psychiatry, 173*(6), 501–513. https://doi.org/10.1192/bjp.173.6.508.
  - Yellowlees, P., et al. (2017). A retrospective analysis of a child and adolescent emental health program. *Journal of the American Academy of Child & Adolescent Psychiatry, 47*(1), 103–107. doi:10.1097/chi.0b013e31815a56a7.
- Improved family functioning and ability to care for the child, as outlined extensively in these write-ups from the WHO:
  - Belli, C., et al. (2005). Investing in children's health: what are the economic benefits? *Bulletin of the World Health Organization, 83*, 777–784.
  - Promoting mental health. A report of the world health organization. http://www.who.int/mental_health/evidence/MH_Promotion_Book.pdf

- Increased satisfaction with follow-up, planning, and patient outcome observed by Dvir et al. for primary care CL:
  - Dvir, Y. (2012). An assessment of satisfaction with ambulatory child psychiatry consultation services to primary care providers by parents of children with emotional and behavioral needs: The Massachusetts child psychiatry access project University of Massachusetts parent satisfaction study. *Frontiers in Psychiatry, 3*, 7. https://doi.org/10.3389/fpsyt.2012.00007.
- Reduced risk of complaints and/or litigation: In fact, in the resource document below, there were no known cases of malpractice. The document also provides a framework on matters to consider in an integrated practice.
  - Resource document on risk management and liability issues in integrated care models. American Psychiatric Association official actions. https://www.integration.samhsa.gov/workforce/Risk_Management_and_Liability.pdf
- Improved timeliness of access to quality mental health care, through primary care-psychiatry collaborations, either face to face, facilitated by a care manager, or involving distance education (e.g., Project ECHO, or Extension for Community Healthcare Outcomes):
  - Kaye, D., et al. (2016). Learn then apply: Increased impact of formal education with consultation support on primary care physician knowledge, skills and confidence in child mental health care. *Journal of the American Academy of Child and Adolescent Psychiatry, 55*(10), S210–S211. https://doi.org/10.1016/j.jaac.2016.09.341.
  - Sarvet, B. (2017). The need for practice transformation in children's mental health care. *Journal of the American Academy of Child and Adolescent Psychiatry, 56*(6), 460–461. https://doi.org/10.1016/j.jaac.2017.04.001.
  - Cheng, K., et al. *Using the project ECHO model to train rural primary care clinicians to deliver child mental health services in Oregon: Poster* presented at 64th American academy of child and adolescent psychiatry annual meeting.
- Improved physician satisfaction and presumably improved retention:
  - Kisely, S., et al. (2006). Collaboration between primary care and psychiatric services: Does it help family physicians? *Canadian Family Physicians, 52*, 876–877.
- Research opportunities: Richardson et al. stressed the importance of ongoing research, as the body of literature is currently limited.
  - Richardson, R., et al. (2017). Research in the integration of behavioral health for adolescents and young adult in primary care settings: A systematic review.

The Journal of Adolescent Health: Official Publication of the Society for Adolescent Medicine, *60*(3), 261–269. https://doi.org/10.1016/j.jadohealth.2016.11.013.

In 2008, Dr. Don Berwick described (in "Triple Aim: Care Health, and Cost") that an improved healthcare system "requires simultaneous pursuit of three aims: improving the experience of care, improving the health of populations, and reducing per capita costs of health care." In 2014, Dr. Thomas Bodenheimer (in "From Triple to Quadruple Aim: Care of the Patient Requires Care of the Provider") added "improving the work life of health care providers, including clinicians and staff" as the fourth component. It will become increasingly evident that these aims are more achievable when we work together, and consultation-liaison psychiatry is well-positioned to contribute to these essential improvements in healthcare.

Additional References

Berwick, D., et. al. (2008). Triple aim: Care, health and cost. *Health Affairs*, 27(3). https://doi.org/10.1377/hlthaff.27.3.759.

Bodenheimer, T., & Sinsky, C. (2014). From triple to quadruple aim: Care of the patient requires care of the provider. *Annals of Family Medicine*, *12*(6), 573–576. https://doi.org/10.1370/afm.1713.

Index

A. P. S. Guerrero et al. (eds.), *Pediatric Consultation-Liaison Psychiatry*,
https://doi.org/10.1007/978-3-319-89488-1

D

T

The manufacturer's authorised representative in the EU is Springer Nature Customer Service Centre GmbH, Europaplatz 3, 69115 Heidelberg, Germany. If you have any concerns regarding our products, please contact ProductSafety@springernature.com

Printed and bound by CPI Group (UK) Ltd, Croydon, CR0 4YY
05/10/2026
02228144-0016